INTELLIGIBILITY IN SPEECH DISORDERS

STUDIES IN
SPEECH PATHOLOGY AND CLINICAL LINGUISTICS

SERIES EDITORS

EDITORIAL BOARD

AIMS AND SCOPE

The establishment of this series reflects the growth of both interest and research into disorders of speech and language. It is intended that the series will provide a platform for the development of academic debate and enquiry into the related fields of speech pathology and clinical linguistics.

To this end, the series will publish book length studies or collections of papers on aspects of disordered communication, and the relation between language theory and language pathology.

Volume 1

Raymond D. Kent (ed.)

Intelligibility in Speech Disorders
Theory, measurement and management

INTELLIGIBILITY
IN
SPEECH DISORDERS
THEORY, MEASUREMENT
AND MANAGEMENT

Edited by

RAYMOND D. KENT
University of Wisconsin, Madison

JOHN BENJAMINS PUBLISHING COMPANY
AMSTERDAM/PHILADELPHIA

1992

Library of Congress Cataloging-in-Publication Data

Intelligibility in speech disorders : theory, measurement, and management / edited by Raymond D. Kent.
     p.   cm. -- (Studies in speech pathology and clinical linguistics ; v. 1)
  Includes bibliographical references and index.
  1. Speech disorders. 2. Speech, Intelligibility of. I. Kent, Raymond D. II. Series:
Studies in speech pathology and clinical linguistics ; no. 1.
RC423.I49   1992
616.85'5--dc20   92-4811
ISBN 90 272 4331 X (Eur.)/1-55619-387-4 (US)(alk. paper)   CIP

John Benjamins Publishing Co. · P.O. Box 75577 · 1070 AN Amsterdam · The Netherlands
John Benjamins North America · 821 Bethlehem Pike · Philadelphia, PA 19118 · USA

Contents

Introduction

Raymond D. Kent
University of Wisconsin

The intelligibility of speech is a paramount issue in speech pathology. One of the members of our research group at Wisconsin calls intelligibility "the behavioral standard of communication." This description rightfully acknowledges that an immediate principal criterion by which we judge a communicative attempt is the intelligibility of the talker. Despite the obvious importance of intelligibility in speech pathology, it apparently has not been the subject of a book-length treatment. The only available discussions are in various journal articles and book chapters. In the belief that there is sufficient interest and activity to warrant a larger and more integrated discussion, several authors experienced in intelligibility issues in speech pathology or related fields were invited to write chapters to reflect their work and thinking. The resulting set of chapters describes the basic dimensions by which speech intelligibility can (and perhaps *must*) be understood. These dimensions are: auditory perceptual, linguistic, acoustic and physiologic. The dimensions, in turn, are applied to the fundamental problems of definition and theory, measurement, and clinical management.

Definition, theory and measurement are not trivial matters. Intelligibility is part of a more general concern that we might call *communicative competence*, which can be studied with several different methods, including those of sociolinguistics and speech act theory. But even if the best attempts are made to distinguish intelligibility from other aspects of communicative competence, it quickly becomes clear from a study of the literature that intelligibility is not a monolithic phenomenon. Intelligibility has been studied on different levels and with a variety of techniques. Therefore, although two persons may share some common idea of what intelligibility is, they may use very different methods to measure it and understand its correlates in the act of speaking.

The common clinical procedures for intelligibility assessment involve listener ratings of speech samples. Rating procedures have been popular for many reasons, not the least of which is the relative ease of assessment. However, ease is not the only property by which an assessment procedure should be judged. At the minimum, one should consider issues of validity and reliability. Remarkably, the psychophysical issues of intelligibility scaling have been rather neglected until recently. Nicholas Schiavetti and colleagues have turned our attention to this matter in an important series of papers on scaling methods and results. In the first chapter of this book, Dr. Schiavetti summarizes this work and discusses it as it pertains to the clinical and research needs for intelligibility assessment. He concludes that neither interval scaling nor percentage estimation judgments appear to be satisfactory for the measurement of speech intelligibility in clinical or research applications. Although direct magnitude estimation has greater promise, it suffers from certain drawbacks that limit its successful application. What then remains? Dr. Schiavetti recommends word identification tests and reviews a number of factors that support this recommendation. One of his concluding statements could well be taken as the *raison d'être* for this book: "Obviously, reliable and valid measures of speech intelligibility are necessary for the indexing of severity of speech disorders and for the explanation of intelligibility deficits from both an acoustic and an articulatory standpoint."

Intelligibility implies the retrieval of linguistic decision units. Therefore, intelligibility is necessarily bound within the properties of language. In Chapter 2, Rida Bross proposes an intelligibility measurement based on the principles of structural linguistics, specifically, the Aspectual Theory of George L. Trager and Henry Lee Smith, Jr. This approach considers the structural units of segmentals and suprasegmentals at the phonological *and* morphological levels. The unit of morphophone is defined at the higher of these two levels as a "calibration" unit by which alternate phonemic expressions of the same lexical items are recognized. Bross incorporates the Aspectual analysis in a test called the Quantitative Rating of Performance (QRP) test, which elicits all structural contrasts of the system. She demonstrates the application of this tool in an assessment of the intelligibility of esophageal speakers using two different electromechanical larynges. An important consequence of Bross' approach is that it defines intelligibility at the morphological or word level, thus emphasizing the linguistic function of speech behaviors.

Impairments of speech intelligibility associated with neurologic disorders have received long overdue attention in the last decade. A special focus has been the development of procedures for the quantification of the intelligibility reduction. Kathryn Yorkston and David Beukelman, working at the University of Washington, were leaders in this effort. Other recent contributions have been made by Wolfram Ziegler and associates in West Germany and by a group of investigators at Wisconsin (Raymond Kent, John Rosenbek and Gary Weismer).

Directions of this research are examined by Gary Weismer and Ruth Martin, who suggest that an analysis model designed to explain intelligibility deficits should be sufficiently broad to include various speech disorders that involve intelligibility impairment. To make their task manageable, they concentrate on speech intelligibility in one class of speech disorders, dysarthria. A major goal of their chapter is to present analytic methods for the interpretation of intelligibility impairments. Drs. Weismer and Martin describe a rationale for the determination of variables that should be useful in an explanatory model of speech intelligibility. They also describe the problem of reduced intelligibility from a perspective that is rarely addressed, that of the listener. Drs. Weismer and Martin suggest that the disordered speech signal may present more difficulties to the listener than might be expected from a "mismatch" between acoustic-phonetic events. This perspective recognizes that intelligibility is not just a speaker characteristic; rather it is a joint characteristic of a speaker-listener dyad. For the listener, disordered speech can be much more than a disturbance of the acoustic characteristics of individual segments. It may represent a significant departure from the kind of speech signal for which normal processing strategies have been adapted. That is, a speech disorder, especially a severe one as it affects intelligibility, may thwart the speech perception strategies that work efficiently for normal speech signals.

A particularly interesting result of the regression analysis performed by Weismer and Martin is that although intelligibility involves a number of potential phonetic dimensions, only a small number of these dimensions may be needed to predict a speaker's level of intelligibility. From Weismer and Martin's analysis of the data for speakers with dysarthria associated with amyotrophic lateral sclerosis, it appears that only two or three phonetic contrasts provide a reasonable basis to predict word recognition intelligibility. Similar results have been reported by others. For example, Billman (1986), in a study of 15 phonologically disordered children, determined that intelligibility was most highly correlated with two processes. Interestingly, the two processes, prevocalic singleton omission and backing, were relatively infrequent. Although the phonologically disordered children exhibited more frequently occurring processes (such as liquid deviation), the less frequently occurring processes seemed to be more senstive to intelligibility differences among the children. Billman also reported that the largest differences between the least and most intelligible groups of her subjects occurred for the processes of stridency deletion and consonant sequence reduction. These results, and those described by Weismer and Martin, may point the way to sensitive and efficient intelligibility testing along phonetic or phonological directions.

It is commonly supposed that speech intelligibility rests almost entirely on supralaryngeal functions. This supposition is reflected in the literature as an overwhelming emphasis on articulatory correlates of intelligibility. Lorraine Ramig's chapter helps to correct for the neglect of laryngeal functions in speech intelligibility. As Dr. Ramig comments, "in most of the studies of disordered speech and intelligibility, the significant support roles of the laryngeal and respiratory systems have been simply assumed." She goes on to assert that the role of phonation in speech intelligibility should be understood in respect to three major functions: (a) as an aerodynamic and acoustic source for speech production, (b) as a generator of suprasegmental features, and (c) as an articulator. She reviews each of these functions in relation to the intelligibility reductions experienced by alaryngeal speakers, persons with motor speech disorders, hearing-impaired individuals and others with communicative disorders. As a demonstration of the contribution of phonatory function to speech intelligibility, Ramig reports a study of the relationship between improved vocal fold adduction and speech intelligibility in patients with Parkinson's disease. The study involved intensive voice therapy given to seven patients with idiopathic Parkinson's disease. The therapy was followed by improvements in vocal function, as confirmed by acoustic and kinematic measures, and also by improvements in articulatory variables. Ratings of post-therapy intelligibility were closely related to ratings of reduced monotony and shakiness of speech. This provocative study shows that therapy directed to improve speech intelligibility in patients with Parkinson's disease should not neglect phonatory function. This principle may apply to other communicative disorders as well.

Both the Weismer-Martin and Ramig chapters refer to acoustic as well as perceptual data. An acoustic-perceptual understanding of speech intelligibility impairment is emerging. The road has been difficult, in part because of the extraordinary richness of the acoustic signal of speech. There are simply too many possible measures. However, research on speech perception, voice quality, acoustic phonetics and speech disorders has helped in the selection of acoustic measures that are most highly correlated with intelligibility. As Weismer and Martin point out, the mean slope of second-formant (F2) transitions has been reported to be highly correlated with the word-recognition intelligibility scores of dysarthric individuals with amyotrophic lateral sclerosis. The emergence of a single acoustic measure that is highly correlated with intelligibility carries promise of clarifying the acoustic-perceptual interpretation of intelligibility deficits. This work is an obvious preliminary to the large-scale application of automatic (machine-based) procedures for the assessment of speech intelligibility.

It remains to be seen how well automatic procedures will work for speech-impaired populations, but early indications are promising. Carlson and Bernstein (1988) reported that a template-based speech recognizer had better recognition performance than human listeners for about 25% of their 81 speech-impaired subjects. This result was obtained for a 300-word vocabulary with context. The speech-impaired subjects included persons with hearing impairment and cerebral palsy. Although these two groups were about equal in intelligibility, the machine recognized more words for the hearing-impaired speakers. The authors concluded that the hearing-impaired subjects produced more repeatable and distinct utterances. Carlson and Bernstein also reported a brief analysis of the acoustic properties of the speech of two subjects, one hearing-impaired and the other cerebral-palsied. The hearing-impaired subject, who was more recognizeable by machine than intelligible to listeners, had a number of consistent segmental errors. The cerebral-palsied subject, who was more intelligible to listeners than recognizeable by machine, had inconsistent errors in duration, pitch and energy. This result, although limited to only two subjects, suggests directions for the continued study of acoustic properties of speech in relation to intelligibility and machine recognition.

Carlson and Bernstein foresaw application of their results to telecommunication systems for speech-impaired persons, but another important application of this technology is speech training. An example of such work is the Indiana Speech Training Aid (ISTRA) described by Watson, Reed, Kewley-Port and Maki (in press) and by Kewley-Port, Watson, Elbert,

Maki and Reed (in press). ISTRA consists of a microcomputer, a low-cost, speaker-dependent speech recognizer, and a series of programs to be used in speech training. The system provides feedback to the client based on a multidimensional acoustic comparison between a new utterance and a stored template formed from previous utterances of the client. A rationale behind this system is that speech intelligibility can be enhanced by reinforcing successive syllable, word, or phrase approximations to a target utterance. New templates are made for the various phases of training, so that the client works toward progressively improved speech patterns.

James Flege addresses the important issue of second language (L2) learning. In particular, he evaluates a speech learning model that proposes to account for the adjustments, or the lack of adjustments, in the phonetic system of a second language learner. An hypothesis of the speech learning model is that the processes and mechanisms that enable children to learn their first language (L1) are influential throughout the lifespan. Following a review of the literature on phonetic adjustments in L2 learners and a presentation of the speech learning model, Dr. Flege reports a study of English vowel production by native Dutch talkers and native speakers of British English. He discusses a number of important concepts in speech learning, including the sensitive period hypothesis, the relationship between speech production and perception, phonetic category prototypes, the perception of L2 sounds and factors influencing vowel intelligibility. These concepts are relevant not only to the learning of L2 phonetic systems but to the general acquisition and maintenance of language abilities. Indeed, many of these factors loom large in the next chapter on speech intelligibility in the hearing impaired.

Intelligibility implies oral communication, and it is therefore to be expected that intelligibility is a primary means by which the oral communication of hearing-impaired speakers can be evaluated. In her chapter on speech intelligibility in the hearing impaired, Mary Joe Osberger discusses methods of measuring intelligibility, the effects of speech errors on intelligibility, and the development of speech training and assessment procedures. In addition to her review of intelligibility tests, Dr. Osberger comments on a scale that is designed to evaluate the speech of hearing-impaired children in everyday situations. The scale, the Meaningful Use of Speech Scale (MUSS), evaluates not only speech but overall communicative functioning. Specifically, MUSS is used to determine if (a) a child uses speech unsupported by other communicative modalities (gestures, signs or other nonvocal cues), (b) the child's use of speech is contingent on listener familiarity with the child's speech, and (c) the child appropriately uses repair and clarification strategies when problems in understanding arise. This scale is an important extension of intelligibility assessment per se and helps to put the child's communicative strategies in a social context. A scale of this kind may have broad application for the clinical assessment and management of individuals with intelligibility deficits.

Dr. Osberger stresses the importance of context and listener experience in the assessment and management of intelligibility problems. When properly viewed, the factors of context and listener familiarity are not just nuisances that stand in the way of reliable and valid intelligibility measurement. Rather, they can become valuable dimensions in both assessment and management.

Clinical applications of intelligibility measurement in the area of dysarthria are explored by Kathryn Yorkston, Patricia Dowden and David Beukelman. They consider the ways in which intelligibility tasks are used to make clinical intervention decisions. The points under discussion fall into three major areas: tasks that are used to measure the level and pattern of disability; tasks that can identify factors important to improving functional performance; and the nature of the complex interactions among the factors that determine intelligibility. These authors, like Osberger, draw attention to the important roles of listener and context in the assessment and management of speakers with impaired intelligibility. Their discussion also embraces the important factors of speaking rate, prosthetic management, behavior modification and partner training. In the final section of their paper, "Toward an intelligibility-based model of intervention," the authors present two case studies that exemplify the combination of factors that influence the intelligibility of a dysarthric individual.

It is instructive (and encouraging) to note the parallels and convergences in the chapters considered so far. Although intelligibility is a complex phenomenon, it is yielding its secrets to careful research. Refinements have been introduced in the measurement of intelligibility, and important progress has been made in the understanding of factors that determine intelligibility. Perhaps no single intelligibility test will satisfy every need, but valuable alternatives are available. It may be that no single test will ever satisfy research and clinical needs. If so, a choice will have to be made among the alternatives, or a process of *triangulation* might be used. Triangulation, as used in ethnograpy, is similar to the concept of the same name used in fixing a geographic position, as in surveying. The ethnographer, recognizing that any single data source may be inadequate, relies on multiple data sources to study cultural phenomena. In like fashion, the study of intelligibility might be undertaken with several tools, including word-intelligibility tests, sentence-intelligibility tests, rating scales, and others as appropriate (Kent, 1990).

The last two chapters in the book relate to the physiological level of speech production and intelligibility. William Hardcastle and Susan Edwards present data on apraxic speech errors derived from electropalatography (EPG). This noninvasive technique permits a look into the actual patterns of articulatory contact during speaking tasks. The EPG data underscore the importance of careful observation. The four subjects under study were all considered to be apraxic, but they had individual profiles of error types. The error types included misdirection, distortion, seriation errors, large spatial or temporal variability, omission, and repetition. Clearly, many things can go wrong in the motor act of speaking. Techniques such as EPG should lead to a useful clinical taxonomy to undergird the assessment of speech disorders. Apraxia of speech is an interesting disorder in this respect because it is poorly understood and has been variously interpreted as a phonological disorder, a motor programming disorder, a motor sequencing disorder, and so on. A taxonomy of motor performance in speaking is needed to resolve the many uncertainties of data interpretation that converge in the speech disorder called apraxia of speech. The same taxonomy could be usefully applied to a number of speech disorders, including the dysarthrias and the aphasias.

Rapid advances in the brain sciences are bringing many human behaviors, even complex ones, into the provinces of neurophysiological research. Steven Barlow considers the prospects for neurophysiological studies to address issues in speech intelligibility. He reviews research on neural systems that have been implicated in the control of animal vocalizations. These studies complement research on humans, and are particularly valuable in showing the effects of selected lesions on vocal behaviors. The neurophysiological requirements of speech are complicated, but Dr. Barlow suggests that they culminate in a requisite precision of the spatial-temporal organization of structural forces along the vocal tract. The effects of various disorders, including neurologic disorders such as dysarthria, may be largely to disrupt the precision of the force patterns. The neurophysiological interpretation of impaired speech intellibility, then, rests on both an understanding of the normal control of force patterns in speech and an understanding of the ways in which these patterns are altered through neurologic disease.

It may seem to some that speech intelligibility is far removed from animal vocalizations. However, studies of animal vocal behaviors have revealed a number of phenomena that may inform the understanding of the neurophysiological basis of human speech and language. Bauers (1989) pointed out that recent studies of nonhuman primates present evidence of language-like capacities for "referential signaling" (Seyfarth, Cheney and Marler, 1980), "representational signaling" (Gouzoules, Gouzoules, and Marler, 1984; Marler, 1985), and "syntactic structure" (Robinson, 1984). These studies were based on only three of the approximately 185 (Jolly, 1985) living primate species. Obviously, the field for potential research is vast. In her own research, Bauers noted interesting similarities between some of the vocalizations used by stumptail macaques (especially those used in friendly, close encounters) and isolated syllables of human speech.

Studies of avian communication also are of great interest in this respect. Many birds learn conspecific songs through a process of exposure and imitation; moreover, the auditory-motor interactions that underlie song learning are being studied in association with the neural processes that control vocalization (Williams, 1989). The continued investigation of these brain-behavior relationships in avian song may suggest principles for the understanding of the neural regulation of human speech.

Intelligibility is the *sine qua non* of spoken language. Disorders that impair intelligibility are among the most serious disorders of communication. Regrettably — and remarkably — few, if any, books have been published on intelligibility concerns in speech pathology, even though intelligibility is a common, if not foremost, issue in this clinical field. Only relatively recently has there been significant progress in formal intelligibility assessment. Perhaps there is no single intelligibility assessment that can be used across the spectrum of ages, abilities and assessment needs encountered in the population of speech and language disordered individuals. But a relatively small number of tests might suffice. Recent progress is a hopeful sign. Several researchers have introduced promising methods for intelligibility assessment and management. It is hoped that this book represents the topic of intelligibility in a way that encourages further invention in research and clinical efforts relating to this essential aspect of speech and language performance.

References

Bauers, K.A. 1989. *The Role of Vocal Communication in the Intra-group Social Dynamics of Stumptailed Macaques*. Unpublished Ph.D. dissertation, University of Wisconsin-Madison, Madison, Wisconsin.

Billman, K.S. 1986. "Phonological processes and intelligibility of spontaneous utterances in young children." Unpublished Master's thesis, San Diego State University, San Diego, California.

Carlson, G.S. and Bernstein, J. 1988. "A voice-input communication aid." Final Report of Contract N01-NS-5-2394 submitted to the National Institute of Neurological and Communicative Disorders and Stroke (April, 1988). SRI International, Menlo Park, California.

Gouzoules, S., Gouzoules, H., and Marler, P. 1984. "Rhesus monkey (Macaca mulatta) screams: Representational signaling in the recruitment of agonistic aid." *Animal Behavior* 32, 182-193.

Jolly, A. 1985. *The Evolution of Primate Behavior*. New York: Macmillan.

Kent, R.D. 1990. "Speech intelligibility and communicative competence in children." Paper presented at the Conference on the Social Use of Language: Pathways to Success, sponsored by the National Institute of Child Health and Human Development, and the John F. Kennedy Center, Peabody College, Vanderbilt University, Nashville, Tennessee, June 20-22, 1990.

Kewley-Port, D., Watson, C.S., Elbert, M., Maki, and Reed, D. (in press). "The Indiana Speech Training Aid (ISTRA) II: Training curriculum and selected case studies." *Clinical Linguistics and Phonetics*.

Marler, P. 1985. "Representational vocal signals of primates." *Fortschritte der Zoologie*. 31.211-221.

Robinson, J.G. 1984. "Syntactic structures in the vocalizations of wedge-capped Capuchin monkeys, Cebus olivaceus." *Behavior* 90, 46-79.

Seyfarth, R.M., Cheney, D.L., and Marler, P. 1980. "Vervet monkey alarm calls: Semantic communication in a free-ranging primate." *Animal Behavior* 34, 1450-1468.

Watson, C.S., Reed, D, Kewley-Port, D., and Maki, D. (in press). "Indiana Speech Training Aid (ISTRA) I: Comparisons between human and computer-based evaluation of speech quality." *Journal of Speech and Hearing Research*.

Williams, H. 1989. "Multiple representations and auditory-motor interactions in the avian song system." In M. Davis, B.L. Jacobs and R.I. Schoenfeld (eds.), *Modulation of Defined Vertebrate Neural Circuits. Annals New York Academy of Sciences* 563, 148-164.

Chapter 1

Scaling procedures for the measurement of speech intelligibility

Nicholas Schiavetti
State University of New York

Introduction

For decades, speech intelligibility measurements have served a number of different purposes for a variety of professionals with various goals in mind. Communication engineers began this work with their use of speech intelligibility tests to evaluate the distortion of speech passed through different transmission systems, especially telephones (Fletcher, 1953). Audiologists later employed intelligibility measures to evaluate the speech discrimination or recognition abilities of hearing impaired persons (Penrod, 1985). Speech intelligibility measurements may also be important to linguists in determining whether two related speech varieties are to be considered as different dialects of the same language or as two different languages on the basis of the mutual intelligibility of the two speech varieties (Comrie, 1987).

Of most concern to readers of this volume, speech pathologists have adopted speech intelligibility measurement as one criterion for the assessment of the severity of speech disorders (Metz, Schiavetti, and Sitler, 1980). Using speech intelligibility as a severity criterion follows from Van Riper's long held notion that "speech is defective when it is conspicuous, unintelligible, or unpleasant" (Van Riper & Emerick, 1984:34). Recent work by Weismer, Kent, Hodge, and Martin (1988) suggests that intelligibility measurement may transcend the mere indexing of severity of speech disorder and be useful for explaining the basis of a speech disorder in terms of specific articulatory deficits. In addition, Monsen (1981) has suggested several uses for speech intelligibility assessments of deaf children, including monitoring student progress in speech therapy, comparing methods of speech training, and evaluating candidacy for mainstreaming. Yorkston and Beukelman (1981) have also suggested that speech intelligibility measurement is useful because results of intelligibility testing can be easily communicated to the speaker's family and to other professions. Furthermore, they concluded that their finding (Beukelman & Yorkston, 1979) of a strong relationship between intelligibility scores and information transfer indicated that speech intelligibility measures can provide a functional index of communicative performance. Subtelny (1977) expressed a similar opinion about the value of intelligibility measures for the speech of the hearing impaired population, but added a strong methodological caution, when she stated:

> Intelligibility is considered the most practical single index to apply in assessing competence in oral communication. For many years the difficulties and limitations in evaluating the intelligibility of deaf speech have been recognized. This basic fact has necessitated considerable study to establish the reliability and validity of the intelligibility assessments and to define the variables influencing intelligibility. Without this effort, the term "intelligibility" cannot be used with confidence for research, academic, social, or vocational purposes. (1977:183)

Subtelny's remarks point out the importance of careful attention to methodological considerations in the use of speech intelligibility measures with any speech disordered population. It is crucial to understand that any measure of speech intelligibility is a measurement of the interaction between a speaker, a transmission system, and a listener. Therefore, it is important to quantify the parameters that concern the speaker's production, the quality of the transmission system, and the listener's response. Thus, the audiologist wishes to hold constant the parameters affecting the speaker and transmission system to study the effects of the listener's hearing impairment on the intelligibility of normal speech presented through a high quality transmission system to a hearing impaired listener. In a similar vein, the communication engineer holds the normal speaker and normal listener constant and varies the parameters of the transmission system to evaluate the effects of transmission system parameters (e.g., signal-to-noise ratio, bandwidth, etc.) on speech intelligibility. (The audiologist might also hold the speaker and the listener constant and vary the transmission system quality by comparing the responses of one hearing impaired listener trying out several different hearing aids.) Finally, the speech pathologist wishes to hold constant the transmission system and listener parameters in order to evaluate the effect of variations in speaker parameters on speech intelligibility. The speech pathologist might, for example be concerned with the influence of the speaker's prosodic errors, in addition to segmental phonemic errors, on speech intelligibility (Parkhurst & Levitt, 1978). Therefore, regardless of the purpose of any speech intelligibility measurement, the interaction of speaker, transmission system, and listener must be considered in making the measurement.

Definition of speech intelligibility

Speech intelligibility, therefore, may be defined as the match between the intention of the speaker and the response of the listener to the speech passed through the transmission system. When all of the words in the listener's response list match all the words intended to be produced by the speaker, speech intelligibility is perfect. When none of the words in the listener's response list match the words intended to be produced by the speaker, speech intelligibility is zero. In between these extremes of perfect and zero speech intelligibility lies a continuum on which we may quantify the degree to which the response list of the listener matches the intended productions of the speaker.

The major question to be asked is: How shall we quantify our measurements of the degree of match between speaker intention and listener response along this continuum of speech intelligibility? Will the match be measured with word identification tests that allow us to line up the listener's words against the speaker's words for comparison? Or will the match be measured with a scaling procedure that allows the listener to make a judgment about the match between the listener's and speaker's list of words? As Stevens (1966a: 385) has said:

> The core of the act of judgment is the process of matching....In the process
> of judging, he (the listener) selects from one domain an item that matches,
> in some respect or other, an item drawn from another domain.

Stevens (1966b, 1968) has shown that magnitude *estimation* scaling procedures (such as those available for the measurement of speech intelligibility) typically ask the observer to match each stimulus to be judged with a number that represents some characteristic of the stimulus. Alternatively, in a magnitude *production* or cross-modality task, the observer can adjust the value of some other stimulus until it corresponds to the value of the characteristic to be judged. In any case, then, a variety of procedures exists to measure the match between speaker intention and listener response and the major question to be addressed is how to make this measurement of speech intelligibility.

Measurement

To answer this question, we should first define what we mean by measurement and specify the properties of measurement required for valid quantification of the continuum of speech intelligibility. Stevens (1946: 677) presented a succinct definition of measurement when he stated:

> ...measurement, in the broadest sense, is defined as the assignment of numerals to objects or events according to rules. The fact that numerals can be assigned under different rules leads to different kinds of scales and different kinds of measurement. The problem then becomes that of making explicit (a) the various rules for the assignment of numerals (b) the mathematical properties (or group structure) of the resulting scales, and (c) the statistical operations applicable to measurements made with each type of scale.

Stevens (1946, 1951) specified four levels of measurement on the basis of the operations performed in assigning numerals to objects or events: nominal, ordinal, interval, and ratio levels of measurement. The nominal level of measurement is achieved when objects or events are classified into mutually exclusive categories by determination of the equality of the characteristic to be measured for the members of a category. For example, speakers could be classified into the categories of "intelligible" vs. "unintelligible" speakers. The ordinal level of measurement is achieved when objects or events are put into a relative ranking by determination of a greater or lesser value of the characteristic to be measured. For example, a group of speakers could be ranked from the most to the least intelligible. The interval level of measurement is achieved by determination of the equality of intervals or differences between the objects or events on the value of the characteristic to be measured. For example, a seven-point equal-appearing interval scale could be used to assess the degree of intelligibility of speakers. Finally, the ratio level of measurement is achieved by determination of the equality of ratios between the objects or events to be measured on the value of the characteristic to be measured. For example, a ratio scaling procedure such as magnitude estimation could be used to assess the degree of intelligibility of speakers or a word identification test could be used to count the number of a speaker's words correctly heard by a listener.

In general, when a choice is available, a preferable order of selection of level of measurement to be used is: ratio, interval, ordinal, and nominal. The reason for this order of preference is that more statistical operations are permissible with ratio than with interval, with interval than with ordinal, and with ordinal than with nominal (Stevens, 1951, see especially Table 6, p. 25). As Stevens (1958: 384) has said:

> Each of these scales has its uses, but it is the more powerful ratio scale that serves us best in the search for nature's regularities.... Why, it may be asked do we bother with the other types of scales? Mostly we use the weaker forms of measurement only *faute de mieux*. When stronger forms are discovered we are quick to seize them.

When possible, then, one strives to reach the highest level of measurement available (i.e., ratio), but practical limitations may force one to drop back to a less preferable level in order to make the most feasible measurement available. It would be desirable, therefore, to employ measures of speech intelligibility at the ratio level, but if circumstances preclude this, then one would try to make the measurement at the interval level. Barring the interval level, one would then try the ordinal level, and then the nominal level. Because feasible methods are available for making ratio level measurements, the highest level of measurement should be our practical goal in the assessment of speech intelligibility.

Intelligibility measurement methods

There are basically two kinds of tasks that have been used to measure speech intelligibility: (1) word identification tests in which the listener is required to write down what the talker says and (2) scaling procedures in which the listener makes judgments about the talker's intelligibility using a technique such as an equal appearing interval scaling procedure or direct magnitude estimation. Word identification procedures provide a frequency count of the number of words on the listener's response list that match the words on the speaker's list of intended words. This frequency count is usually converted to a percentage or a proportion of matched words relative to the total word list as the metric of speech intelligibility. Scaling procedures basically ask the listener to judge in some way how well his/her responses could match the speaker's list of intended words and yield a value on some predetermined scale such as a constrained 7-point interval scale or an unconstrained magnitude estimation scale. Such scale values do not correspond to a traditional unit of measure of intelligibility such as percent or proportion of correctly matched words. However, scaling procedures may also be used by the listener to estimate what percent of the words on the listener's response list would match the words on the speaker's intended list . In other words, a scaling procedure could be used by the listener to estimate what percent of words they believe they could hear correctly by listening to this speaker (Beukelman & Yorkston, 1980).

Word identification tests have been used almost exclusively to measure speech intelligibility for the evaluation of the efficiency of speech transmission by communication engineers and for the evaluation of speech recognition ability of the hearing impaired by audiologists. Speech pathologists, on the other hand, have been divided between the use of word identification procedures and scaling procedures to measure speech intelligibility for the evaluation of severity of disordered speech. This division may reflect a number of factors, including personal preference, previous experience with the measurement technique, implications of previous research findings, or practical considerations. The important factors to review here are the practical considerations and the implications of previous research findings.

Use of scaling procedures in communication disorders

Scaling procedures have been applied to the measurement of many parameters in communication disorders. Typically, scaling procedures have been applied to the measurement of some aspect of a speaker's behavior that is considered a *dependent variable*, i.e. a behavior that is influenced by the manipulation of an independent variable or that is a criterion variable used to compare the performance of subjects in different group classifications such as deaf vs. hearing speakers. The utility of scaling procedures in communication disorders resides in two major advantages (Schiavetti, 1984). First, the scaling of many dimensions of disordered communication is considered by some writers to be the most direct assessment for a particular dimension. For example, Young (1969: 135) has said:

> ...a measurement of a speech disorder is primarily a perceptual event, and
> the observer's response necessarily represents the "final" validation for
> any measurements.

Because many terms such as "speech defectiveness", "hoarseness", "severity of stuttering", or "speech naturalness" may be denoted by listener reactions to speech, direct measurement of the degree of these aspects that are
present in a given talker's speech may be obtained by asking listeners to
scale these parameters. Of course, many such parameters also have other
metric counterparts that could qualify as valid measures; for example stuttering severity could be quantified by counting the number of nonfluencies
in a speech sample. An important consideration, then, is the determination
of when scaling is a more direct measure of a parameter in question than
some other available metric. Such is the case in deciding to use a nonf-
luency count vs. scaled stuttering severity or a word identification test vs.
scaled speech intelligibility. Nevertheless, many aspects of disordered communication can be measured directly with scaling and this is a primary
reason for the historically common use of scaling procedures in communication disorders research and clinical measurement.

A second advantage resides in the relative simplicity of the use of scaling procedures. Scaling can often be used as an appropriate alternative to a
more time-consuming, expensive, or cumbersome measurement procedure.
For example, Metz, Schiavetti, and Sitler (1980) pointed out that although
word identification tests appear to have better face validity than scaling of
speech intelligibility, many people have adopted scaling procedures
because of their relative ease, efficiency, economy, and because the use of
scaling requires fewer listeners than word identification tests. Also, scaling
is available to a wide range of users in clinical settings because it usually
requires a pencil-and-paper format rather than expensive equipment. Guilford (1954: 297) has listed several advantages of rating scale procedures,
including their economy of time, the ability to maintain the interest of the
raters, the ability to use naive raters with a minimum of training, and the
usefulness of scaling with large numbers of stimuli.

Use of scaling to measure speech intelligibility

The communication disorders literature contains a number of studies that
have used scaling procedures instead of, or in addition to, word identifica-

tion tests to measure speech intelligibility. The most commonly used scaling method has been the equal-appearing interval scaling technique. The purpose and methods of these studies are varied as seen in the following examples.

Platt, Andrews, Young, and Quinn (1980) used word identification tests and interval scaled intelligibility of a prose reading passage in a study designed to compare intelligibility and articulatory impairment of spastic and athetoid cerebral palsied adults. Hanson and Metter (1980) used interval scaled prose intelligibility, in conjunction with speaking rate and vocal intensity measures, to assess the effectiveness of delayed auditory feedback as an instrumental treatment for an adult with dysarthria. An often-cited study by Jensema, Karchmer, and Trybus (1978) examined the relationships between interval scaled speech intelligibility of deaf children and a number of variables such as degree of hearing loss, age, hearing aid usage, type of educational program, ethnic background, income, and communication method. McGarr and Osberger (1978) used interval scaled speech intelligibility in a study of pitch deviancy and other aspects of speech production of deaf children. Subtelny (1977) reviewed in detail an interval scaling technique for assessment of speech intelligibility of deaf adults and Kelly, Dancer, and Bradley (1986) assessed the relationship between this scale and the SPINE test of speech intelligibility developed by Monsen (1981).

Substantial reliability has been reported for the scaling of speech intelligibility in a number of studies. Subtelny (1977) examined interjudge agreement with a 5-point interval scale of intelligibility used with deaf adults and found 95.3% agreement within 1 scale point among the judgments of 5 speech pathologists rating 467 different speakers. Her measure of intrajudge reliability with a re-rating of 50 speakers showed a test-retest correlation coefficient of +0.97. Samar and Metz (1988) examined interrater and intrarater reliability for the same scale. They found test-retest correlations for spontaneous speech ratings of +0.96 and for oral reading of +0.94 and intrarater coefficients of +0.98. and +0.97 for the same two speech tasks. Darley, Aronson, and Brown (1969) reported intraobserver and interobserver reliability data for 7-point interval scaling of the intelligibility of dysarthric speakers. Their results indicated perfect agreement or agreement within 1 scale point on the scaling of intelligibility and a number of other dimensions approximately 85% of the time.

Comparison of scaling procedures

Numerous scaling procedures are available for the assessment of a dimension such as speech intelligibility. As Guilford (1954: 263) has said:

> Of the psychological-measurement methods that depend upon human judgment, rating scale procedures exceed them all for popularity and use.

Although there are many varieties of paired comparison, ordinal judgment, interval scaling, and ratio production and estimation procedures available, the methods of equal-appearing interval scaling and direct magnitude estimation have been the most widely used procedures for scaling variables such as speech intelligibility in the communication disorders literature. Procedural details for the use of the large variety of scaling techniques available and methods for scaling data reduction and analysis can be found in Guilford (1954), Engen (1971), Marks (1974), Nunnally (1967), Senders (1958), and Snodgrass (1975). Discussion of all the variations of scaling method and data processing is beyond the scope of this chapter which will focus on the interval scaling and magnitude estimation procedures most commonly used to scale speech intelligibility.

Interval scaling

The method of equal-appearing interval scaling is the most common method of interval scaling seen in studies of speech intelligibility. With this method a listener is required to assign a number to each stimulus sample in order to place the stimulus along a linear partition of the continuum to be scaled, in this case the intelligibility of the speech sample listened to by the rater. Various sizes of the partition have been used, most commonly 5-point, 7-point, or 9-point scales. Odd numbered scales are typically used to provide a middle number as well as end points. Some researchers have simply asked the listeners to partition the intelligibility into the N intervals without descriptions of each interval whereas others have provided descriptors for each number along the scale. Stevens (1975) and Guilford (1954) have reviewed numerical scales and descriptive scales and found little substantive psychometric difference between them. The scale developed at the National Technical Institute for the Deaf (NTID) provides descriptors for each of the 5 numbers used to partition intelligibility. End point descriptors such as "1 = Speech is completely unintelligible" and "5 = Speech is completely intelligible" are used with intermediate descriptors. Samar and Metz

(1988) report the NTID descriptors for scaling intelligibility of oral reading passages and spontaneous speech. In addition, Subtelny (1977) indicated that "since ratings may be made at half-intervals between integers, the scale actually involves 9 points."

Listeners are presented with a number of speech samples of varying intelligibility and asked to rate each sample with a number on the interval scale. Speech samples should be arranged in a random order to minimize the biasing of listeners with an ascending or descending series of speech intelligibility in the samples. Typical speech samples used for scaling have included recordings of oral reading of paragraphs such as the "Rainbow Passage" or "My Grandfather" that are made familiar to the listeners through a prior reading. Also, listeners are usually familiarized with the range of speech intelligibility to be scaled by presentation of a few examples that fall along the range from low to high intelligibility. The arithmetic mean of the interval scale values assigned to each speech sample by the various listeners usually is computed as the metric of intelligibility for each speech sample. Guilford (1954) has written a detailed analysis of scaling procedures and data reduction and analysis methods for equal-appearing interval scaling and similar rating methods.

Direct magnitude estimation

Unlike the interval scaling procedure, direct magnitude estimation does not constrain listeners to fit their rating numbers into a linear partition of the speech intelligibility continuum with fixed maximum and minimum numbers at the extreme ends of the continuum. Instead, direct magnitude estimation allows each listener to judge each speech sample with a number that is proportional to the perceived ratios of speech intelligibility among the speech samples.

Direct magnitude estimation may be accomplished in one of two ways: with or without standard/modulus. In the first variety, the listener scales each speech sample relative to a *standard* speech sample that is assigned a *modulus* or standard subjective value of intelligibility by the experimenter. The experimenter may select the standard from the lower, middle, or upper portion of the intelligibility range and may assign any modulus number to it. Standard samples are typically selected from the middle of the range and the modulus number is customarily 10 or 100. A detailed discussion of the effects of various standard positions and moduli is given by Poulton (1968).

Direct magnitude estimation may also be accomplished with no standard or modulus imposed on the listener by the experimenter. The free-modulus direct magnitude estimation variation permits each listener to begin with any number to assign to the first speech sample and then to assign numbers to subsequent speech samples that correspond to the ratios of the perceived magnitudes of the intelligibility of the various speech samples. A correction for the inter-listener variation in choice of modulus number should be applied to the data prior to analysis (Lane, Catania, & Stevens, 1961). Engen (1971) has written a detailed analysis of scaling procedures and data reduction and analysis methods for both variations of direct magnitude estimation.

Scaling prothetic vs. metathetic continua

Many important theoretical and methodological issues have been raised over the years concerning selection of appropriate scaling procedures for the measurement of different variables. Yet one issue, first discussed by Stevens and Galanter (1957), has repeatedly emerged in the literature with regard to the selection of the direct magnitude estimation vs. interval scaling procedures discussed above: the issue of appropriate methods for scaling prothetic vs. metathetic continua. The research of Stevens and his colleagues over a number of years has demonstrated that there are serious differences in the validity of direct magnitude estimation and interval scaling for the measurement of the two classes of prothetic and metathetic continua (Stevens, 1975).

According to Stevens, a prothetic continuum is additive, whereas a metathetic continuum is substitutive and he has described them as follows:

> The prototypes of the two kinds of perceptual continua are exemplified by loudness and pitch. Loudness is an aspect of sound that has what can best be described as degrees of magnitude or quantity. Pitch does not. Pitch varies from high to low; it has a kind of position, and in a sense it is a qualitative continuum. Loudness may be called a prothetic continuum, and pitch a metathetic one. The criteria that define those two classes of continua reside wholly in how they behave in psychophysical experiments....(1975: 13)

A tabulated summary of prothetic and metathetic continua in a number of different sensory modalities is given in Snodgrass (1975: 52)

Stevens (1975) has summarized experimental evidence which indicates that observers can easily partition a metathetic continuum (such as pitch) into equal intervals and that their interval scale judgments are linearly related to direct magnitude estimates of the same set of stimuli. Although many psychophysicists prefer direct magnitude estimation to interval scaling for a number of other reasons (Engen, 1971; Stevens, 1975), the linear relation of the two sets of scale values may be construed as evidence that either interval scaling or direct magnitude estimation may be valid for use with a metathetic continuum (Snodgrass, 1975). Stevens concluded, however, that interval scaling is invalid for measurement of a prothetic continuum because experimental evidence has repeatedly demonstrated that observers cannot partition a prothetic continuum into equal intervals. If observers attempt to partition a prothetic continuum into equal intervals they typically demonstrate a systematic bias toward subdividing the lower end of the continuum into smaller intervals than the upper portion of the continuum. Engen (1971), Snodgrass (1975), and Stevens (1975) have summarized evidence that the apparent inequality of intervals along a prothetic continuum may be the result of variations in the observer's discriminal ability along the continuum.

Stevens (1975) has summarized his efforts to develop a procedure for comparison of interval scale and direct magnitude estimation values to determine operationally whether a particular continuum is prothetic or metathetic. A set of stimuli falling along the dimension in question is presented to two different groups of observers, one of which uses direct magnitude estimation and the other of which uses equal-appearing interval scaling to judge the stimuli. The arithmetic means of the interval scale values are plotted against the geometric means of the direct magnitude estimates for each stimulus sample. Marks (1974) and Stevens (1975) have suggested the geometric mean as the appropriate measure of central tendency for direct magnitude estimates because the distribution of scale values for a typical set of stimuli is skewed in a log-normal fashion. If the relationship between the two sets of scale values is linear, the observers can partition the continuum into equal intervals and the continuum is metathetic. However, if the two sets of scale values form a downward-bowed (i.e., negatively accelerating) curve they would exhibit the typical inequality of intervals due to unequal discriminal ability that is characteristic of a prothetic continuum. Stevens and Galanter (1957) examined a dozen perceptual continua with this method and later research by Stevens (1966c, 1968) examined continua from a number of areas of behavioral research, including important social, opinion, and legal variables.

The serious problem with interval scales applied to prothetic continua is that the intervals are not, in reality, equal for the observers when they try to partition the continuum. Therefore, a true interval level of measurement cannot be obtained through the use of such scaling procedures with prothetic continua. As stated earlier, preference is expressed for the highest level of measurement obtainable in a given situation because of the greater variety of permissible statistical operations available for the higher levels of measurement. What results from the attempt to partition a prothetic continuum into equal intervals is really an ordinal scale without the benefit of equal distances or differences between the numbers on the so-called equal-appearing interval scale. Obviously, the ratio level of measurement resulting from direct magnitude estimation of a prothetic continuum would be preferable. For this reason authors such as Stevens (1974) and Snodgrass (1975) have referred to interval scaling as "category" scaling since the numbers really identify an ordered series of categories or adjectives (e.g., "very soft", "soft", loud", "very loud") for rating the stimuli. Guilford (1954) has also discussed a method called the method of successive categories, an essentially ordinal scaling method which makes no assumptions regarding the equality of intervals between numbered categories. With regard to the use of such scaling procedures, Stevens (1974: 374) has stated:

> ...the human being, despite his great versatility, has a limited capacity to effect linear partitions on prothetic continua. He does quite well, to be sure, if the continuum happens to be metathetic, but, since most scaling problems involve prothetic continua, it seems that category and other forms of partition scaling generally ought to be avoided....

Stevens called this conclusion "inescapable for the purposes of serious perceptual scaling" and, indeed, a serious reconsideration must be given to the widespread use of equal-appearing interval scaling in light of his findings.

Evidence against the use of scaling procedures for the measurement of speech intelligibility

Evidence against the use of scaling procedures for the measurement of speech intelligibility comes from three sources. First is the consideration of the construct validity of interval scaling of speech intelligibility in light of the foregoing comparison of scaling techniques. Second is the evidence concerning the criterion validity of interval scaled speech intelligibility when

compared to the direct metric of the speaker-listener match, the word identification test. Third is the issue of the practical applicability of scaled
speech intelligibility vs. word identification tests of speech intelligibility.

With regard to the first consideration, Schiavetti, Metz, and Sitler
(1981) investigated speech intelligibility scaling procedures with hearing
impaired speakers in order to determine whether the continuum of speech
intelligibility falls on a prothetic or a metathetic continuum. Direct magnitude estimates and 7-point equal appearing interval scale judgments were
made by two groups of 20 listeners of the speech intelligibility of 20 hearing
impaired talkers whose intelligibility ranged from 0.8% to 99% as measured by word identification tests. Each listener scaled three sets of speech
samples (short sentence, long sentence, and Rainbow Passage spoken by
each talker) presented in counterbalanced orders with talker order randomized within each set of speech material. Stevens' method of plotting
the arithmetic means of the interval scale judgments against the geometric
means of the direct magnitude estimates revealed the downward bowed
curvilinear relationship that is characteristic of a prothetic continuum for all
three sets of speech material. Curvilinearity tests revealed a greater proportion of variance in the data accounted for by a curvilinear than a linear
regression formula and the negatively accelerating exponential formulae
that were used to fit the three functions for the three sets of speech samples
accounted for 98 to 99% of the variance in the three curves.

These results clearly indicate that equal appearing interval scaling is
inappropriate for the measurement of speech intelligibility. Because the
continuum is prothetic, listeners cannot effect a linear partition of the
dimension with the result that the intervals used to scale speech intelligibility are not equal. Therefore, attempts to use interval scaling result in an
ordinal, rather than an interval, level of measurement. Direct magnitude
estimation, therefore, has better construct validity in relation to Stevens'
formulations for the scaling of speech intelligibility and would result in an
intelligibility measure at the ratio level of measurement.

In addition to this problem of construct validity, serious concern has
been raised by Samar and Metz (1988) regarding the criterion validity of
interval scale measures of speech intelligibility. Based on their logical
analysis of the face validity of word identification testing of intelligibility,
they used a word identification test as a validating criterion for the NTID 5-
point intelligibility rating scale. Although a previous study by Subtelny
(1977) had shown relatively high correlations between the NTID scale and

word identification measures, Samar and Metz identified methodological and interpretive problems with the Subtelny study, including a lack of suitable percentage score transformations, curvilinearity in the supposedly linear correlational data, and a lack of an attentuation correction in the validity criterion. By computing confidence intervals across the intelligibility range for the prediction of word identification test intelligibility from scaled intelligibility, Samar and Metz showed that the NTID scale intelligibility measures provided a prediction of the criterion variable with a wide overlap of the range of prediction error among the rating scale categories. The widest confidence intervals were evident in the clinically important midrange of intelligibility where it is quite common to find many hearing impaired students. For example, the 95% confidence interval for the word identification percentage scores associated with the NTID spontaneous speech rating scale score of 3 was 64 percentage points wide, a clearly unacceptable margin of error.

Samar and Metz's comparison of their data to those of Subtelny (1977) showed a similar problem in the midrange of her intelligibility data. Subtelny's (1977: 185, Figure 1) data comparing the NTID scale to sentence context word identification intelligibility scores indicated small standard deviations of intelligibility scores among the subjects with the highest and lowest NTID scale scores (approximately 5% for a rating of "5" and 10% for a rating a "1") but rather large standard deviations of intelligibility scores among the subjects with the three middle ratings (approximately 20% for ratings of "2", "3", or "4"). Samar and Metz pointed out a similar problem in the data of Kelly, Dancer, and Bradley (1986) who compared the NTID scale to Monsen's (1981) SPINE test of intelligibility, a word identification test. Examination of their data (Kelly et al., 1986: 148, Figure 1) by Samar and Metz revealed a wider variability of SPINE scores for subjects in the midrange of the NTID scale than for subjects at the end points. A consistent pattern seems to emerge from Samar and Metz's analysis, in which subjects at either extreme of the NTID scale are relatively homogeneus with respect to word identification test measures of intelligibility but in which speakers at the midrange values of the NTID scale are heterogeneous groups of subjects even within one rating category.

Thus, the work of Samar and Metz suggests that the apparently high correlations seen between word identification tests and rating scale measures of intelligibility in their study and the studies of Subtelny (1977) and Kelly, Dancer, and Bradley (1986) may be spurious indicators of the validity of rating scales because linear correlational analyses often do not take into account the possibility of sigmoidal relationships along the entire intelligibility range, nor do they typically calculate confidence intervals surrounding the predicted criterion variable for all points along the interval scale measure. In addition to highlighting the problems of interpreting the true relation of scaled intelligibility to the criterion variable, Samar and Metz also pointed out other advantages of word identification tests over the NTID rating scale procedure. These include the potential for constructing word identification tests that contain distinct dimensions of speech for analysis of linguistic dimensions of intelligibility, an idea that blends quite well with the suggestions of Weismer et al. (1988) for identifying an "explicit acoustic basis for a single-word intelligibility test." Samar and Metz concluded (1988: 315):

> The foregoing considerations lead us to conclude that there is little justification for the continued use of rating scales in most clinical and research settings. The write-down procedure appears to be a decidedly superior alternative.

In addition to studies of interval and magnitude estimation of speech intelligibility, research has considered the use of a judgment procedure in which listeners audit a paragraph-sized sample of speech and then assign a percentage intelligibility score to the speaker based on the listeners' impressions of how well they could understand the speaker from the overall reading of the passage. Beukelman and Yorkston (1980) studied the relationship of word identification tests completed by naive listeners to the results of such a judgment procedure in which sophisticated listeners (speech pathologists) estimated the intelligibility of speakers by assigning a percent intelligibility score to each speaker after auditing the speaker's reading of the grandfather passage. In assessing mild, moderate, and severe dysarthric speech samples, speech pathologists estimates of their intelligibility consistently overestimated the word identification intelligibility scores derived from transcriptions by inexperienced listeners. In addition, wide variability was evident among the judges, especially for the moderate and severe speech samples, the areas of severity of most importance clinically.

Beukelman and Yorkston further evaluated the speech samples to determine if the differences between actual percent scores (i.e., word identification tests) and estimated percent scores (i.e., judgments of intelligibility) were the result of listener familiarity with the reading passage or listener sophistication in auditing dysarthric speech (i.e., speech pathologists vs. naive listeners). Their results indicated that increased familiarity with the reading passage increased the intelligibility percentage estimates assigned by listeners, especially to dysarthric speakers in the clinically important mid-range of intelligibility. The intelligibility estimates from initially naive listeners who were later highly familiarized with the passage were similar to the estimates from the experienced speech pathologists, suggesting that a large part of the discrepancy between intelligibility percentage estimates and actual word identification scores may stem from listener familiarity with the reading passage.

It is interesting to note that most, if not all, scaling procedures employed in the literature to assess speech intelligibility have used a passage familiarization task to ensure uniformity among listeners in judging the intelligibility of the speech samples. This apparent control procedure may have actually introduced another artifact into the listeners' judgments of intelligibility by causing all listeners to overestimate intelligibility on whatever scale they used because of their familiarity with the passage. Thus, although the control procedure might produce an experimental group of listeners who are uniform with respect to passage familiarity, it might also produce an experimental group of listeners that is *too* familiar with the passage to generalize their results to unfamiliarized listeners. In other words, external validity may have been sacrificed in many studies to improve internal validity, a common problem in experimental and quasi-experimental research (Campbell & Stanley, 1966).

Thus, it appears that neither interval scaling nor percentage estimation judgment of speech intelligibility is a viable technique for the clinical or research measurement of speech intelligibility. Direct magnitude estimation could be a viable scaling procedure if a scaling procedure were necessary. However, it should be pointed out that, although direct magnitude estimation has a long history of successful use in research measurement of a number of dimensions (Stevens, 1975), it may not be the most practical method for clinical measurement of speech intelligibility for a number of reasons. For example, direct magnitude estimation yields a scaled value of intelligibility without a common unit of measure such as percent correct words heard. This lack of an easily interpreted unit of measurement reduces the clinical utility of direct magnitude estimates for communicating intelligibility data to other professionals or laypersons. Also, the direct magnitude estimation procedure can be somewhat cumbersome to use in that it requires the use of either a standard speech sample assigned a modulus value or the difficult modulus equalization technique to remove inter-listener variance in selection of a modulus value for the free-modulus procedure. Finally, direct magnitude estimation is best employed for the measurement of a dimension when a relatively large number of stimulus samples along the dimension are to be scaled so its use is contraindicated when only one or a relatively few speakers are to be measured in a single instance.

It could be argued that it is not necessary to employ a scaling procedure to measure speech intelligibility because of the availability of word identification tests. Although word identification tests may, in some cases, be considered less efficient than scaling procedures, their distinct advantages outweigh whatever inconvenience their use might cause. The next section, then, reviews some of the reasons for the adoption of word identification tests of speech intelligibility.

Evidence for the use of word identification tests for the measurement of speech intelligibility

In addition to the problems mentioned above regarding the use of scaling procedures (particularly interval scale methods) for the measurement of speech intelligibility, there are compelling advantages to the use of the alternative procedure of the word identification test of speech intelligibility.

First of all, word identification tests produce a metric of speech intelligibility that is more readily usable by the researcher or clinician in a form that can be communicated to other professionals and to laypersons. The word identification score is typically calculated as a percentage of words correctly heard or as a proportion that can be easily converted to a percentage. Indexing speech intelligibility with a percentage makes a certain degree of intuitive sense for informing someone of the degree to which they can expect to understand the speech produced by a disordered speaker. Scaling procedures for the most part do not result in a metric that uses percentage of words correctly heard as the unit of measure. And those judgment procedures that do yield a percentage score have been shown to be overestimates of speech intelligibility (Beukelman & Yorkston, 1980).

Secondly, Beukelman and Yorkston (1979) have shown a close relationship between information transfer and word identification test intelligibility scores with dysarthric speakers. A measure of information transfer was taken in which listeners audited recordings of a dysarthric speakers reading a prose paragraph and then answered 10 questions about the content of the paragraph. This information transfer measure was then compared to both isolated word and contextual speech intelligibility measures for the same speakers. The information transfer measure was highly correlated with both isolated word and contextual word speech intelligibility measures, indicating good criterion validity for the two word identification test intelligiiblity measures.

Thirdly, the claims that have been made for the superiority of scaling procedures in efficiency, economy, and ease of use may not be as powerful as once thought (Metz, Schiavetti, and Sitler, 1980). Samar and Metz (1988) reported that their per-capita administration and scoring time for word identification testing was essentially equivalent to the time required for the NTID rating scale. Another putative efficiency advantage of scaling is the use of fewer listeners who are already familiar with the reading passage to be scaled. Yet the research of Beukelman and Yorkston (1980) indicates that this advantage may be a disadvantage in disguise as it yields overestimates of intelligibility relative to word identfcation tests, especially in the midrange of intelligibility.

In regard to ease of use, it should be mentioned that isolated word and contextual word identification tests of intelligibility present a contrast of validity and administrative advantages. It has been pointed out by Schiavetti, Sitler, Metz, and Houde (1984) that although isolated word intelligibility tests are much easier to administer and score, contextual speech intelligibility tests have more external validity as measures of real-world speech intelligibility. However, Sitler, Schiavetti, and Metz (1983) have summarized data indicating a complex relation between contextual speech and isolated word intelligibility measures in which context only improves intelligibility under favorable listening conditions. The problem of whether to use the easier isolated word or more valid contextual word measure has been substantially reduced by the work of Boothroyd (1978, 1985) in developing curvilinear transforms for predicting the more valid contextual measure from the easier to use isolated word measure. Schiavetti, Sitler, Metz, and Houde (1984) have demonstrated the power of Boothroyd's approach for making the more easily administered and scored isolated word intelligibility measure and then predicting the more externally valid contextual word intelligibility measure.

A fourth point concerns the reliability of word identification tests of speech intelligibility. Samar and Metz (1988) reported on the interscorer and intrascorer reliability of contextual word identifcation test results with hearing impaired speakers and found substantial correlations of +0.985 in both instances. Metz, Samar, Schiavetti, Sitler and Whitehead (1985) reported reliabilities for both isolated word and contextual word identification tests of intelligibility with hearing impaired speakers. Interlist reliability for the CID sentence lists C and J was +0.95 and split-half (odd-even) reliability for CID W22 list 1A was +0.93. Yorkston and Beukelman (1978) reported intra- and inter-listner reliabilities for both scaling and word identification tests of the speech intelligibilty of dysarthric speakers. Their results indicated good intra- and inter-listener agreement for both types of measures, with somewhat better consistency for the word identification tests than for the scaling procedures. Word identification tests, then, can provide speech intelligibility measures that are at least as reliable as those yielded by scaling procedures.

A fifth reason concerns the relationship of word identification test data to acoustical characteristics of speech. Monsen (1978) and Metz, Samar, Schiavetti, Sitler, and Whitehead (1985) have analyzed the relationships among acoustical characteristics of the speech of hearing impaired talkers and measures of their intelligibility and found reasonably good ability to predict intelligibility from acoustic parameters, especially measures of consonant voicing contrast such as VOT differences among voiced/voiceless pairs. This research is important as a step toward the development of an acoustical description of unintelligible vs. intelligibile speech that may one day result in automated instrumental measurement of speech intelligibility for disordered populations. Metz et al. (1985) found much better prediction of word identification test than direct magnitude estimation scaling measures of speech intelligibility from their acoustical parameters. In addition, the work of Weismer, Kent, Hodge, and Martin (1988) and Kent, Weismer, Kent, and Rosenbeck (1989) discussed below suggests that these preliminary attempts at predicting speech intelligibility will ultimately require specifically designed word identification tests that are sensitive to the kinds of speech errors made by specific speech-impaired populations with intelligibility deficits.

Finally, and perhaps most importantly, it has been suggested that word identification tests of speech intelligibility may transcend the mere indexing of severity of speech disorder and be useful in the efforts aimed at the explanation of intelligibility deficits. Weismer, Kent, Hodge, and Martin (1988) began the development of such an explanatory test of speech intelligibility for dysarthric speakers with their study of acoustic "signatures" for intellgibility test words. They described formant trajectories and segment durations for male and female normal geriatric speakers for seven test words. Acoustic signatures might be developed from such data as normal ranges of segment duration with a criterion specified for the distance of a dysarthric speaker from an empirically derived signature boundary (e.g., a confidence interval for normal segment duration). In addition to these acoustic data, Kent and Weismer (1989) have begun collection of x-ray articulatory motion data to develop articulatory as well as acoustic signatures for intelligibility test words. A major goal in both cases would be the specification of both intraspeaker and interspeaker variability in articulatory and acoustic parameters to determine the usefulness of normative signature values in explanatory intelligibility testing with speech disordered populations. Kent, Weismer, Kent, and Rosenbeck (1989) have proposed a multiple-choice and a paired-word intelligibility test that include test words that incorporate acoustic/phonetic contrasts that are both sensitive to dysarthric impairment and contribute to speech intelligibility. The development and validation of explanatory word identification tests of speech intelligibility would satisfy the need for a metric to transcend the mere indexing of severity of speech disorder and produce a test of unlimited utility for description of disordered speech and documentation of therapeutic change.

In conclusion, it is important to heed the words of Monsen (1983) in his call for further research and development concerning the measurement of the speech intelligibility of hearing imopaired speakers and to consider his comments in a more general call for improvement of intelligibility measurement with all apporpriate populations. Monsen (1983: 287) stated:

> Despite the generally acknowledged importance of speech intelligibility, most hearing-impaired children grow to adulthood and graduate from a variety of special education programs without ever having their speech intelligibility measured by anything other than a nonstandardized rating system (e.g., "very intelligible," "intelligible," ... "unintelligible")....The need for objective measures of speech intelligibility is particularly important at a time when a variety of claims are being made for different teaching methods that are being implemented in different educational settings.

Obviously, reliable and valid measures of speech intelligibility are necessary for the indexing of severity of speech disorders and for the explanation of intelligibility deficits from both an acoustic and an articulatory standpoint. Such measures would provide important data for the description of disordered speech and for the documentation of gains provided by treatment procedures.

References

Beukelman, D.R., & Yorkston, K.M. 1979. "The relationship between information transfer and speech intelligibility of dysarthric speakers." *Journal of Communication Disorders* 12, 189-196.

Beukelman, D.R., & Yorkston, K.M. 1980. "The influence of passage familiarity on intelligibility estimates of dysarthric speech." *Journal of Communication Disorders* 13, 33-41.

Boothroyd, A. 1978. "Speech perception and sensorineural hearing loss." In M. Ross & T. Giolas (eds), *Auditory Management of Hearing Impaired Children*. (pp 117-144). Baltimore, MD: University Park Press.

Boothroyd, A. 1985. "Evaluation of speech production of the hearing impaired: Some benefits of forced-choice testing." *Journal of Speech and Hearing Research* 28, 185-196.

Campbell, D.T., & Stanley, J.C. 1966. *Experimental and quasi-experimental designs for research*. Chicago, IL: Rand-McNally.

Comrie, B. 1987. *The world's major languages*. NY: Oxford University Press.

Darley, F.L., Aronson, A.E., & Brown, J.R. 1969. "Clusters of deviant speech dimensions in the dysarthrias." *Journal of Speech and Hearing Research* 12, 462-496.

Engen, T. 1971. "Psychophysics II. Scaling methods." In J.W. Kling & L. Riggs (eds.), *Woodworth and Schlossberg's Experimental Psychology*, 47-86). New York: Holt, Rinehart, & Winston.

Fletcher, H. 1953. *Speech and Hearing in Communication*. Princeton, NJ: Van Nostrand.

Guilford, J.P. 1954. *Psychometric Methods*. New York: McGraw-Hill.

Hanson, W.R., & Metter, E.J. 1980. "DAF as instrumental treatment for dysarthria in progressive supranuclear palsy: A case report." *Journal of Speech and Hearing Disorders* 45, 268-276.

Jensema, C., Karchmer, M., & Trybus, R. 1978. *The rated speech intelligibility of hearing impaired children: Basic relationships and a detailed analysis*. (Series R, Number 6) Washington, DC: Gallaudet College, Office of Demographic Studies.

Kelly, C., Dancer, J., & Bradley, R. 1986. "Correlation of SPINE test scores to judges' ratings of speech intelligibility in hearing impaired children." *Volta Review* 88, 145-150.

Kent, R.D., & Weismer, G. 1989, May. Articulatory and acoustic signatures of selected monosyllabic words. Paper presented at the meeting of the Acoustical Society of America, Syracuse, NY.

Kent, R.D., Weismer, G., Kent, J.F., & Rosenbeck, J.C. (1989). "Toward phonetic intelligibility testing in dysarthria." *Journal of Speech and Hearing Disorders* 54, 482-499.

Lane, H.L, Catania, A.C., & Stevens, S.S. 1961. "Voice level: Autophonic scale, perceived loudness, and effects of sidetone." *Journal of the Acoustical Society of America* 33, 160-167.

Marks, L.E. 1974. *Sensory Processes.* New York: Academic Press.

McGarr, N.S., & Osberger, M.J. 1978. "Pitch deviancy and intelligibility of deaf speech." *Journal of Communication Disorders* 11, 237-247.

Metz, D.E., Samar, V.J., Schiavetti, N., Sitler, R.W., & Whitehead, R.L. 1985. "Acoustic dimensions of hearing-impaired speakers intelligibility." *Journal of Speech and Hearing Research* 28, 345-355.

Metz, D.E., Schiavetti, N., & Sitler, R. 1980. "Toward an objective description of the dependent and independent variables associated with intelligibility assessments of hearing impaired adults." In J. Subtelny (ed.), *Speech Assessment and Speech Improvement for the Hearing Impaired*, 72-81. Washington, DC: A.G. Bell Association for the Deaf.

Monsen, R.B. 1978. "Toward measuring how well hearing impaired children speak." *Journal of Speech and Hearing Research* 21, 197-219.

Monsen, R.B. 1981. "A usable test of speech intelligibility of deaf talkers." *American Annals of the Deaf* 126, 845-852.

Monsen, R.B. 1983. "The oral speech intelligibility of hearing-impaired talkers." *Journal of Speech and Hearing Disorders* 48, 286-296.

Nunnally, J.C. 1967. *Psychometric theory.* New York: McGraw-Hill.

Parkhurst, B.G., & Levitt, H. 1978. "The effect of selected prosodic errors on the intelligibility of deaf speech." *Journal of Communication Disorders* 11, 249-256.

Penrod, J.P. 1985. "Speech discrimination testing." In J. Katz (ed.), *Handbook of Clinical Audiology*, (3rd ed.), 235-255. Baltimore, MD: Williams & Wilkins.

Platt, L.J., Andrews, G., Young, M, & Quinn, P. 1980. "Dysarthria of adult cerebral palsy: I. Intelligibility and articulation impairment." *Journal of Speech and Hearing Research* 23, 28-40.

Poulton, E.C. 1968. "The new psychophysics: Six models for magnitude estimation." *Psychological Bulletin* 69, 1-19.

Samar, V.J., & Metz, D.E. 1988. "Criterion validity of speech intelligibility rating-scale procedures for the hearing-impaired population." *Journal of Speech and Hearing Research* 31, 307-316.

Schiavetti, N. 1984. "Scaling procedures for quantification of speech, language and hearing variables." In R.G. Daniloff (ed.), *Articulation Assessment and Treatment Issues*, 237-253. San Diego, CA: College-Hill Press.

Schiavetti, N., Metz, D.E., & Sitler, R.W. 1981. "Construct validity of direct magnitude estimation and interval scaling of speech intelligibility: Evidence from a study of the hearing impaired." *Journal of Speech and Hearing Research* 24, 441-445.

Schiavetti, N., Sacco, P.R., Metz, D.E., & Sitler, R.W. 1983. "Direct magnitude estimation and interval scaling of stuttering severity." *Journal of Speech and Hearing Research* 26, 568-573.

Schiavetti, N., Sitler, R.W., Metz, D.E., & Houde, R.A. 1984. "Prediction of contextual speech intelligibility from isolated word intelligibility measures." *Journal of Speech and Hearing Research* 27, 623-626.

Senders, V.L. 1958. *Measurement and statistics*. New York: Oxford University Press.

Sitler, R.W., Schiavetti, N., & Metz, D.E. 1983. "Contextual effects in the measurement of hearing-impaired speakers' intelligibility." *Journal of Speech and Hearing Research* 26, 30-34.

Snodgrass, J.G. 1975. "Psychophysics." In B. Scharf (ed.), *Experimental Sensory Psychology*, 17-67. Glenview, IL: Scott Foresman.

Stevens, S.S. 1946. "On the theory of scales of measurement." *Science*, 103, 677-680.

Stevens, S.S. 1951. "Mathematics, measurement, and psychophysics." In S.S. Stevens (ed.), *Handbook of Experimental Psychology*, 1-49. New York: Wiley.

Stevens, S.S. 1958. "Measurement and man." *Science* 127, 383-389.

Stevens, S.S. 1966a. "On the operation known as judgment." *American Scientist* 54, 385-401.

Stevens, S.S. 1966b. "Quantifying the sensory experience." In P.K. Feyerabend & G. Maxwell (eds) *Mind, Matter, and Method: Essays in Philosophy and Science in Honor of Herbert Feigl*, 215-233. Minneapolis, MN: University of Minnesota Press.

Stevens, S.S. 1966c. "A metric for the social consensus." *Science* 151, 530-541.

Stevens, S.S. 1968. "Ratio scales of opinion." In D.K. Whitla (ed.), *Handbook of Measurement and Assessment in Behavioral Sciences*, 171-199. Reading, MA: Addison-Wesley.

Stevens, S.S. 1974. "Perceptual magnitude and its measurement." In E.C. Carterette & M.P. Friedman (eds.), *Handbook of Perception (Vol.II)*, 361-389. New York: Academic Press.

Stevens, S.S. 1975. *Psychophysics*. New York: Wiley.

Stevens, S.S., & Galanter, E.H. 1957. "Ratio scales and category scales for dozen perceptual continua." *Journal of Experimental Psychology* 54, 377-411.

Subtelny, J. 1977. "Assessment of speech with implications for training." In F. Bess (ed.), *Childhood Deafness*, 183-194. NY: Grune & Stratton.

Van Riper, C., & Emerick, L. 1984. *Speech Correction*, 7th Ed. Englewood Cliffs, NJ: Prentice-Hall.

Weismer, G., Kent, R.D., Hodge, M., & Martin, R. 1988. "The acoustic signature for intelligibility test words." *Journal of the Acoustical Society of America* 84, 1281-1291.

Yorkston, K.M., & Beukelman, D.R. 1978. "A comparison of techniques for measuring intelligibility of dysarthric speech." *Journal of Communication Disorders* 11, 499-512.

Yorkston, K.M., & Beukelman, D.R. 1981. *Assessment of Intelligibility of Dysarthric Speech*. Tigard, OR: C.C. Publications.

Young, M.A., (1969. "Observer agreement: Cumulative effects of rating many samples." *Journal of Speech and Hearing Research* 12, 135-143.

Chapter 2

An application of structural linguistics to intelligibility measurement of impaired speakers of English

Rida S. Bross
Biomedical Metatechnology, Inc.

Introduction

The methods of structural linguistics have been demonstrated to be an effective means of obtaining an accurate description of the language of normal speakers. The same methods have been applied with equal success to speech samples of impaired speakers to provide descriptions of the structural deviation of pathological forms of English. The precise results of objective procedures required by the discipline have an immediate relevance to the diagnosis, treatment, and evaluation of these speakers.

In studies of impaired speakers, the purpose of the investigation dictates the pertinent units and levels of language to be examined. Such studies customarily focus upon phonetic detail for information about articulation features, or on phonemic classes for a wider perspective of phonological damage. In many instances, there is a confusion as to whether the production of the speakers is accurate, acceptable, and intelligible, with no clear distinction between these factors and how they relate to language structure. The Aspectual theory of structural linguistics encompasses within its theoretical framework the various levels and strata of language structure that very clearly differentiate between these factors.

Linguistics was established as a scientific discipline early in the 20th century with investigations of the American Indian languages. The rigorous procedures for the objective study of languages in their own terms, without preconception, became a hallmark of the American school of structural, or descriptive, linguistics. With the empirical approach to the complex behavior exhibited by language, techniques of elicitation, transcription, and analysis were developed. These rigorous techniques were confirmed as valid by their successful application to a variety of linguistic systems by subsequent investigators.

With the emergence of an American school of structural linguistics, several structural theories evolved. The basic assumption which is characteristic of these theories is that language has an hierarchic structure, and that the structure can be described. The various structural theories diverge in perspective, in concepts of the nature of the language hierarchy, and in identifying the units, levels, and relationships of the hierarchy.

The Aspectual theory of structural linguistics was developed by George L. Trager and Henry Lee Smith, Jr. within the tradition of American descriptivism as a comprehensive theory of language. Applying to the English language the rigorous procedures which had been found appropriate for the exotic languages, Trager and Smith produced an authoritative description of English structure commended by colleagues and considered a classic in the discipline. The Trager-Smith (T-S hereafter) analysis of English structure (1961) serves as a standard for all dialects of the language, and as a basis for comparison for non-standard varieties and for pathological forms of impaired speakers.

The T-S analysis of English structure has stood the test of time and been found to be sound.

> Trager and Smith's *Outline of English Structure* presents the system which has most generally been used by linguists in the last few years. ... After years of searching criticism, Trager and Smith's analysis remains without close competition as the most workable available. (Gleason, 1961: 490-492)

Customary testing of impaired speakers involves examination of the phonological system to determine problems of articulation. Errors are manifest in phonetic and phonemic segments. Diagnosis and treatment for these speakers are dependent on close scrutiny of the phonological levels of language structure. At a higher level of language structure, an Aspectual analysis addresses the problem of intelligibility by close scrutiny of morphological structures to identify the morphophone unit. The morphophone is the abstract structural unit by which different pronunciations of the same words, produced by different phonemes, are accepted by speakers of the same language as being the same. It is by means of the morphophone that speakers are judged to be intelligible.

The key to intelligibility is the concept of "calibration". All speakers experience this phenomenon. A frequent example is that of Americans first encountering Australian speech. At first, this variety of English appears to be almost unintelligible. However, after some conversation, the Australian speaker may miraculously *become* intelligible. What is the mechanism by which this takes place? The Australian speaker has not changed his ingrained speech habits and is producing the same sounds. Therefore, intelligibility is not entirely a matter of the sounds produced by a speaker.

Both speaker and listener are necessarily involved in intelligibility. In linguistic terms, the listener has calibrated the speaker's variety, or dialect, of English. Listeners apparently have the remarkable ability to make rapid correlations. It appears that listeners automatically correlate the different sounds or phonemes of other dialects that serve the same linguistic function as the phonemes of their own dialect.

The mechanism of this instantaneous calibration involves the unit of the morphophone. The calibration between dialects, or between speaker and listener, may not be perfect. There are degrees of intelligibility even when the individuals are not impaired. Non-native speakers of English may be unintelligible because they fail to produce variants of morphophone units which can be calibrated. Listeners habitually calibrate "out of awareness", that is, without their conscious knowledge of the mechanism. But for linguists, the morphophone is the objective means of calibration which permits the measurement of mutual intelligibility.

This unit of structure, unique to Aspectual theory, is established by a rigorous set of procedures identifying contrasts in lexical items. For the purpose of obtaining a measure of degree of intelligibility of a speaker, the morphophone inventory provides the basis for a quantitative measurement. While the key to intelligibility is calibration, the key to calibration is the morphophone.

Theoretical frame of reference

Assumptions

The Aspectual theory of structural linguistics is a comprehensive and integrated theory of language. The basic assumption, as with other structural theories, is that language has an hierarchic structure which can be described. In addition, Aspectual theory holds that all languages have three properties: *sound*, *shape*, and *sense*. That is, all languages have a sound system; the sounds of a language distribute into recognizable shapes which make sense to the speakers of that language.

What is language?

Communication is defined by Aspectualists as an interaction between three distinct modalities: *language, paralanguage*, and *kinesics* (Smith, 1969: 93; 1976: 111). Each of these modalities has its own system and can be analyzed in its own terms. Language, the principle vehicle of communication, is of primary importance to the linguist. Accompanying language proper are those idiosyncratic features called paralanguage which serve to identify a speaker as a member of a social, generational, or professional group and to provide information about his emotional and physical state. Paralinguistic features are often referred to as "tone of voice" or "vocal quality" and include factors such as over-loud or over-soft delivery, and such habits as laughing, crying, belching, sighing, etc. during speech (Trager, 1958b). Kinesics is the modality concerned with gestures and body movements during speech.

The subject of microlinguistic analysis is the modality of language. Paralinguistic and kinesic phenomena are not identified as events within the tripartite Aspectual model of language structure. They are not considered a part of microlinguistic study which is the province of the linguist. Disciplines representing applications of linguistics and related to language study, such as acoustic measurements of the speech signal and physiological studies of the individual during speech, are considered prelinguistic in nature, and not a part of microlinguistics. In similar fashion, those disciplines concerned with the relationship of the linguistic system to other cultural systems, as in sociology, psychology, or philosophy, are considered to be metalinguistic. The three divisions of study: prelinguistics, microlinguistics, and metalinguistics constitute the field designated macrolinguistics. The Aspectual framework discriminates between the linguistic system and those communication systems and physical events peripheral to, but uniformly accompanying, language.

Aspectual model of language structure

The Aspectual model of language structure, applicable to all languages, is tripartite, consisting of strata, levels, and aspects. In the tripartite hierarchy, the sound system of language is analyzed at the ∝ stratum, Phonology; the shapes into which sounds are distributed are examined at the β stratum, Morphology; the sense of the language is described at the ɤ stratum, Semology. Each stratum is composed of three levels, which in turn consist of three aspects. A complete language description would, therefore, include analysis of twenty-seven aspects of language structure. This theoretical frame of reference, and the methods and procedures developed by Trager and Smith for linguistic study, have been proven valid by their successful application to the analyses of a variety of Indo-European and non-Indo-European languages. Such diverse languages as English, Czech, Russian, German, Chinese, Japanese, American Indian languages have been described in terms of this model.

The strata and levels of the Aspectual framework entering into the ensuing discussion can be presented in a simplified schema.

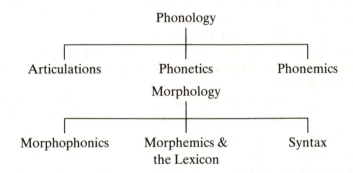

An important advantage of this approach to linguistic analysis is that it keeps like kinds of data together. This facilitates comparisons between systems, permitting observations to be made at specific points within the structure. The presentation of data following this framework proceeds from the least complex data to more complex structural units. With this hierarchy it is possible to make a rigorous distinction between what is language and what is not.

Analysis by levels

The organization of language data within the Aspectual model presents the results of analysis in a progression of aspects, levels, and strata. Each level is unique, the data for each distinct. Mixing of levels is quickly exposed (and condemned).

Initially, the first aspect of the α stratum uses prelinguistic, physiological information about the organs of speech, including the pathology of these organs, for consideration of sound production. The aspects which follow are concerned with inventories of articulation features, phones, and phonemes. The final aspect of the stratum specifies distributional data, the permissions and prohibitions of patterning within a syllable, for a phonotactic description. Both segmental and suprasegmental phenomena are accounted for at these levels of description.

The morphophone inventory is presented at the initial level of the β stratum. The entry point for the analysis of the β stratum is the morpheme, the unit identified in the lexicon of the language. The basic unit of the morpheme is the morphophone (analogous to the relationship of the phone to the phoneme at the α stratum). These structural units are identified at different levels of the linguistic system, but they are interrelated. Morphemes are represented in morphophones; morphophones are expressed in the phonemes of a speaker's dialect, but they are actually realized in the phones of that speaker's idiolect. People speak in phones, not in phonemes or morphophones.

A rigorous procedure is followed in identifying the units of each level of structure (phone, phoneme, and morphophone). Distinctions are made between levels by notational convention as well as by terminology. At the phonetic level of discussion, data are presented in square brackets ([ ]), and segmentals are referred to by the terms "contoid" and "vocoid"; phonemes are presented in diagonals (/ /) and are designated by the terms "consonant", "vowel", and "semi-vowel"; morphophones are noted by a symbol followed by a period (C., V., S-V.), and segmental morphophones are called "consonantal", "vocalic", or "semi-vocalic" (see Appendix 1).

The data differ on each level of the linguistic system, so that the terms and notational symbols applied to the varying levels are not interchangeable. Phonetic segments are noted with all observable detail of production. All phones do not achieve phonemic status. Phonemes are defined as classes of sound oppositions, established by significant contrasts in minimal pair lexical items. In the course of determining phonemic classes, each phone is assigned to one, and only one, phonemic class. As members of a phonemic class, they are allophones of the phoneme. The allophones of a phoneme exhibit the characteristics of phonetic similarity, and non-contrastive, complementary distribution. The members of each phoneme class, the allophones, pattern congruently with the members of other, similar phonemic classes. Establishing morphophones employs systematic contrasts in minimal pair lexical items, similar to the procedure for determining phonemes. However, at this level of the linguistic structure, free variation is accounted for, so that one phoneme may be assigned to two different morphophone units as overlapping variants. Depending on the aspect and level of observation of the data, it can be said that "sames" at one level of structure become "differents" at another.

This perspective of language structure and the successful application of Aspectual analysis to English achieved recognition in the discipline.

> The highly technical Trager-Smith *Outline of English Structure* ... has been extraordinarily influential among structuralists, especially for its insistence on a separation of "levels" in analysis and for its report on how we use suprasegmental morphemes to determine constructions. (Faust, 1964: 96)

Establishing the morphophone

Intelligibility is directly related to the unit of the morphophone at the morphological level of language structure. Morphophone units are established by a set of procedures as rigorous as that for phonemes. The morphophone unit, a communication concept without counterpart in other linguistic theories, was defined as

> ... a sort of "holding company" or "super-family" of different phonemes which are *non-contrastive in the same words.* (Smith, 1967: 311)

It is at the level of the morphophone that differences between phonemic expressions of the same lexical item are resolved. With only a phonological (i.e. phonetic or phonemic) perspective of language data, a problem arises in accounting for the mechanism by which contrasting phonemes, binding on all speakers of the language, are accepted by all speakers as renditions of the same lexical item.

An example of this problem is that of the lexical item *either*. All speakers of English contrast the two words *peek* and *pike* (/píyk/ ≠ /páyk/). Consequently, the phonemic contrast /i/ ≠ /a/ is said to be binding on all speakers of the language. Yet, the word *either* is produced by some speakers as /iýðir/, by some as /áyðir/, and some produce both. All are accepted as being the same lexical item. The question of how different phonemic units are accepted as equivalent in the same lexical item is answered in the mechanism of the morphophone unit.

The morphophone unit is the explanatory notion used to account for mutual intelligibility of different dialects of the same language. While phonological units of the structure are pertinent to the speaker's production, the morphophone involves the listener in calibration of that production.

Morphophone units are identified by contrasts in specific positions in the utterance. Procedures for establishing phonemes require contrasts in minimal pairs which are not predictable by environment; not all such contrasts establish morphophones. In the T-S analysis of SE (1961), there are thirty-three segmental phonemes and twelve suprasegmentals for a total of 45. The Smith inventory of SE morphophones (1968) defines 42 segmental morphophones and 7 suprasegmental for a total of 49 units.

The difference in totals is evident from a comparison of the inventories (Table 1):

Table 1

		Phonemes			Morphophones
Segmental					
1.	Consonant	21	1.	Consonantal	21
2.	Semi-vowel	3	2.	Semi-vocalic	3
3.	Vowel	9	3.	Vocalic	18
				a. short-7	
				b. long-11	
Suprasegmental					
1.	Pitch	4	1.	Pitch	2
2.	Stress	4	2.	Stress	2
3.	Juncture	4	3.	Juncture	3
Total:		45			49

Procedures for morphophone analysis begin with scrutiny of the idiolect of a single speaker followed by a survey of other dialects of the language to establish the minimum number of units necessary to account for all phonemic contrasts (Smith, 1967: 23). Morphophones are established by primary contrasts in pristine environment, and by secondary contrasts in non-pristine environment. Phonemes entering into primary and secondary contrasts are known as the principal variants of the morphophones.

For segmental morphophones, the vocalic pristine environment is defined as that preceding vl. stops, /p/, /t/, /k/, in monosyllabic lexical items (e.g. /pít/ ≠ /pét/ ≠ /pǽt/). In this environment for SE, the vowel nucleus is shortest. Secondary contrasts in non-pristine environment are those in monosyllabic minimal pairs with final consonants other than vl. stops (e.g. "halve" ≠ "have", "can" n. ≠ "can" v., "bomb" ≠ "balm").

Semi-vocalic morphophones are established only in initial position in minimal pairs (e.g. "yen", "hen", "wen").

The pristine environment for consonantals is initial position in minimal pairs. Consonantal secondary contrasts occur in medial and final positions (Hoffman, 1970: 17). Not all phonemes enter into primary or secondary contrasts to establish morphophone units. Where there is free variation between two phonemes in the same lexical item, and the phonemes can be assigned to two morphophone units, these are *overlapping variants* of morphophone units and constitute tertiary contrasts.

> A tertiary contrast, then, is one made by phonemes which are assignable *within the dialect* under examination to two morphophone units and with the phonemes always in free variation with those constituting the principal variants of each of the two units. (Smith, 1968: 25)

Since the morphophone inventory for SE is the total pattern for the language as a whole, it is expected that no single dialect will include all units. For the consonantal inventory, not all dialects include the secondary units #31 ž. and #34 ŋ.. The vocalic inventory ranges from a minimum of fourteen to a maximum of seventeen units.

> From a survey of dialects from all over the English-speaking world, it would appear that very few, if any, have fewer than fourteen of the fifteen primary units plus the one secondary unit 5a. oh. .... . Of all dialects so far studied in detail, the writer's southern variety of the Central Atlantic Seaboard dialect shows the maximum number of units, fifteen primary units, and the secondary units 3a. eh. and 6a. ah.. (Smith, 1968: 28)

Suprasegmental morphophones are established by an equally rigorous procedure of primary contrasts in intonation patterns. The pristine environments for identification of stress, pitch, and juncture morphophones are the point of primary stress, the point of highest pitch, and the point of termination of the intonation pattern. The details of this complicated procedure can be found in Bross (1983: 69-80).

Comparison of IPA and T-S notation

With the widespread use of the IPA notational system for transcription, the correlation of the IPA symbols with the T-S system may be of assistance in the discussion to follow. The diacritics and notation used in the discussion are presented in Appendix 2, and the correlations are shown in Tables 2 and 3.

The two systems are based on the principle of recording raw data with one symbol representing one sound, and there is a close relationship between the two systems. To summarize Trager (1972: 300), the complete IPA alphabet of segmental symbols with diacritics is in close agreement with the Trager-Smith system of phonetics, although it is not as extensive a system. The transcription system developed by Trager was originally prepared for the Foreign Service Institute of the U.S. State Department for the purpose of training in phonetic transcription.

Most of the consonant symbols are the same for the two systems. However, the differences between the symbols are listed below. The IPA symbols are from Fairbanks (1960: 10), and the segments referred to in the examples are underlined (Table 2).

IPA transcription at times interchanges phonemic and phonetic symbols without distinguishing between the two different levels of language structure. It should be noted that while the affricates in the two examples, *choke, joke,* ([tʃ], [dʒ] = /č/, /ǰ/) occur within morphemes, where two morphemes are adjacent, the transcription for T-S and IPA would use a sequence of thwo phonemes. An example is the phrase *heart shaped* /hárt + šeỳpt/.

Phonetically, the vocoid transcription of the T-S system is also similar to that of the IPA, but some amplification is required to relate the IPA diphthong symbols to the T-S analysis of English vowels and semi-vowels.

While the IPA diphthong is transcribed with two syllabic vocoid symbols, (i.e. [eɪ] fa<u>il</u>), the T-S system notes the non-syllabic feature with the diacritic [Y̯], [eⁱ]. Non-syllabics occur as on-glides or off-glides, depending

Table 2

IPA Phonetic symbols	Example	T-S Phonemic equivalents
Consonants		
[ʃ]	a<u>sh</u>	/š/
[ʒ]	a<u>z</u>ure	/ž/
Semi-vowels		
[j]	<u>y</u>acht	/y/
Phonetic combinations		
[tʃ]	<u>ch</u>oke	/č/
[dʒ]	<u>j</u>oke	/j/
[hw]	<u>wh</u>at	/hw~w/
[ju]	<u>you</u>th	/yuw/

on their position in relation to the syllabic vocoid. The phonetic, non-syllabic glides occur as front, central, or back vocoids. At the phonemic level glides are called "semi-vowels", since they pattern like consonants but are produced like vowels. The English semi-vowels are /y/, /h/, and /w/. Several of the IPA symbols for simple, vocoid nuclei correspond to this T-S analysis of vocoid plus off-glide (Table 3).

Table 3

IPA	Example	T-S Phonemic equivalent
[i]	b<u>ea</u>t	/iy/
[e]	b<u>ai</u>t	/ey/
[o]	b<u>oa</u>t	/ow/
[u]	f<u>oo</u>l	/uw/
[eI]	f<u>ai</u>l	/ey/
[aI]	f<u>i</u>le	/ay/
[ɔI]	f<u>oi</u>l	/ɔy/
[oU]	f<u>oa</u>l	/ow/
[aU]	f<u>ow</u>l	/aw/

The T-S analysis of the English vowel system is one of nine vowel phonemes serving as simple syllable nuclei which have the potential of combining with the three semi-vowels to form twenty-seven complex (vowel plus semi-vowel) nuclei. The IPA notation of on-glides as [w], [h], [j] and off-glides as [I], [U] correspond to the T-S symbols /w/, /h/, /y/ (with no corresponding IPA symbol for the central off-glide [ə]).

> Initial /h/ starts voiceless and with some friction noise, but is otherwise an onglide from central position: *hit, head, hot* have [$ḭ^{y+}$, $ə̣^{+}$, $ə̣^{y+}$].
> The prevocalic and postvocalic allophones of these three phonemes are almost exact mirror images of one another: *woo, ye, hah* are phonemically /wuw, yiy, hah/; when they are recorded on tape and the tape played backward, they sound almost the same as they do in normal sequence. (Trager, 1972: 44)

One other distinction between the IPA and T-S systems is seen in the T-S emphasis in recording suprasegmental phenomena in a different system from that of segmental. Two IPA vocoids have variant symbols for their occurrence in weak stressed syllables (Table 4).

Table 4

IPA Phonetic symbols	Example	T-S Phonemic equivalent
Primary stress (strong)		
[ʌ]	abo̱ve	/ə́/
[3ˀ]	wo̱rd	/ə́(h)/~/ɨ́(h)/
Weak stress		
[ə]	a̱bove	/ə̆/
[əˀ]	onwa̱rd	/ə̆(h)/~/ɨ̆(h)/

The IPA and the T-S phonetic transcription systems each represent a method of recording the reality of speech behavior, and the differences between the two systems can mostly be reconciled. Ultimately, the record depends on the facility of the observer in using the system.

The emphasis of the T-S procedures and analysis is on consistency and economy. The same speech sound is consistently represented by the same phonetic symbol. Modifications of the sounds are indicated by diacritics. For example, the T-S system consistently notes front, central, and back phonetic glides as non-syllabics ([I̞], [ə̣], [U̞]; these are phonemically, /y/,

/h/, /w/) whether they occur preceding or following the syllabic vocoid. Economy results from this practice, and, therefore, there is no unnecessary multiplying of entities.

An aspectual analysis of alaryngeal speech

Purpose

Since the Aspectual frame of reference is valid for analysis of the language of normal speakers, it was believed that these same methods and procedures could be fruitfully applied to speech samples of laryngectomees to evaluate methods of rehabilitation. Two artificial larynges were to be evaluated to determine which instrument performed more efficiently. It was believed that a linguistic approach would provide a more comprehensive and precise evaluation of the speech performance than might be obtained by other procedures. The design of the study was primarily to ascertain the extent and range of damage to the structural units of the linguistic system of alaryngeal speakers using artificial larynges.

Speakers

It is customary in studies of anthropological linguistics to identify the population studied by numbers of speakers as well as by geographical location. The population of laryngectomees in the United States is one that is expanding. The group currently numbers approximately 40,000, with a ratio of 7 males to 1 female (Buffalo News, 1989: C-5). Primarily in an age range of 40-65 years, it is increased annually by approximately 3,000 individuals, and is decreased in the same period by an almost equal number of deaths. Total excision of the larynx by surgery usually occurs as treatment for laryngeal cancer, with about 12,000 new cases occurring yearly in the United States. The growth of this group is evident from the statistics from 1971. At that time the population of laryngectomees was estimated at 25,000, with a ratio of 10 males to 1 female (The Inter. Assoc. of Laryngectomees, 1971: 2).

Following standard linguistic procedures, field work provided a set of observations which were recorded for analysis. Speakers were selected to serve as informants for the study. With the kind cooperation of Dr. Donald

P. Shedd, chief of the department of head and neck surgery at The Roswell Park Memorial Institute for Cancer Research in Buffalo, New York, two male laryngectomees were permitted to participate as informants. Both were native speakers, of similar age and education, and resident speakers of the Western New York dialect area. An advantage to the study of this group of impaired speakers is that the informants had been normal speakers prior to the onset of the disease. The competence of the speakers in the linguistic system was not in question.

The two patients selected had undergone laryngectomy for cancer of the larynx as well as extensive pharyngeal surgery, so that development of esophageal voice, the preferred means of rehabilitation, was precluded. A variety of instruments has been designed for rehabilitation of laryngectomees, and new devices featuring mechanical refinements are frequently marketed. Selection of the most appropriate instrument from all available can pose unforeseen difficulties.

Instruments

For the study, the two speakers used pneumatic reed artificial larynges (hereafter instruments A and B). The pneumatic reed artificial larynx is an external instrument, activated by air expelled from the lungs through the stoma directly into a tube. The expelled air stream vibrates after passing over a membrane which duplicates the function of vocal cords in the normal speaker. The vibrating air stream continues through the tube, enters a surgically created fistula leading to the pharynx, and passes into the oral cavity. Here the articulators, which have not been altered by surgery, function in the normal way to produce speech. The difference in design of the instruments lies in the position of the vibrating membrane. In instrument A, the membrane is in the external portion of the instrument, in the tube between the stoma and the fistula; in instrument B, the membrane is in the fistula. Both speakers were accustomed to the instruments so that errors of production were not attributed to unfamiliarity of operation.

The speakers were interviewed in two sessions of about one hour each, allowing sufficient time for each to rest occasionally or to clean or adjust the instruments if necessary. Each speaker was presented with elicitation material prior to the taping of the session and encouraged to question unfamiliar items included in the elicitation schedule. The purpose of the sessions was to obtain an adequate speech sample for analysis, and not to test familiarity of vocabulary or speed of response. The informant sessions were taped for the analysis to follow. Instructions given were for the speaker to read each item in the usual manner and to repeat each item once after a brief pause. The complete elicitation schedule could be administered easily within one hour without tiring the patients.

Elicitation material

A two-part test was devised for elicitation. The first purpose was to elicit a corpus which would provide inventories of all structural units found in the standard language--segmental and suprasegmental. Segmental units were obtained from contrasts in initial, medial, and final positions in minimal pair lexical items. Suprasegmental contrasts of pitch, stress, and juncture were elicited in minimal pair intonation patterns occurring in sets of phrases and sentences. The first section of the test material provided all principal inventories. All phonetic, phonemic, and morphophone inventories could be obtained from analysis of a total of 88 vocabulary items and 10 phrases and sentences (see Appendix 3).

The resulting inventories include segmental contoids, consonants, consonantals; phonetic on- and off-glides, semi-vowels, and semi-vocalics; vocoids, vowels, and vocalics in medial positions in monosyllabic lexical items. Analysis of pitch, stress, and transitional phonemes identifiable in pertinent positions of word phrases and sentences provided the suprasegmental inventories.

The schedule can be easily administered and quickly scored to provide a quantitative rating of performance for the speaker in the form of a numerical score designated the QRP. Reviewing the performance on the QRP test in depth provides accurate and precise diagnostic information concerning the range and extent of damage to the speaker's system, pinpointing specific segments for further review. These errors in performance can be confirmed by the remainder of the elicitation schedule. It is important in examining language behavior to determine not only that all structural units are present, but also whether the units distribute appropriately.

The second purpose of the elicitation was to obtain a phonotactic description of the distribution of phonemic units in syllables. For this section of the material, lexical items were selected to include vowel nuclei in initial and final positions and all consonant clusters in initial and final positions. The total elicitation schedule includes 295 lexical items and 18 phrases and sentences.

QRP scoring

Following the microlinguistic analysis which determined the articulatory, phonetic, phonemic, and morphophone inventories, a contrastive analysis was conducted comparing the structural systems of the speakers and the norm. By examining the types of errors, quantity of errors, and patterns of occurrence throughout, it was possible to judge one instrument as clearly superior in performance.

Responses to the QRP Test were examined to determine whether the results confirmed the conclusions resulting from the exacting microlinguistic and contrastive analyses. Linguistic factors were weighted in a scoring system to obtain a numerical value for accuracy of production of the principal variants of morphophone units.

The QRP numerical score is arrived at by a system of weighting which totals 100 points possible for a perfect performance. The weighting system includes:

> 57 points scored for 19 three position consonants;
> 4 points scored for 2 two position consonants;
> 9 points scored for 3 three position consonants;
> 18 points scored for 9 vowels (double weighted for occurrence in medial position);
> <u>12</u> points scored for 12 suprasegmentals
>
> 100 points.

Normal speakers are expected to score in the 90's. Since no dialect is expected to have all phonemic units for the language as a whole, it is possible for a speaker to have a seven unit vowel system (lacking /i/ and /ɔ/), and an absence of the 2 two position consonants, /ŋ/ and /ž/. In these dialects [ŋ] is an allophone of /n/ preceding velar stops /k/ and /g/; /ž/ occurs as the sequence /zy/; [i] is an allophone of /ə/ and [ɔ] is an allophone of /o/. These examples illustrate the importance of discriminating between phonetic and phonemic data. In this situation, the speaker would score 92 on the QRP with all other units present.

The scores achieved on the QRP by the speakers confirmed the conclusions of the more complicated microlinguistic and contrastive analyses. After obtaining the QRP scores, further tests determined the statistical significance of the results. An important question frequently posed when numerical scores are presented is whether the linguistically determined differences are statistically significant. It is important to verify whether the results of the test are due to a real difference between the instruments being evaluated, or whether the results are due to random variation or inherent experimental error. To answer this question, three statistical tests were applied: the Analysis of Variance, the Sign test, and the t-test. All statistical tests indicated that the results were statistically significant.

Methods and procedures

The elicitation material devised was structurally sound in that it reflected the structure of the language at the strata which were to be examined, and was comprehensive in containing all structural units of the pertinent levels of interest. The raw data were transcribed in the notation system defined by Trager (1958a) with diacritics appropriate for microlinguistic analysis (see Appendix 2). Standard linguistic procedures were followed. The resulting analysis determined whether all structural units were present, whether the units distributed in the expected patterns, as well as the presence and positions of production errors.

Following the Aspectual framework, analysis of the α stratum, Phonology, at the first aspect of the first level, Articulations, identifies the effects of the pathology of the speaker's organs of speech. The second aspect of this level establishes an inventory of articulation features, and at the third aspect, bundlings of articulation features within the segment of a phone are specified. The second level of the stratum is that of Phonetics. At the first aspect of this level, kinds of phones are identified (i.e., "stops", "spirants", etc.); at the second aspect, phones are classified in phonetic tables according to the traditional features of place and manner of articulation, and voicing. The third aspect of the Phonetic level provides an inventory of phones and identifies the deviation of the segmental phones from cardinal positions of the phonetic table by means of diacritic symbols (i.e., [p'-], [sp̲-]).

At the third level of the stratum, Phonemics, phonemic classes are determined. Segmental phonemes of consonants, vowels, and semi-vowels are identified by minimal pairs of lexical items. Suprasegmental phonemes of stress, pitch, and juncture are identified by contrasts in intonation patterns co-occurring with segmental minimal pairs. Analytic procedures require that each phone be assigned to one and only one phonemic class on the basis of phonetic similarity, congruent patterning, and non-contrastive, complementary distribution. At the final aspect of the Phonemic level, the systems of relations describe permissions and prohibitions of distribution for segmental and suprasegmental phonemes. Initial and final consonant clusters are described, and simple and complex nuclei are defined.

The stratum of Phonology presents the sound system of the speakers which is pertinent to determining accuracy of production in pathological linguistic structures. For structural information about the intelligibility of the speakers, attention moves to the function of the phonological units at the β stratum, Morphology. At the first level of Morphology, Morphophonics, phonemic variants are examined to determine the morphophone inventory, where phonemic differences are calibrated within lexical items and judgments of the intelligibility of the speakers are appropriate.

Results

The QRP scores serve two purposes: the scores are indicative of the speaker's deviation from the norm, and of the difference in capability of rehabilitative instruments. The speaker with instrument A achieved a QRP score of *87*, while the speaker with instrument B scored *68*. The score of 87 would indicate relatively good intelligibility, compared to the normal range with a minimum of 92, while the score of 68 could at best be rated as fair intelligibility. The considerable differences in the QRP scores paralleled the substantial differences between instruments in numbers of errors in the extended corpus. Applying statistical tests to determine the validity of the QRP scores, on the Analysis of Variance the results were statistically significant at the 5% level; on the t-test and the Sign test, the results were statistically significant at the 1% level.

Relating the performance to the Morphophone level, it was found that the inventory of morphophone units for the speakers included all segmental consonantal units for both, the full complement of vocalics (fifteen primary and one secondary), but instrument B was deficient in the semi-vocalic #39. h., while instrument A included all semi-vocalics. Damage to the suprasegmental system was severe, with both speakers having a loss of the pitch 4. (/4/), used primarily for emphasis in SE, and instrument B having a loss of the rising juncture unit, double bar, ||.. Alaryngeal speech is frequently characterized as monotonous or monotonal, and loss of the pitch and juncture units would indicate the reason for this effect.

In the comparison of the inventories, instrument A had a loss of one morphophone unit, while instrument B lost three. The differences between the inventories in terms of lost units are indicators. The instrument with the larger number of units absent from the inventory is predictably the less intelligible. Where morphophone units are absent, calibration of differences cannot take place, and it is expected that the speaker using that instrument will be less comprehensible.

The QRP score presents an immediate interpretation of the speaker's relative level of intelligibility. The simplest scoring procedure is a judgment of *correct-incorrect* for the target segments, preferably by a native speaker. For diagnostic purposes, this would be followed by a close examination of the phonemic variants. Direct observation of the variants is essential to determine the failure of specific units which prompt the judgment of *incorrect* for target segments. Responses were scored as *incorrect* and counted as errors if they could not be reconciled as dialect variations, or if there was no correction in the repetition of the item. Details of the responses uncover patterns of production errors in terms of position and structural level of occurrence.

Diagnostics

Production errors are defined in the traditional way as

(1) *Excrescence* — an intrusion of a phoneme in the lexical item where it is neither expected nor required.
(2) *Substitution* — the replacement of the expected unit by another in the system.
(3) *Loss* — an absence of the required unit.
(4) *Unintelligible* — a segment which cannot be identified as a speech sound by the customary parameters.
(5) *Non-English* — a segment which is clearly identifiable by the customary procedures but is not a part of the SE system.

In transcription, errors were noted as follows:

Excrescence — $\underline{C}$, $\underline{V}$
Substitution — $C_1 \leftarrow C_2$ (C_1 replaces C_2)
Unintelligible — [X]

Excrescence errors

Excrescences are widespread for normal speakers but do not have morphophonic status since they are not binding on all speakers of the language.

They may occur, however, as a dialect variety, and, thus, are binding on all speakers of a dialect. Some of the more frequent examples of excrescences are /wórš/ *wash*; /órfənt/ *orphan*; /kə́mpf + təbɨl/ *comfortable*. The most frequent excrescent error for both instruments was the central vowel schwa /ə/. The varying position of this segment demonstrated a real difference in performance between the two instruments. Instrument A had most excrescences in initial position, /h-/ before vowels, and /ə-/ before consonants. For instrument B, most of the schwa excrescences appeared in final position, with additional syllables appearing in those lexical items for both speakers. The initial excrescences prevalent for instrument A with /ə-/preceding consonants, and /h-/preceding vowels tends to support the Trager-Smith analysis of /h/ as a central non-syllabic vocoid.

There is a widespread misconception that laryngectomees are unable to produce the phoneme /h/. This unit is defined by Jones (1967: 1) as being "pure breath", produced in the glottis by air passing from the lungs through the vocal cords. The /h/ of the SE system is described by Trager-Smith (1961: 20) as a glide to a central, unrounded position, with the tongue in motion during the passage of air through the oral cavity. Speaker A produced a strong, clear, distinct /h/ with considerable friction in initial position. This may be identified as a pharyngeal spirant in initial position ([ḥ]); it is analyzed as an allophone of /h/ in complementary distribution with the central glide, occurring medially (often preceding /l/ and /r/ in SE), or in final, post-vocalic position.

Examples of excrescent errors are

A	B
#28. rival /ɝ́ráyvəl/	#38. zinc /zíŋkə̆/.

The number of excrescences was similar for both instruments. From the distribution of this error, there is an indication that one instrument is more difficult to activate, requiring more effort, while the second instrument is more difficult to arrest.

Substitution errors

Substitutions are the most numerous errors for both instruments, with instrument B producing more than twice the number than A. Speaker A displayed a surprising tendency to back front vowels. This is considered idiosyncratic rather than a flaw of the instrument in maintaining place of articulation in vocoid production. Instrument B exhibited a very serious difficulty with the voicing feature, and apparently the speaker was unable to devoice at will. In effect, vd. ≠ vl. did not occur as required, with the vd. counterpart usually substituted for the vl. opposition.

Substitution examples for the speakers include

	A	B
(1) u. ← i.		
#19. chin	/čún/	
#20. gin	/jún/	
(2) ə. ← e.		
#21. etching	/ə́čɪ̆ŋ/	
(3) ž. ← š.		
#47. ruche		/rúwžə̠/
(4) z. ← s.		
#37. sink		/zí[X̱]kə̠/ .

A special type of substitution is that of the non-English speech sound. For instrument A, there was a severe problem with the production of velar stops [k] and [g] in all positions. These were regularly replaced by the medio-velar, slit spirants [x] and [ɣ]. While this substitution was sometimes corrected with the repetition, occasionally the second response contained the error. Usually, both responses were incorrect. The substitution of the spirants for the stops entered into contrasts and were phonemic.

Instrument B produced only a single non-English segment, the lax, high back, unrounded vocoid [Ï] in #12. cot and #13. got. These occurrences were predictable by environment and were assigned to the phoneme /a/. Examples of the non-English occurrences for both instruments are

	A	B
#13. cot		[gÏt] /gát/
#14. got	/xát/	[gÏdᵈ] /gád/
#18. bag	/bǽɣ/	

This substitution demonstrates a serious problem with instrument A's ability to maintain the correct manner of articulation for the production of velar stops. As variants of the morphophones, #18.k. and #21.g., these non-English variants are not easily calibrated, and there is a consequent loss of intelligibility with their occurrence.

Loss errors

Losses for both instruments, at the phonetic level, include the glottal stop
[ʔ], which has a predictable, non-phonemic distribution in SE. This phone
appears in pre-vocalic position, initial in intonation patterns. Its absence is
to be expected for speakers who have had the physical structure, the glottis,
excised.

This error type also demonstrated a great difference in performance
between the two instruments. Where instrument A had few segmental losses, instrument B exhibited loss of a variety of consonantals, most often in
final position. Unlike instrument A, B could not produce /h/- initial.

There was also a large group of segments which were phonetically
unidentifiable and untranscribable. These unintelligible segments constitute
a class of loss errors and were noted in transcription by the symbol [X].
Instrument A produced very few unintelligibles. However, this was a frequent error for B, usually occurring in initial position and not specific to
place or manner of articulation.

Among the suprasegmentals, both instruments lost the high pitch /4/
(4.), indicating SE emphasis. For instrument A, emphasis was exhibited by
juncture, /#/, preceded by a change in tempo to very slow, which is paralinguistic. In the item testing for the emphasis response,

#10. What're we having for dinner? STEAK????,

instrument A produced

$$\frac{/\overset{2}{s}téyk\overset{1}{\#}/}{te > > >}$$

Instrument B was unable to produce either the rising juncture ||., or
the pitch 4., in spite of cueing. For the emphasis test, the item was demon-
strated as /stéyk⁴/ ||. The speaker produced /stéyk↑/, and it is therefore
assumed that both morphophones 4. and ||. are absent from the inventory.

The importance of testing units in all positions in which segmentals
occur in the standard language can be seen by the distribution of errors for
these speakers. If initial position alone is the basis for comparing performance, no difference can be seen between the two instruments. However,
the superiority of performance by instrument A is evident from the distribution of errors in other positions. Total number of errors for consonants
and semi-vowels in the QRP test were distributed in the following manner:

	Initial position	Medial	Final
Instrument A	6	2	1
Instrument B	8	9	5

According to this distribution, both instruments were equally poor in initial position. Instrument A performed more accurately than B in other positions, and therefore achieved a higher intelligibility rating.

Summary and conclusions

The Aspectual methods of analysis of pathological forms of the language are an effective means of providing relevant data pertaining directly to the linguistic system rather than to factors peripheral to the system. The Aspectual conceptual frame of reference clearly distinguishes between microlinguistic phenomena and paralinguistic features accompanying language. With varying methods of rehabilitation of the speakers of pathological forms of the language, assessing damage to the linguistic system and the effect of remedial measures is of interest.

Purpose

In an investigation of laryngectomees, speech samples were examined for the purpose of evaluating the language of these speakers using artificial larynges. The objective was to examine the systems of the speakers using standard linguistic techniques to determine the deviation of the speech sample from that of the standard language of the normal speaker, and to develop an objective method of rating proficiency of alaryngeal speakers on the basis of linguistic factors.

Theoretic orientation

The theoretical orientation for the study was that of the Aspectual theory of structural linguistics developed by George L. Trager and Henry Lee Smith, Jr. In Aspectual theory, language is viewed from the perspective of a tripartite, hierarchic structure composed of aspects, levels, and strata. All languages exhibit the same properties of sound, shape, and sense. The tripartite, hierarchic structure addresses these properties in the strata of Phonology, Morphology, and Semology. The sound system of language is examined at the stratum of Phonology; the sounds of language distribute into recognizable shapes which are identified at the stratum, Morphology; the shapes of the linguistic system make sense to the speakers of the language, and this property is examined at the stratum, Semology.

The usual focus of attention is on the production of impaired speakers — the sound system. At the aspects and levels of this stratum, the system is examined in terms of articulation features and structural units of segmentals and suprasegmentals which are relevant to diagnosis and treatment of these speakers. It is via the aspects and levels of the stratum of Morphology that the functioning of these structural units can be examined to determine level of intelligibility. At the first level of this stratum, the structural unit of the morphophone, a unit unique to Aspectual theory, is identified. The morphophone functions to calibrate phonemic differences of the same words of the language, so that different pronunciations of the vocabulary of the language by speakers of different dialects are recognized and accepted as being the same. It is at this level that the impaired speaker is judged as intelligible by listeners.

In past studies of laryngectomees, it was not unusual for judgments of intelligibility to rest on opinions of panels of listeners, or on mechanical measurements of the speech signal, or on performance on possibly inadequate test materials. In contrast, for this investigation, elicitation material was designed to ensure a structurally sound corpus which would contain all structural units of the standard language. The subsequent microlinguistic analysis resulted in an accurate and precise statement of the speakers' structural system, serving a diagnostic purpose in distinguishing where that system was intact, where it was deficient, and how the system failed. It is therefore a more objective means of determining relative level of intelligibility than statements of opinion.

Analysis

The elicitation text consisted of word lists and sentences which would provide inventories of the alaryngeal speakers' articulation features, phonetic, and phonemic units of the phonological system according to standard techniques of Aspectual analysis. Following the microlinguistic analysis, an error analysis was completed identifying types of error production. Errors were classed in the traditional way as excrescence, substitution, and loss — with non-English speech sounds and unintelligible segments constituting special classes of substitution and loss. Errors of production were identified by type and distribution and were related to the appropriate structural level as phonetic, phonemic, or morphophonic phenomena. A contrastive analysis comparing speakers' systems to the standard language indicated the extent and range of damage to the linguistic system, and a judgment of proficiency of the instruments tested could be made on the basis of the performances of the rehabilitative devices.

QRP

To facilitate evaluation of speakers of a pathological form of the language with similar precision, but without undergoing a lengthy microlinguistic analysis, a concise test procedure was developed, the Quantitative Rating of Performance test. The QRP test, based on linguistic factors, elicits all structural contrasts of the system and provides the results in the form of a numerical score indicative of the speaker's relative level of intelligibility. The QRP is diagnostic in revealing type and position of error, and analytic in providing an inventory of structural units of the pathological system.

Because of the ease of administration, this procedure can be conducted by non-technical personnel, who only judge the targeted response as *correct* or *incorrect*. A numerical score can be obtained which assesses intelligibility relative to a normal speaker. It is possible to compile diagnostic information such as a list of morphophones absent from the speaker's inventory. This indicates whether the calibration of phonemic variants has occurred. The procedure can be largely automated.

Results

Applying the QRP test to the alaryngeal speakers, their scores confirmed the results of the contrastive analysis — one instrument performed substantially more accurately. The results of the QRP test were found to be statistically significant on the basis of three statistical tests. These confirmed that the resulting QRP scores were due to a real difference in performance of the two rehabilitative devices, and were not due to chance or random error. The speakers involved in this investigation represent examples of the extreme, requiring extensive surgery. As a consequence, rehabilitative measures were restricted. In spite of this limitation, one speaker achieved a good level of speech performance and intelligibility with an auxiliary device which permitted a resumption of normal activities and a return to former employment.

Applications

Newer, small, easily concealed, or implanted devices are frequently designed and marketed, and new methods of surgery are developed in the treatment and rehabilitation of laryngectomees. While evaluations of new instruments and surgical procedures invariably report achieving "good" or "excellent" voice in a short period of time, the QRP represents a comprehensive and precise method of evaluating these new rehabilitative procedures in terms directly related to the communication system. This test procedure is applicable in this innovative area and represents a simple but effective method of evaluating the degree of intelligibility of these speakers.

Threshold of intelligibility

The unit of the morphophone, the structural unit whereby phonological differences function as morphological equivalences, accounts for mutual intelligibility among speakers of different dialects of the same language. It is by means of this abstract, theoretical unit that a linguistic problem may be resolved — determining when two dialects of the same language diverge to become two distinct languages. If two linguistic systems cannot resolve phonological differences within the morphophonic system, the conclusion must be drawn that there exist two separate systems and two distinct languages.

In the same measure, for impaired speakers, examination of the morphophone system reveals damage to the units of calibration or the loss of units. In pathological forms of the language, the kind of damage that occurs at the phonemic level is important in the effect on the morphophone level. Loss of a morphophone unit may inhibit calibration, while changes in the principal variants may not have so drastic an effect on calibration. A question of linguistic interest is: How much damage can the morphophone system sustain before a speaker is considered unintelligible? Further research in this area may determine the tolerance level for specifying a *threshhold of intelligibility* at the morphophone level.

References

Bross, Rida S. 1983. *A Linguistic Analysis of Alaryngeal Speech*. Unpubl. dissertation. Buffalo: SUNYaB.

Fairbanks, Grant. 1960. *Voice and Articulation Drillbook*, 2nd ed. New York: Harper & Row.

Faust, George P. 1964. "Something of Morphemics." *Readings in Applied Linguistics*" (2nd edition), ed. by Harold B. Allen, 92-97. New York: Appleton-Century-Crofts, Division of Meredith Publ. Co.

Gleason, H.A., Jr. 1961. *An Introduction to Descriptive Linguistics* (revised edition). New York: Holt, Rinehart and Winston.

Hoffman, Melvin J. 1970. *The Segmental and Suprasegmental Phones, Phonemes, and Morphophones of an Afro-American Dialect*. Unpubl. dissertation. Buffalo: SUNYaB.

Jones, Daniel. 1967. *The Pronunciation of English*, 4th ed. Cambridge: Cambridge University Press.

Smith, Henry Lee Jr. 1967. "The concept of the morphophone." *Language* 43:1, 306-341.

————. 1968. *English Morphophonics — Implications for the Teaching of Literacy*. Monograph No. 10. Oneonta, N.Y.: N.Y. State English Council.

————. 1969. "Language and the total system of communication." *Linguistics Today*, ed. by Archibald A. Hill, 89-102. New York: Basic Books Inc. Publishers.

————. 1976. "Linguistics as a behavioral science." *Forum Linguisticum* 1, 95-121.

The Buffalo News. June 12, 1989. "Your Health — New treatment for cancer of larynx saves voice." C-5. Buffalo, N.Y.

The International Assoc. of Laryngectomees. 1971. *Rehabilitating Laryngectomees*. New York: IAL.

Trager, George L. 1958a. *Phonetics: Glossary and Tables. Studies in Linguistics*. Occasional Papers 6. Buffalo, N.Y.: Dept. of Anthropology and Linguistics, Univ. of Buffalo.

————. 1958b. "Paralanguage: A first approximation." *Studies in Linguistics* 13, 1-12.

————. 1972. *Language and Languages*. San Francisco: Chandler Publishing Co.

————. and Henry Lee Smith, Jr. 1961. *An Outline of English Structure* (4th printing). *Studies in Linguistics*. Occasional Papers 3. Washington, D.C.: American Council of Learned Societies.

Appendix 1. *Standard English Morphophone Inventory.*

I. Segmentals

A. Vocalic		B. Consonantal		C. Semivocalic
Primary	*Secondary*	*Primary*	*Secondary*	
1. i.		16. p.		37. y.
2. e.		17. t.		38. w.
3. æ	3a. eh.	18. k.		39. h.
4. u.		19. b.		
5. o.	5a. oh.	20. d.		
6. a.	6a. ah.	21. g.		
7. ə.		22. č.		
8. iy.		23. j.		
9. ey.		24. f.		
10. ay.		25. Θ.		
11. uw.		26. s.		
12. ow.		27. š.		
13. aw.		28. v.		
14. yuw.		29. ð.		
15. oy.		30. z.	31. ž.	
		32. m.		
		33. n.	34. ŋ.	
		35. r.		
		36. l.		

II. Suprasegmentals

A. Stress
    ´. strong
    ˘. weak
B. Pitch
    4. high
    1. low
C. Juncture
    #. double cross--falling
    ||. double bar--rising
    |. single bar--sustained

(from Smith 1967)

Appendix 2. *Diacritics and Notation*

Notation

C	Consonant
V	Vowel
[ ]	Phonetic
/ /	Phonemic
C., V.	Morphophone
≠	in contrast with
( )	optional
	Free variation:
~	within the language
≈	within the dialect
≈	within the idiolect of a single speaker
te > > >	Paralanguage: decreased tempo

Diacritics

Symbol	*Articulation Feature*
C̬, V̬	fortis, tense
C, V	lenis, lax
C>, V>	backed from cardinal position
C<, V<	fronted from cardinal position
C^, V^	raised from cardinal position
C˅, V˅	lowered from cardinal position
C̬, V̬	voiceless
C˙	released
C˺	unreleased
C'	aspirated
$_w$C	rounding
V·, V:	length
Ṽ	nasalized
V̰	non-syllabic
V+	spirantization

Appendix 3. *QRP TEST*

A. Segmental targets

Consonants

1. pit	31. thigh	61. all
2. bit	32. thy	62. or
3. dapper	33. ether	*Semi-vowels*
4. dabber	34. either	63. ye
5. cap		64. he
6. cab	35. wreath	65. we
7. tip	36. wreathe	66. flyer
8. dip	37. sink	67. ahead
9. bitter	38. zink	68. flower
10. bidder	39. muscle	69. law
11. pat	40. muzzle	70. low
12. pad	41. fuss	*Vowels*
13. cot	42. fuzz	71. pit
14. got	43. shoot	72. pet
15. bicker	44. Zhukov	73. pat
16. bigger	45. mesher	74. putt
17. back	46. measure	75. pot
18. bag	47. ruche	76. put
19. chin	48. rouge	77. taught
20. gin	49. more	78. taut
21. etching	50. nor	79. peat
22. edging	51. simmer	80. pate
23. batch	52. sinner	81. pout
24. badge	53. singer	82. kite
25. fail	54. ram	83. Hoyt
26. vale	55. ran	84. toot
27. rifle	56. rang	85. tote
28. rival	57. late	86. cute
29. waif	58. rate	87. bomb
30. wave	59. teller	88. balm
	60. terror	89-90. Rosa's roses

B. Suprasegmental targets (underlined)

Stress
1. He has a permit to permit him to leave.
2. Every white house is not The White House.

Pitch
3. What're we having for dinner, Mother? (vocative)
4. What're we having for dinner, Mother? (annoyance)
5. What're we having for dinner? Mother? (facetious, tentative answer)
6. What're we having for dinner? STEAK??? (surprise and emphasis)

Juncture
7. I scream for ice cream.
8. What's that in the road ahead.
9. What's that in the road? A head?
10. What's that in the road? A head!

Chapter 3

Acoustic and perceptual approaches to the study of intelligibility

Gary Weismer and Ruth E. Martin
University of Wisconsin (Madison)

Introduction: The concept of intelligibility

The concept of speech intelligibility, which had it's origins in the 1920s, comes from the telephony literature. This literature was concerned with the quality of voice transmission systems, and the means by which that quality could be best assessed. Within the framework of a simple, three-part model of communication, consisting of a speaker, medium, and receiver, the emphasis in this early literature was clearly on the effects of medium characteristics on speech intelligibility. In 1949, Wood focussed on the 'speaker' side of this model when he assessed the speech intelligibility of children with articulation disorders. His idea was to use the percentage intelligibility score as a metric of severity of an articulation disorder. Many later evaluations of speech intelligibility in disordered speakers, to be discussed in more detail below, have not deviated much from the idea that speech intelligibility scores may serve as an index of severity.

In this chapter, we discuss the current status of speech intelligibility tests as they are used to gain insight to speech disorders. We evaluate critically the various approaches to testing the speech intelligibility of disordered speakers, and suggest that advances in this area must go past simple estimates of severity to seek *explanations* of intelligibility deficits. Some preliminary ideas and data that are driving the development of an explanatory test of speech intelligibility (Kent, Weismer, Kent, & Rosenbek, 1989) will be discussed throughout the chapter. Ideally, an analysis model that would generate explanations of intelligibility deficits should be broad enough to cover the variety of speech disorders for which intelligibility testing is useful. Because the task of developing such a model is imposing, we have chosen to focus our efforts on speech intelligibility in dysarthric persons. No claims are made here that the suggested approach would be useful in evaluation of the speech of, say, the hearing impaired or second language learners. Detailed treatment of speech intelligibility issues in the latter populations are found in the chapters by Osberger and Flege, but we also provide a brief review of the literature on the hearing impaired, as it bears on the themes of our work.

We also include a discussion of the rationale for, and the form of, variables that may eventually find use in an explanatory model of speech intelligibility. Part of this discussion is based on the current status of work done in our laboratory (e.g. Kent et al., 1989; Kent, Kent, Weismer, Martin, Sufit, Brooks & Rosenbek, 1989; Kent, Kent, Weismer, Sufit, Rosenbek, Martin & Brooks, in press; Weismer, Kent, Hodge, & Martin, 1988), but a good deal is highly speculative. The purpose of this speculation is to provide a coarse outline of the issues that may need to be studied to construct the most productive model of speech intelligibility.

Finally, we will present some ideas on the contribution of the listener to speech intelligibility deficits in persons with dysarthria. A typical, if not near universal, view of an intelligibility deficit is that the speaker is the primary, if not lone, 'source' of the communication difficulty. We will argue that there is much in the speech perception literature to suggest that the listener has more trouble with a disordered speech signal than would be predicted solely from the mismatch between 'normal' and degraded acoustic-phonetic events. In this sense, it is possible that speech intelligibility deficits are as much in the ear of the listener as they are in the mouth of the speaker.

Review of dysarthric intelligibility studies

The original work on speech intelligibility of dysarthric speakers was performed by Tikofsky and Tikofsky (1964). A set of single words was developed that could be used to estimate intelligibility of dysarthric persons; a later item analysis of the original 160 words (Tikofsky, 1970) suggested a restricted word set that would be maximally effective in differentiating dysarthric from normal speakers. One of the findings from the item analysis was that spondees (such as *lifeboat*, *northwest*) produced more frequent errors than monophthongal words. This suggested the potential of an in-depth phonetic treatment of intelligibility data, but no further work on this data base was reported. Platt and his associates (Platt, Andrews, Young, and Neilson, 1978; Platt, Andrews, Young, and Quinn, 1980) reported an analysis of phonetic errors in spastic and athetoid adults, as well as overall intelligibility scores from a single-word intelligibility test. Unfortunately, the construction of the word items did not allow a systematic analysis of the relationship of phonetic errors to intelligibility deficits; our own reanalysis of a portion of those data, however, suggested that this approach could help identify the *origins* of an intelligibility problem (see Kent, Weismer, Kent, & Rosenbek, 1989).

Kent et al. (1989) developed a systematic approach to evaluating the phonetic underpinnings of intelligibility deficits. Target words are grouped

Table 1: *Phonetic contrasts and selected acoustic correlates in the word intelligibility test of Kent et al. (1989).*

CONTRST	ACOUSTIC CORRELATE(S)
1. Front vs. back vowels	Range of F2 frequencies
2. High vs. low vowels	Range of F1 frequencies
3. Long vs. short vowels	Duration of vocalic nuclei; formant pattern
4. Voiced vs. voiceless initial consonant	Vocie onset time
5. Voiced vs. voiceless final consonant	Duration of preceding vowel
6. Alveolar vs. palatal consonant	Spectrum type
7. Place of articulation: stops	Burst spectrum type; transitions
8. Place of articulation: fricatives	Noise spectrum type; transitions
9. Fricative vs. affricate	Closure duration; noise duration
10. Stop vs. fricative	Presence of stop interval
11. Stop vs. affricate	Duration of noise interval
12. Stop vs. nasal	Presence of nasal F-pattern
13. Initial /h/ vs. initial vowel	Presence of noise energy with aspiration-type spectrum
14. Presence vs. absence of initial consonant	Indication of spectral energy associated with any consonant
15. Presence vs. absence of final consonant	Same as 14
16. Initial singleton vs. initial cluster	Temporal or spectral evidence of one vs. two segments
17. Final singleton vs. final cluster	Same as 16
18. [r] vs. [l]	F-pattern at constriction interval; transition types
19. [r] vs. [w]	Same as 18

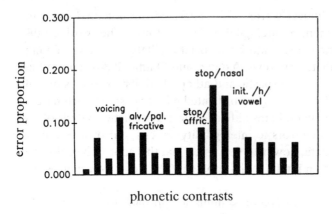

Figure 1. *Proportions of errors within phonetic contrasts for ALS males (N=25)*

with foils that have a minimal-pair, or near-minimal pair, relationship to the target. The pairs differ according to specific phonetic dimensions, summarized in Table 1, which are chosen to reflect the types of errors that are commonly observed in dysarthric speech, and are deemed likely to have a major impact on speech intelligibility.

For example, the phonetic contrast *stop-nasal* is evaluated by means of the confusability between word pairs such as *beat-meat, bill-mill, dock-knock, side-sign*, and so forth. In the actual administration of the test there are three foils for each target word, and a listener is presented all four choices for each presentation of a word. The analysis of all test words according to phonetic contrasts yields results like those shown in Figure 1.

These data (Kent et al., 1990) were based on word productions of 25 male patients with amyotrophic lateral sclerosis (ALS), and the listening responses of ten women. The key observation from this 'error profile' is that the set of phonetic contrasts is not uniformly affected by the intelligibility deficit. Rather, certain contrasts seem to contribute much more heavily than other contrasts to the word-identification errors that define an intelligibility deficit. In the case of this group of male ALS subjects, it appears that the stop-nasal and initial glottal-null contrasts are transmitted relatively less effectively than many other contrasts, such as the front-back distinction for vowels. From our perspective, an observation such as this is important because it may serve to identify the primary articulatory bases of

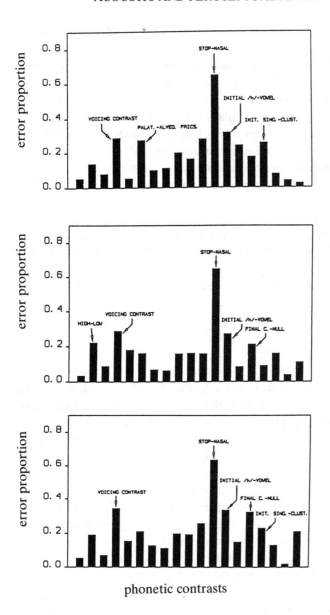

Figure 2. *Phonetic contrasts errors in three ALS subjects*

an intelligibility deficit, and also may drive well-defined hypotheses concerning the acoustic and physiological underpinnings of the contrast errors.

Figure 2 illustrates another reason why an explanatory component of intelligibility tests is desirable. Error profiles are shown for three ALS subjects whose overall intelligibility scores were similar (between 40-53%). The interesting aspect of these displays is that the error profile is not the same for each speaker. Whereas this is hardly a conceptual breakthrough for clinicians who have treated many individuals with motor speech disorders, and who know that speakers can be highly unintelligible in many different ways, the profile analysis provides a principled approach to describing this variation.

Ziegler, Hartmann, and von Cramon (1988) have been developing a similar type of explanatory intelligibility test for German-language speakers with dysarthria. Preliminary data from this test, which was derived from 32 dysarthric subjects with varying etiology, suggest that polysyllabic words were misidentified more often than monosyllabic words, and that the initial consonant position of words was more affected than the medial or final positions (see below, *Influence of normal perceptual processes on speech intelligibility*). Ziegler et al. also present data that demonstrate similar, overall intelligibility deficits having varying articulatory bases.

Yorkston and Beukelman (1981a) and Enderby (1983) have described intelligibility tests that are designed with the dysarthric speaker in mind. Neither of these tests, however, provides more than the estimate of severity noted above. Kent et al. (1989) have pointed out that the Frenchay Test (Enderby, 1983) contains word items that are highly variable with respect to syllable number (recall Tikofsy, 1964) and shape, making it difficult to understand the sources of variability in an intelligibility score. Yorkston and Beukelman (1981a) base the construction of their test on a fairly extensive research program (see, for example, Yorkston and Beukelman, 1978, 1981b), and make two new claims concerning the utility of the instrument. First, the results of the single word test are said to predict sentence intelligibility and 'information transfer' with a high degree of accuracy (Yorkston and Beukelman, 1978, 1981b). Second, Yorkston and Beukelman (1981b) introduce the concept of 'communication efficiency ratio', which captures the fact that in a connected speech sample two speakers who produce an identical number of intelligible words may do so at different rates. The speaker who produces more intelligible words per unit time is regarded as a more efficient communicator.

Both of these claims, however, can be criticized on important grounds. First, the experimental results that were taken to demonstrate predictability of sentence intellibility, or information transfer, from single word intelligibility tests (Yorkston and Beukelman, 1978, 1981b) actually show little more than the classical 'third variable' effect in correlational analysis. Yorkston and Beukelman (1978, 1981b) chose their dysarthric subjects to span a wide range of severity, which virtually guaranteed the high correlations between single word scores and either sentence intelligibility or information transfer. In other words, the purposeful choice of subjects who have widely varying degrees of severity will mean that each of the speech intelligibility measures will be highly correlated with severity, and so with each other. The proper test of predictability of sentence intelligibility from single word measures would require that groups of subjects be blocked according to their single word intelligibility scores, with the prediction of similar subject blockings for sentence intelligibility scores. The most clinically relevant and stringent test of this idea would be to train single word intelligibility, and observe the effect on (untrained) sentence intelligibility. Unfortunately, the literature on motor speech disorders does not include these kinds of studies. Frearson (1985) reported a study in which the Yorkston-Beukelman sentence intelligibility scores were found to be approximately 8.5% higher than intelligibility scores derived from the spontaneous speech of twenty dysarthric speakers. Although Frearson concluded that "...sentence intelligibility scores may not be representative of a dysarthric client's spontaneous speech" (1985: 13), her results should be interpreted with a certain amount of caution for the following reasons. First, examination of the published data (Frearson, 1985, Table 2) shows that only five of the twenty subjects had substantially different (i.e., greater than 10%) intelligibility scores in the Yorkston-Beukelman sentences and in spontaneous speech. Secondly, Frearson (1985) did not control for context differences between the two kinds of speech material. It has been known for many years that the intelligibility of connected discourse produced by normal speakers is a function of the amount of context available to the listener (Pollack and Pickett, 1963). Recently, Kreider (1987) demonstrated the same effect in dysarthric and apraxic speakers. Because Frearson did not control or describe context differences between her two types of speech material, it is impossible to interpret her findings in a straightforward way.

The second claim, concerning the communication efficiency ratio, is not necessarily flawed in concept, but has no independent support. That support should be in the form of an independent demonstration of a relationship between rate of intelligible words and the construct, 'communication efficiency'.

As a footnote to this section, it should be pointed out that there has been one major effort to measure speech intelligibility of seven groups of dysarthric speakers by means of equal-appearing interval scales. Darley, Aronson, and Brown (1975) used a seven-point scale and reported that the worst speech intelligibility was associated with their pseudobulbar palsy group (Mean= 3.44), and the best intelligibility with their cerebellar group (Mean= 2.09). These data are difficult to interpret in the absence of corresponding data from traditional speech intelligibility tests; for example, how does the mean difference in scale value between the least and most intelligible groups (mean difference= 1.35) relate to percentage differences in a typical word-identification test? Moreover, can a scaled estimate of speech intelligibility be related to, or predicted by, other scaled estimates of speech dimensions? Note that this latter question is an 'explanatory' issue, in the sense that a scaled estimate of intelligibility should be viewed as a composite of the full set of dimensions that may describe disordered speech production. Ideally, the Darley et al. (1975) analysis should have consisted of regression analyses wherein various combinations of independent variables (e.g., scaled estimates of *imprecise consonants*, *distorted vowels*, *breathy voice*, and so forth) were evaluated for their ability to predict the scaled estimate of intelligibility. Because the Darley et al. (1975) analyses were not conducted in this way, the reported intelligibility scalings only provide a very crude notion of severity.

There has been one attempt in the literature to relate acoustic dimensions to the kind of perceptual dimensions employed by Darley, Aronson, and Brown (1975). Ludlow and Bassich (1984) reported that, in general, acoustic measures did not have strong predictive utility for the scale values of perceptual dimensions associated with hypokinetic dysarthria. It is possible that this negative finding relates either to the predominance of 'prosodic' acoustic variables (i.e., variables that bear minimally on segmental integrity) in the Ludlow and Bassich (1984) study (see below), or the focus on a disorder (Parkinson's disease) wherein the speech deficit tends to be minimized in situations that are highly structured and non-propositional (see, for example, Weismer, 1984a). Although we will not deal with scaling issues further in this chapter, additional work along the lines of the Ludlow and Bassich study should be pursued (see also, Southwood, 1990).

Review of literature on intelligibility of deaf speech

Individuals with severe to profound hearing impairment typically exhibit deficient speech production and reduced speech intelligibility (Smith, 1975). The relationship between these two associated symptoms of deafness has been of interest to researchers and clinicians for many years. In fact, a major theme in the hearing-impaired literature has been the extent to which various perceptual and/or acoustic characteristics of deaf speech result in reduced speech intelligibility. Studies addressing this issue have been justified on the grounds that the perceptual and acoustic correlates of intelligibility must be understood in order to develop speech training programs which are likely to promote enhanced intelligibility (Nickerson and Stevens, 1980).

Curiously, although dysarthric speakers also suffer from reduced intelligibility, and increasing intelligibility is a primary goal of dysarthria rehabilitation, few studies have attempted to elucidate the phonetic and acoustic factors that contribute to the intelligibility deficits seen in this population. In this respect, the studies of deaf speech and dysarthric speech have followed quite different historical paths.

Three general experimental approaches have been employed in attempts to determine the relationship between various phonetic and/or acoustic variables and the intelligibility deficit associated with deaf speech. The most common method involves determining correlations between some metric of speech intelligibility and certain speech parameters. Typically, intelligibility has been quantified by means of 1. word identification tests and 2. scaling procedures such as interval scaling and direct magnitude estimation (for a discussion, see Schiavetti, Metz and Sitler, 1981). A number of speech parameters have been studied in relation to intelligibility, including frequency of consonantal and vocalic errors as determined by phonetic transcription (Hudgins and Numbers, 1942; Markides, 1970; Smith, 1975; Levitt and Stromberg, 1983), ratings of suprasegmental factors (Hudgins and Numbers, 1942; McGarr and Osberger, 1978; Parkhurst and Levitt, 1978), and a variety of temporal and spectral acoustic attributes (Monsen, 1976a; Monsen, 1978; Whitehead, 1986). Training studies also have been reported (John and Howarth, 1965; Stevens, Nickerson and Rollins, 1983). In these, the deaf speaker participates in a speech training program aimed at modifying one specific speech characteristic and intelligibility scores pre- and post-training are compared. Finally, the relationship between intelligibility and various acoustic variables has been explored by means of "speech transformation" (Bernstein, 1977; Huggins, 1977; Osberger and Levitt, 1979; Maassen and Povel, 1984a,b; 1985). Specific acoustic parameters of natural or synthetic speech are manipulated orthogonally by means of digital signal processing techniques and the effects on intelligibility are determined.

The effects of both segmental and suprasegmental variables on the intelligibility of deaf speech have been addressed. Whereas the complex interrelationships between segmental and suprasegmental characteristics of speech have been discussed (Kent, 1983; Smith, 1975), the typical approach in the deaf speech literature has been to study these two types of variables from a dichotomous perspective. That is, attempts have been made to examine the effects of *either* segmental or suprasegmental effects on intelligibility, but few studies have been directed toward studying the *combined* effects of concurrent segmental and suprasegmental modifications (but see Maassen and Povel, 1985).

Segmental characteristics

Several studies have reported moderate negative correlations between intelligibility and the frequency of perceptually-identified segmental errors (Hudgins and Numbers, 1942; Markides, 1970; Smith, 1975). Hudgins and Numbers (1942) found correlations of -.70 and -.61 between the frequencies of consonantal and vocalic errors and intelligibility. Smith (1975) reported a correlation of -.80 between the frequency of segmental errors and intelligibility. Error types most strongly associated with reduced intelligibility include omission of word-initial phonemes (Hudgins and Numbers, 1942; Levitt, Stromberg, Smith, & Gold, 1980), voicing errors and errors of consonant clusters (Hudgins and Numbers, 1942), consonant substitutions involving manner, substitutions of non-English phonemes and unidentifiable distortions (Levitt et al, 1980). While Hudgins and Numbers (1942) and Markides (1970) reported that consonantal errors contributed more to reduced intelligibility than vocalic errors, Smith (1975) found a stronger association between vocalic errors and intelligibility. Levitt and Stromberg (1983) noted that although deaf childrens' speech varied markedly in terms of intelligibility, the types and relative frequencies of errors were highly consistent across children. Only children with extremely low intelligibility scores exhibited qualitatively different error profiles, including glottal substitutions and unidentifiable substitutions.

Correlations between intelligibility and the acoustic attributes of segments also have been reported. Monsen (1976a) examined the relationship between speech intelligibility and vowel space in a group of 36 deaf children. Vowel space was defined as the difference between the maximum and minimum values of each of formants 1 and 2 (F1 and F2) for the vowels /i/, /a/ and /o/. Monsen reported correlations of .74 and .45 between sentence intelligibility and the spectral ranges of F2 and F1 respectively and suggested that restricted vowel space contributes to reduced intelligibility of both vocalic and consonantal segments. Monsen (1976b) also studied the F2 vowel transitions in the speech of 6 deaf adolescents. He reported that transitions were characterized by reduced frequency extents and speculated that this acoustic attribute also may contribute to reduced intelligibility.

As Nickerson and Stevens (1980) note, the results of these correlational analyses are difficult to interpret. Because speech is an aggregate of interrelated variables, it is difficult to know whether a change in intelligibility is the result of a change in the particular attribute under study or whether this attribute simply varies with intelligibility by virtue of its positive correlation with some other 'deterministic' variable. In spite of their inherent ambiguity, however, Nickerson and Stevens (1980) advocate the use of correlational analyses in the study of intelligibility as a means of providing guidelines for subsequent research.

One means of gaining greater insight into the complex relationship between speech dimensions and intelligibility involves the use of multivariate analyses in which correlations are determined not only between intelligibility and various phonetic or acoustic variables but also among the variables themselves. In this vein, Monsen (1978) used a stepwise multiple regression analysis to examine the relationship between intelligibility and 9 acoustic variables in the speech of 37 hearing-impaired adolescents. The 9 variables, which were measured spectrographically, included the VOT differences between /p/ and /b/, /t/ and /d/, and /k/ and /g/, evidence of liquid and nasal productions, the spectral ranges of F1 and F2, the F2 frequency change associated with the diphthong /aI/, mean sentence duration and mean fundamental frequency. Of these 9, 3 variables yielded a multiple correlation of .85 with intelligibility, accounting for 73% of the variance in intelligibility scores: the VOT difference between /t/ and /d/; F2 difference between /i/ and /o/; and the ability to produce liquids and nasals.

Although Monsen (1978) noted that several of the acoustic predictor variables bore high intercorrelations, he did not report these correlation values. This is unfortunate, since the results of stepwise regression may be ambiguous in the absence of information about the specific intercorrelations among predictor variables. For example, as Metz, Samar, Schiavetti, Sitler and Whitehead (1985) note, if the 3 voicing contrasts studied by Monsen (1978) (the VOT differences between /p/ and /b/, /t/ and /d/, and /k/ and /g/) are based on a common process, then they would be expected to yield high intercorrelations. If these 3 variables were entered as predictor variables in a stepwise regression analysis aimed at predicting speech intelligibility, it is possible that only the single VOT variable with the highest simple correlation with intelligibility would be selected as a significant predictor variable. The other VOT variables could be rejected, due to their shared variance with the selected VOT variable. To interpret this pattern of results, however, as support for the notion that one VOT variable contributes to reduced intelligibility while the other two do not, could be erroneous. Knowledge of the intercorrelations between predictor variables would provide greater insight into the extent to which the results of the stepwise regression analysis reflect the relationships between the criterion and predictor variables versus the relationships between predictor variables themselves.

Metz et al (1985) have discussed the problems in developing theories based on the results of multiple regression analyses when the predictor variables are highly intercorrelated. They note that high intercorrelations among predictor variables suggest that the variables reflect a smaller set of more fundamental parameters. In attempts to elucidate these fundamental factors, Metz, et al. (1985) studied the relationships between 3 measures of intelligibility (based on single-word identification, contextual word identification and direct magnitude estimation) and 12 predictor variables in the speech of 20 hearing-impaired adults. The 12 variables included 7 of those previously studied by Monsen (1978) (3 VOT measures, 2 formant difference measures, F2 movement in /aI/, mean sentence duration), as well as the standard deviations of the VOT and sentence duration measures. Metz, et al. (1985) submitted these 12 variables to a principal component analysis, with the result that 4 factors emerged which accounted for 78% of the variance in the original 12 variables. When these 4 factors subsequently were used as predictors in a stepwise multiple regression analysis, the primary predictor of intelligibility was a factor reflecting the temporal and spatial control for segmental events. A secondary factor was interpreted as reflecting speech prosody and stability of production for the temporal integrity of certain segmental events.

Nickerson and Stevens (1980) have advocated an alternate approach to the study of the intelligibility of deaf speech. They suggest that, by performing detailed phonetic and acoustic analyses of speech samples which vary in degree of intelligibility, it may be possible to identify those variables that account for reductions in intelligibility. Further, they state that the particular acoustic variables analyzed should be chosen based on our knowledge of speech perception. For example, because points of rapid spectral change and syllabic nuclei both have been implicated as important acoustic cues in the perception of normal speech, it would be of interest to elucidate the relationship between these acoustic events and intelligibility.

Suprasegmental variables

A number of different suprasegmental attributes have been examined in relation to the intelligibility of deaf speech, including rhythm (Hudgins and Numbers, 1942), durations of speech sounds and pauses, stress, fundamental frequency, fundamental frequency contours, intonation and voice quality (Osberger and McGarr, 1982; Stevens et al., 1983). In fact, individual studies typically have focussed on different sets of suprasegmental variables. For example, while Hudgins and Numbers (1942) examined a global timing variable which they termed 'rhythm', more recent studies have addressed more specific temporal variables such as vowel durations (Monsen, 1974; Whitehead, 1986). Similarly, various speech transformation studies have manipulated different elements of the speech signal. While Maassen and Povel (1984a) manipulated the relative durations of phonemes, no corresponding manipulation was performed in an earlier study by Osberger and Levitt (1979). As a result, it is somewhat difficult to compare the findings of several studies in order to determine their reliability or to construct a comprehensive model of the effects of suprasegmental factors on the intelligibility of deaf speech.

Correlational studies have suggested that suprasegmental factors may contribute significantly to the intelligibility deficit associated with deaf speech. In one of the earliest such studies, Hudgins and Numbers (1942) reported a correlation of .73 between rhythm and intelligibility. This was as strong a relationship as that found between the frequency of consonantal errors and intelligibility and stronger than that between vocalic errors and intelligibility.

Smith (1975) also commented on the importance of suprasegmental factors to intelligibility. She noted that deaf children whose intelligibility scores were lower than would be predicted based on their segmental error profiles tended to have greater frequencies of suprasegmental errors. In an analysis of various suprasegmental factors, she found that 50% of the variance in intelligibility scores was accounted for by two variables, one of which reflected poor phonatory control (including intermittent phonation, inappropriate variation of pitch and loudness and excessive variation in intonation) and the other reflecting rate of speech.

Parkhurst and Levitt (1978) attempted to determine the relationship between intelligibility and a number of suprasegmental parameters which were categorized as adventitious sounds, excessive durations, pitch breaks and pauses. Based on a multiple regression analysis, they reported that intelligibility was significantly predicted by (1) unexpected adventitious sounds, (2) long sound prolongations, and (3) unexpected pitch changes. Further, they noted that while segmental errors appeared to predict intelligibility more accurately than suprasegmental errors for most subjects, there were a few young children with severe prosodic distortions for whom intelligibility scores were predicted better by suprasegmental errors. McGarr and Osberger (1978) also examined the association between intelligibility and phonatory characteristics in a group of deaf children. They found that subjects who were unable to sustain phonation and whose speech was characterized by pitch breaks and large pitch fluctuations obtained the lowest intelligibility scores.

Stevens, et al. (1983) reported correlational data suggesting a tendency for intelligibility scores to increase as the fundamental frequency range and the ratio of stressed to unstressed vowel durations approached values characteristic of normally-hearing speakers. However, they also noted that a wide range of intelligibility scores was associated with any given value of either of these suprasegmental factors, suggesting the simultaneous effects of a number of other factors on intelligibility.

Monsen (1974) discussed the relationship between intelligibility and inherent and context-dependent vowel durations in the speech of the deaf. Specifically, Monsen studied the durations of the vowels /i/ and /I/ and the effects on vowel duration of the voicing feature of the following consonant. Whereas /i/ is relatively longer than /I/ in speech produced by normal talkers, /i/ and /I/ differed in absolute duration in deaf speech. Further, the tendency for vowels to be longer preceding a voiced as opposed to voiceless consonant, characteristic of normal speech, was not evident in the speech of the deaf. Monsen suggested that these durational factors contribute to reduced intelligibility, however, he did not test this hypothesis. In a more recent study, Whitehead (1986) extended Monsen's work by examining context-conditioned modification of vowel duration in normal speakers and in two groups of hearing-impaired speakers whose speech was judged as either intelligible or semi-intelligible. He reported that, while the normal and intelligible hearing-impaired speakers exhibited similar modifications of vowel duration preceding voiced versus voiceless consonants and fricative versus plosive sounds, the semi-intelligible subjects failed to demonstrate these trends.

Training studies have yielded conflicting results regarding the impact of suprasegmental factors on the intelligibility of deaf speech. John and Howarth (1965) found an increase in the intelligibility of deaf children who participated in a training program aimed at correcting timing errors. However, Stevens et al (1983) failed to find any increase in intelligibility associated with training of suprasegmental parameters. The results of training studies are difficult to interpret. Without acoustic analyses of the speech signal pre and post-training, there is no assurance that the speech variable focused on in therapy was the only variable actually modified. Thus, an increase in intelligibility could result from a factor other than the one under study. Further, it is possible that the beneficial effects on intelligibility of training one factor could be offset by the simultaneous detrimental effects of the training on some other variable, with the net result that no increase in intelligibility would be observed.

Whereas correlational studies have suggested an important influence of suprasegmental factors on the intelligibility of deaf speech, investigations involving digital manipulation of the acoustic speech signal have suggested that such factors have only a modest effect on intelligibility. Bernstein (1977) found no decrease in the intelligibility of speech produced by normal subjects when it was resynthesized with timing errors typical of deaf speech. In contrast, Huggins (1977) studied the intelligibility of synthesized sentences produced with abnormal timing and/or pitch contours. He found that, whereas 86% of words were correctly identified in sentences with normal prosody, 63%, 52% and 48% of words were identified in sentences synthesized with abnormal pitch contours, abnormal timing, and abnormal pitch and timing respectively. Huggins suggested that these prosodic dimensions influenced intelligibility by providing the listener with sufficiently misleading information that he/she was unable to make use of the segmental information present. Given that the prosodic patterns employed by Huggins are not typical of those produced by human subjects, however, the generalizability of his findings to the intelligibility of deaf speech is questionable.

Osberger and Levitt (1979) studied the effect of correcting timing errors on the intelligibility of sentences produced by 6 deaf children. They created 6 versions of the sentences, which involved (1) no modifications, (2) correction of pauses, (3) correction of the relative durations of stressed and unstressed vowels, (4) correction of absolute syllable durations, (5) correction of relative timing and pauses, and (6) correction of absolute timing and pauses. Only the correction of the relative timing of stressed and unstressed vowels resulted in an increase in intelligibility, the magnitude of which was roughly 4%. Further, the extent to which intelligibility was altered as a result of these suprasegmental modifications was related to the frequency of segmental errors in the sentences.

A study reported by Maassen and Povel (1984a) confirmed Osberger and Levitt's (1979) findings. They performed a number of temporal modifications on sentences produced by 10 deaf Dutch children including modifications of absolute and relative syllable durations and absolute phoneme durations and elimination of pauses from these first three modification conditions. They reported that the correction of relative phoneme durations resulted in the largest increase in intelligibility, of approximately 5%. Increases in intelligibility were related both to the specific temporal modification made and the characteristics of the sentence being modified.

Maassen and Povel (1984b) also examined the effects of correcting fundamental frequency contours on the intelligibility of the same sentences. They reported a 7% increase in intelligibility when intonation contours were corrected. The specific intonation modification that led to the greatest increase in intelligibility depended on the characteristics of the original sentence. For sentences which initially were not overaccented, the greatest gains in intelligibility resulted when existing accents were marked. In constrast, the intelligibility of sentences which initially were overaccented increased most when incorrect accentuations were removed. In addition, when fundamental frequency modifications were made to sentences which previously had been corrected temporally, additional gains in the intelligibility of those sentences which originally were not overaccented were observed. For overaccented sentences, however, the temporal corrections appeared to mitigate the beneficial effects of the intonation corrections. Thus, the combined manipulations of timing and fundamental frequency affected intelligibility in complex ways.

Maassen (1986) examined the influence on intelligibility of marking word boundaries by inserting pauses between words in the speech of deaf children. In this study, a control condition also was incorporated in which segments were lengthened so that the overall durations of the utterances were equal to those in which pauses had been inserted. While no increase in intelligibility was associated with the control condition, the insertion of pauses between words resulted in a 4% increase in intelligibility. Maassen (1986) interpreted these findings within the context of Marslen-Wilson's (1980) and Marcus' (1984) proposals that the identification of word onsets is a fundamental part of speech perception.

Combined segmental and suprasegmental characteristics

As noted earlier, the general trend in studies of speech has been to examine the effects of segmental and suprasegmental factors on intelligibility independently. Few studies have addressed the question of whether segmental and suprasegmental variables interact during speech perception and, if so, what is the nature of their interaction(s). It would appear that these questions are central to an understanding of the intelligibility deficits associated with deaf and dysarthric speech, however. In running speech, segmental and suprasegmental events are executed simultaneously. Modifications of segmental elements, made intentionally by the speaker or as the result of an inablility to control the speech production mechanism, may influence not only the perception of those particular segments but also the perception of the rhythmic structure of the utterance as a whole. In this sense, the segmental event may contribute to a modification of the prosodic structure. Further, as Monsen (1976b) notes, there may be factors responsible for reduced intelligibility in connected speech which can be characterized as neither segmental nor suprasegmental, for example, formant transitions.

In the speech perception literature, the relationship between segmental and suprasegmental factors has received considerable attention. For example, Martin (1975) discussed this issue in regards to the role of rhythm in speech perception. In one experiment involving a reaction-time paradigm, he increased the durations of stop gaps embedded in sentences by 200 m sec. and then asked subjects to respond to segments that occurred two syllables after the modified stop-gaps. Martin (1975) reported slower reaction times for the temporally modified items and suggested that they resulted because the temporal locations of the target segments did not match the listeners' expectations based on the temporal structure of the sentences. Further, he interpreted these results as support for the notion that segmental and suprasegmental effects 'interact' during the perception of continuous speech.

Maassen and Povel (1985) studied the separate and combined effects of segmental and suprasegmental transformations on the intelligibility of sentences produced by 10 deaf children. They found that complete segmental correction of the sentences resulted in a marked increase in intelligibility of 49% (ie. median values increased from 24 to 73%). Whereas the correction of vowels alone led to a 24% increase in intelligibility, the modification of nasals, stops, fricatives, affricates or /l/, /j/, and /w/ had minimal effects on intelligibility. When temporal and intonation transformations (Maassen and Povel, 1984a,b) were then applied to the original and the segmentally-corrected versions of the sentences, the following results were obtained: whereas the combined temporal and segmental corrections resulted in minimal additional increases in intelligibility over the segmental corrections alone, the combined intonation and segmental corrections led to larger increases (between 17 and 24%, depending on the specific transformation employed). Moreover, when the same intonation and temporal modifications were made to the segmentally uncorrected sentences, an increase in intelligibility of only 3% resulted. Thus, a significant interaction between the segmental and suprasegmental manipulations was demonstrated, suggesting that their effects on intelligibility combine in nonadditive, complex ways.

Summary

The literature on speech intelligibility of persons with motor speech disorders has been largely concerned with tests that provide an index of severity. Tests can be designed, however, to permit interpretations in terms of the phonetic and acoustic bases of an intelligibility deficit. This latter approach has been taken in several studies of deaf speech which have attempted to 'explain' reduced intelligibility by determining its perceptual and acoustic correlates. The development of such intelligibility tests is important because of their potential utility in guiding the decision-making process in remediation. This is particularly true in the case of motor speech disorders, where two patients with the same index of severity can have markedly different types of intelligibility deficits. In the next section, we consider some of the factors that might enter into the development of an 'explanatory' test of speech intelligibility.

Variables in an explanatory test of speech intelligibility

An 'explanatory' test of speech intelligibility presupposes some model that relates acoustic measurements and/or phonetic contrast analysis to overall performance on the test. As discussed in the previous section on speech intelligibility of the hearing impaired, both Monsen (1978) and Metz et al. (1985) have made efforts to derive acoustic models of speech intelligibility from regression analyses. The predictor variables in these analyses were a set of acoustic variables thought to relate to the speech production deficit among hearing-impaired individuals. In this part of the chapter, we attempt to provide detailed consideration of why certain variables would be chosen for either an acoustically- or contrast-based model of speech intelligibility in dysarthria. Moreover, the manner in which the variables should be represented in the model is treated, albeit in a fairly speculative way. An important conclusion to this section is that the most productive model may include a combination of variables derived from both acoustic measurements and phonetic contrast analysis. This discussion will also point to the tremendous gaps in the knowledge base needed to develop a truly principled modeling effort.

The variables that are incorporated into an explanatory test of speech intelligibility should reflect at least two basic considerations. First, the variables should be consistent with knowledge of the articulatory deficit in a target disorder, which in the present case is dysarthria. Second, the variables should capture those phenomena that are thought to contribute in a significant fashion to speech intelligibility.

Selection of variables: considerations from dysarthria

In this section we will consider how knowledge of the speech production deficit in dysarthria may guide the selection of variables for a contrast- or acoustically-based model of speech intelligibility. Table 2 provides a

Table 2. *Survey of dysarthric speech production deficits. Terms such as 're-stricted', 'slow', and so forth, use normal as the reference. PD = Parkinson's disease; AD = ataxic dysarthria; ALS = amyotrophic lateral sclerosis; TBI = traumatic brain injury; CP = cerebral palsy; SpD = spastic dysarthria; TE = transition extent*

STUDY	ARTIC DEFICITS
1. Kent, Netsell, & Bauer (1975)	*restricted ranges of tongue, lip, & jaw movement in different dysarthrias (TBI, AD, CP) *slow articulatory movements *non-uniform velocity patterns
2. Kent & Netsell (1975)	*Restricted A-P tongue movement in one AD
3. Kent & Netsell (1978)	*Large jaw movements, restricted A-P movements of tongue in athetoid CP *Dysynchrony of VP and lingual movements
4. Kent, Netsell & Abbs (1979)	*Equal and excess stress in AD *Loss of duration contrasts between long and short vowels
5. Farmer (1980)	*VOT abnormalities in CP
6. Hirose, et al. (1981, 1982)	*Slightly slower velocities of lip, tongue dorsum, and velar movement in PD *reduced range of movement
7. Hunker, et al. (1982)	*Reduced lip displacement in PD
8. Kent & Rosenbek (1982)	*prolonged acoustic vowel steady states and transitions in AD
9. Ziegler & von Cramon (1983a)	*Artic difficulty when successive gestures conflict in TBI *Spirantization in PD
10. Ziegler & von Cramon (1983b)	*collapsed acoustic vowel space in TBI *lack of acoustic transitions
11. Weismer (1984)	*Spirantization in PD *Short voiceless intervals *Faster than-normal speaking rates
12. Weismer, et al. (1985)	*Reduced transition extents in PD *Reduced transition slopes
13. Weismer, et al. (1986)	*Reduced transition slopes in ALS *Spirantization in ALS *Collapsed acoustic vowel space
14. Ziegler & von Cramon (1986)	*collapsed vowel space in SpD *acoustic evidence of slow movement *difficulty with complex gestures

STUDY	ARTIC DEFICITS
15. Caruso & Burton (1987)	*Longer stop closures & vowels in ALS
16. Darkins, et al. (1988)	*reduced contrasts in PD FO contours that distinguish noun phrases from compound nouns
17. Kent, et al. (1989)	*Reduced F2 slopes in ALS
18. Forrest, et al. (1989)	*minimal jaw movement in PD *reduced articulatory velocities *reductions in TE *most abnormal movements and acoustics in complex gestures
19. Caliguiri (1989)	*reduced displacement and velocity of lower lip elevation for /va/ repetitions in PD

selected list of speech production deficits that have been reported in the literature on dysarthria. The list includes findings from both physiological and acoustical studies, and does not partition the findings according to dysarthria type. Whereas most texts that discuss dysarthria often focus on deficiencies in consonant production, the great majority of findings summarized in Table 2 concern vowel production. The acoustic vowel space may be somewhat collapsed (Weismer, Mulligan, & DePaul, 1986; Ziegler & von Cramon, 1983a), as suggested by Lehiste (1965) over twenty years ago; range of lingual movement may be restricted in both the antero-posterior and inferior-superior dimensions (Kent, Netsell & Bauer, 1975; Kent & Netsell, 1978), with compensatory movement of the jaw creating a major functional deficit for the front-back distinction of vowels (Hirose, Kiritani & Sawashima, 1982; Kent & Netsell, 1978); formant transitions may be reduced in range and slope (Weismer, Kimelman, & Gorman, 1985; Weismer et al., 1986; Kent, Kent, Weismer, Martin, Sufit, Brooks, & Rosenbek, 1989) or may be absent (Ziegler & von Cramon, 1983b); and vowel durations may be too long, short, or inappropriately scaled for the rhythmic, contextual, or phonological characteristics of the utterance (Kent, Netsell, & Abbs, 1979; Weismer, 1984b; Kent & Rosenbek, 1982; Caruso & Burton, 1987). Although the classical view in speech perception theory is that consonants are the 'information-bearing' elements of the speech waveform (e.g., infinite peak clipping has only a negligible effect on speech intelligibility: see Licklider, 1951), the incorporation of vowel variables in a test of speech intelligibility for dysarthric persons is motivated by at least several factors. First, the disortions imposed on vowel articulation by dysarthria do not have the monolithic effect on the signal that is produced by an artificial manipulation such as peak clipping; in fact, dysarthric distortions of vowel production are variable in space and time, and so must be viewed as related to normal productions by (unknown) complex functions, rather than simple functions. Secondly, the potential interaction of vowel and consonant information in speech intelligibility is partially addressed by the inclusion of vowel variables in the test. Because cues to segmental identity are distributed over time (Repp, 1982), vowel information may have a strong bearing on the overall identity of an articulatory sequence, and therefore the intelligibility of the message. Thirdly, there have been empirical demonstrations of the importance of vowel variables to the intelligibility deficit in dysarthria. Ansel (1985) found that three vowel variables (the front-back, high-low, and tense-lax distinctions) were significant predictors of speech intelligibility scores obtained from adults with cerebral palsy, and Ziegler, Hartmann, and von Cramon (1988) claimed that vowel items in their single-word intelligibility test made a *greater* contribution than consonant items to the overall intelligibility scores of dysarthric persons with various diseases. Finally, the work of Maasen and Povel (1985) demonstrated that large gains in speech intelligibility were obtained when LPC resynthesis techniques were used to correct *vowel* errors in the speech of hearing-impaired persons.

In the research tool developed by Kent, et al. (1989), the three vowel contrasts found by Ansel (1985) to be significant predictors of intelligibility deficits are included as the phonetic contrasts that represent vowel production. These contrasts also have well-defined acoustic correlates. Whereas these contrasts appear to cover the dimensions of vowel production found in any discussion of English phonetics (with the exception of the rounding-spreading distinction, which is not phonemic in English), they are not the only manner in which vowel integrity can be represented in an explanatory approach to speech intelligibility deficits. More will be said about this below, in the discussion of formant trajectory characteristics.

Table 2 indicates only two studies (Weismer, 1984a; Farmer, 1980) in which acoustical measurements suggest that voicing information may not be transmitted well by dysarthric speakers. There are perceptual studies (e.g., Logemann & Fisher, 1978; Platt et al., 1980) in which errors of voicing control have been identified in Parkinsonian, spastic, and athetoid dysarthria,

but other types of errors (such as place, or manner) seem to be more frequent in these analyses. There is also evidence from the older speech perception literature (Miller and Nicely, 1955) that voicing information is relatively resistant to signal degradation, although it should be kept in mind
that the types of degradation typically used in these studies (filtering, low
signal-to-noise ratios) are not good models of the natural articulatory
deficits that accompany neurogenic dysfunction of the speech mechanism.
The Kent et al. test includes two contrasts that address the potential influence of voicing errors on speech intelligibility. These are the voicing contrasts for syllable-initial and syllable-final consonants, both of which have
well-defined acoustic correlates (see Table 1). The inclusion of these contrasts in the first version of the test is motivated primarily by the perceptual
data reviewed above as well as clinical intuition, rather than clear evidence
that these kinds of control problems are typical in dysarthric populations
exclusively,[1] or that voicing errors would make a substantial contribution to
an intelligibility deficit.[2]

    Hypernasality is usually thought to be a pervasive feature in much
dysarthric speech (e.g., Darley, Aronson, & Brown, 1975), but the effect of
velopharyngeal dysfunction on *segmental* identity has not been addressed in
any depth. Kent and Netsell (1978) reported dysychrony of velar and lingual movements in athetoid cerebral palsy (see Table 2), which presumably
might result in segmental errors, most likely of the nasal-for-stop variety.
Our own recent work shows that the *stop-nasal* contrast contributes significantly to the overall intelligibility deficit in speakers with ALS (Kent et al,
1989; Kent et al., in press). One reason why there have been so few studies
of the nature of velopharyngeal dysfunction in dysarthria (but see Netsell,
1969) is that there are obvious difficulties in viewing a 'hidden' structure
such as the velopharyngeal port, and acoustic analysis of hypernasality can
be difficult and unreliable. We include a stop-nasal contrast in the test for
the obvious reason that clinical experience suggests, but note here that
other types of variables may capture an important effect of velopharyngeal
dysfunction on speech intelligibility. Some of these are discussed below, in
the context of variables not explicitly concerned with phonetic contrasts.

    Variables that relate to obstruent integrity are logical candidates for an
explanatory test of speech intelligibility, largely because so much of the perceptual literature has focused on obstruent errors or distortions in dysarthria. Studies that have employed transcription techniques (Platt et al.,
1980; Logemann & Fisher, 1978) or scaling of dimensions related to

obstruent production (Darley, Aronson, & Brown, 1975; Carrow, Rivera, Mauldin, & Shamblin, 1974; Joanette & Dudley, 1980) indicate that obstruent articulation is typically deficient in various dysarthrias. Interestingly, the acoustical and physiological literature has not provided much information on obstruent production deficiencies in dysarthria that goes past information available in the perceptual literature. Two acoustical studies (Kent & Rosenbek, 1982; Weismer, 1984a: see Table 2) have demonstrated the presence of spirantization of stops in Parkinson's disease, and one study (Weismer, Mulligan, & DePaul, 1986) reported a high frequency of occurrence of spirantization in highly intelligible, young (29-33 years old) patients with recently-diagnosed ALS.[3] Examination of the findings summarized in Table 2 suggests little else that would implicate specific types of obstruent deficits in dysarthria. The stop-fricative contrast identified in Table 1 will capture perceptual errors that might result from spirantization of stops, but we have reason to believe that spirantization will not make a major contribution to an overall intelligibility deficit. Although Weismer, et al. (1986) and Liss, et al. (1990) found spirantization to occur frequently in ALS and very old males, respectively, the speakers in these studies were typically highly (if not perfectly) intelligible. Moreover, the Parkinsonian speakers in Weismer (1984a) spirantized stops very frequently, but were also highly intelligible in their experimental sentence productions. It is possible, of course, that spirantization patterns in connected speech will be more severe, and therefore more detrimental to overall speech intelligibility, as compared to the spirantization observed in prepared sentences or single words (see Weismer, 1984b, for examples of spirantization in connected speech). Because the present test is based on single words, we maintain our skepticism about the eventual productiveness of this contrast in predicting an intelligibility deficit.

The test includes other contrasts that relate to manner (e.g., fricative/affricate, stop/affricate) and place (e.g., alveolar/palatal fricatives, stop and nasal place) of obstruent articulation. Neither of these types of contrast can be related in a direct way to the findings listed in Table 2, but difficulties with place of articulation among dysarthric speakers might be inferred from observations of restricted antero-posterior tongue movement in this population (Kent, Netsell, & Bauer, 1975; Kent & Netsell, 1978). Although the acoustic phonetics literature can suggest certain measures that might relate to these manner and place contrasts (see Table 1), we would not want to claim that they have well-defined acoustic correlates *for the purposes of a predictive model of speech intelligibility*. At the moment, these contrasts are included in the test because of the indication from perceptual studies and clinical experience that place and manner errors occur in the speech of dysarthric individuals, and the expectation that such errors would contribute in significant way to speech intelligibility deficits.

Table 2 provides one indication (Weismer, 1984a) that the articulatory function of the larynx is impaired in dysarthria. Whereas the short voiceless interval durations[4] found for Parkinson's patients in that study have clear implications for syllable-initial voicing contrasts, discussed above, they also bear on the glottal fricative/null contrast (e.g., *hate/ate*). Four other contrasts that bear on syllable shape (initial consonant/null, final consonant/ null, initial cluster/singleton, final cluster/singleton) are included in the test. Some of these syllable shape distinctions are almost certainly difficult for a variety of dysarthric speakers, but the degree to which such contrast errors affect speech intelligibility scores is an empirical question. The acoustic correlates of these contrasts, listed in Table 1, may not be the only way in which a dysarthric speaker might 'mark' a syllable shape distinction.

Several studies in Table 2 indicate either reduced acoustic transition extents and/or slopes, or slow articulatory movements and reduced range of movement. Because semivowels such as /r/, /l/, and /w/ require a fair amount of rapid movement, especially of the tongue, it is possible to expect problems among dysarthric speakers with /r/-/l/ and/or /r/-/w/ contrasts. The general acoustic correlates of these distinctions are relatively well-understood (see Dalston, 1975) for a limited number of speakers and phonetic contexts (see below).

The issues of restricted range of movement and low articulatory velocity in dysarthria seem to be so global (see Table 2) as to suggest special attention in the formulation of a contrast-based or acoustically-based model of speech intelligibility. Unfortunately, the incorporation of these facts into a contrast-based model of speech intelligibility is not conceptually straightforward. Whereas it is true that semivowel contrasts, as well as certain dipththong contrasts (see Kent and Moll, 1972; Gay, 1968) might be directly sensitive to restricted and slow articulatory gestures, these deficits might have a more global influence on a larger set of contrasts. For example, errors in the stop-fricative manner contrast (Kent et al., 1989: See Table 1) could result from general restriction and slowness of articulatory gestures (e.g., during the approach to the obstruent), rather than from problems associated with actual formation of the constriction.[5] The latter

view is probably the more traditional interpretation of a stop-fricative manner error, but it is easy to imagine how restrictions in lingual range and velocity could result in fricative-for-stop errors. This problem is difficult to for-
malize within the contrast approach adopted by Kent et al. (1989), but can
be handled by means of acoustic variables that can be measured and interpreted independently of the contrast framework.

The acoustic variables are formant transition characteristics that are
easily derived from standard spectrographic displays. By *transition* we mean
the portion of the vocalic nucleus over which an operationally-defined
change in formant frequency occurs. The operational definition is that a
transition begins when at least a 20Hz change in formant frequency occurs
over a 20ms time step, and ends at the first subsequent time step for which
the frequency change is less than 20Hz (Weismer, Kent, Hodge, & Martin,
1988). This definition usually isolates a portion of the vocalic nucleus that
subjectively (visually) appears to have the most linear change in formant
frequency over time. Onsets and offsets of transitions for several words

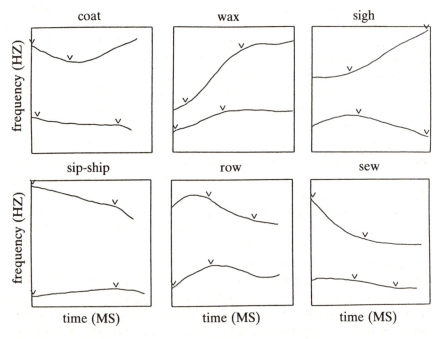

Figure 3. *Vocalic transitions produced by normal geriatric speakers.*

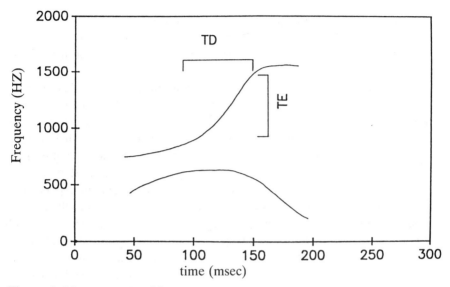

Figure 4. *Measurement of formant transition charactristics.*

produced by normal geriatric speakers are shown in Figure 3 (Weismer et al., 1988), which shows the actual traced F1, F2 trajectories originally traced on spectrograms.[6] As shown in Figure 4, tracings of the first and second formant frequencies throughout the vocalic nucleus of the word '*sigh*' can be measured for transition extent (*TE*) and transition duration (*TD*). TE is the amount of frequency change along the transition, and can be regarded as at least an ordinal metric of amount of change in vocal tract geometry. TD is the duration of the transitional segment. A derived measure, transition rate or slope (*TR*), is given by TE/TD and provides an ordinal estimate of rate of change in vocal tract geometry.

Weismer et al. (1988) investigated these transitional characteristics in single words produced by normal geriatric male and female speakers. They found that the F1, F2 transitions were reproducible across speakers, and in fact might be more stable in more 'complex' vocalic nuclei (e.g., *wax*) as compared to 'simple' vocalic nuclei (e.g., *sip*). Kent, Kent, Weismer, Martin, Sufit, Brooks, and Rosenbek (1989) showed that the overall intelligibility scores of 25 males with ALS was highly correlated ($r = 0.86$) with the averaged F2 slopes (i.e., the TR of F2) from a set of twelve intelligibility words. This finding supports the idea, introduced above, that transition characteristics may reflect something general about the restricted range/ slowness characteristic in dysarthria, and that this characteristic need not be implemented within the contrast framework to have utility in a model of speech intelligibility.

In addition to the indication from the literature that articulatory gestures tend to be slow in dysarthria, there is good evidence (Table 2) that dysarthric speaking rates are often slower — but occasionally faster — than normal. Typically, when a global measure of speaking rate, such as total utterance duration measured from acoustic records, indicates an abnormality, that abnormality is also seen at the segment duration level. Several of the phonetic contrasts in the Kent et al. (1989) test have an explicit temporal component (e.g., *long-short* vowels, syllable-initial and syllable-final *voicing contrast, stop-affricate*), but segment duration measurements could be obtained as acoustic correlates of specific sounds that implement any of the contrasts in the test. Although these acoustic measurements are easy to make and are well understood for normal speakers (see Crystal & House, 1988), we do not believe that they would play a significant predictive role in *single-word* tests of speech intelligibility. As discussed in the final section of the chapter, the role of segment durations might be quite different in models of sentence-level intelligibility.

There are several other variables that cannot be captured easily within a contrast framework, but may have predictive utility in a model of speech intelligibility. These variables include (at least) average fundamental frequency (F0), F0 contour, relative timing of intraword segments, voice quality, and hypernasality. Although it is not known how any of these variables might relate to speech intelligibility, it is certainly reasonable to assume that severe deviations from normal would have some bearing on listeners' ability to understand words. Some of these variables have fairly straightforward acoustic correlates (such as average speaking F0, and jitter/shimmer values and/or signal-to-noise ratios for voice quality), but others are not easily represented by single-valued measures. For example, F0 contours are notoriously difficult to quantify (see, for example, Rose, 1987), and an index of a relative timing pattern in cases where more than two segments are involved has not been developed. The reliability of hypernasality judgments derived from acoustic displays is typically not very good; it is possible, however, that an instrument such as TONAR (Fletcher, 1971) could be used to generate a quantitative estimate of the nasality variable. It is possible that some of these variables might have a greater effect on the intelligibility of phrase- and sentence-level materials than on single words. For example, it is known that mismatches between F0 contours and syntactic structure of an utterance cause decrements in the identification of certain sentences (Geers, 1978). It is also possible that chronic nasality would affect the intelligibility of speech indirectly, by virtue of a distraction or annoyance effect. These issues represent an untapped, but timely, area of research in speech intelligibility studies; the timeliness of the work is due both to the need for complete and quantitative models of speech intelligibility, and the availability of high-quality synthetic speech algorithms for parametric testing of the relevant hypotheses, some of which have been mentioned above.

Selection of variables: General considerations

As indicated above, it might be possible to design, at least in part, a contrast or acoustically-based model of speech intelligibility around factors that are assumed to have general importance to the speech perception process. Before providing an abbreviated discussion of these factors, certain caveats concerning this approach should be mentioned. First, the view that one might design a model of speech intelligibility around the importance of certain features in the speech signal requires that certain of these features be regarded as 'primary'. Presumably, these primary features would be characterized by some degree of consistency across utterances and speakers, in addition to their obvious psychoacoustic and/or linguistic salience. The second formant, for example, which is known to be psychoacoustically salient (because it tends to occupy an auditorily sensitive region in the frequency range) and linguistically salient (because it carries information about place of articulation), will maintain its prominence in normal speech signals as a result of a nonvarying glottal source spectrum and wide range of tongue movements. In disordered speech, however, a variable and noisy source spectrum, variable and excessive hypernasality, and restricted ranges of tongue movement may make F2 a less stable, and therefore less heavily weighted, perceptual cue.

The second consideration is that the highly redundant nature of the speech signal makes it difficult to select those features that might have greater or lesser importance to the process of speech perception, and hence, speech intelligibility. Because cues in the speech signal can trade off against one another (Repp, 1982), it could be that the search for 'primary' cues is a fruitless one. Rather, the listener may always integrate a set of different cues to arrive at a given percept, with primacy assigned to the integrated percept, and not any of the contributing components.

With these caveats in mind, we would suggest that the most likely 'general' variables to include in a model of speech intelligibility would be place contrasts and F2 characteristics. In the traditional way of thinking about acoustic phonetics, place contrasts and F2 characteristics are simply different sides of the same coin (Lieberman, Cooper, Shankweiler, & Studdert-Kennedy, 1967). Errors of place identification seem to be more common than, for example, errors of voicing under various masking and filtering conditions (Miller and Nicely, 1955). Moreover, the speech signal remains fairly intelligible until F2 is removed from the signal (Gay, 1970). If these considerations suggest that F2/place characteristics should be incorporated into an explanatory model of speech intelligibility, the current form of the test described by Kent et al. (1989) and the direction of our thinking reviewed above meets these requirements. The inclusion of explicit place contrasts (see Table 1) and the acoustic focus on F2 trajectories covers this potentially important issue. Fortunately, it seems that in this case the considerations from general intelligibility overlap with considerations from the specific case of dysarthric speech.

Representation (form) of variables for the model

To our knowledge, there has been little or no discussion in the literature concerning the appropriate *form* of variables used in a model of speech intelligibility. In this section of the chapter, we provide one view of how variables should be represented in a model, and illustrate our argument with several cases from the available literature and from our own work. We also consider the issue of redundancy of predictor variables, and suggest certain ways in which research efforts might deal with this pervasive problem.

In a model of speech intelligibility having predictor variables only in the form of phonetic contrasts, it seems fairly straightforward to quantify each contrast in terms of the error rate (or the success rate). Our own approach to this type of analysis, although not yet incorporated into a formal model of speech intelligibility (but see below), has been to express the error rate for a contrast as the proportion of all possible contrast opportunities that are not identified correctly by a panel of listeners. Thus the

0.18 error rate for the stop-nasal contrast in Figure 1 means that 18% of all possible stop-nasal contrasts were misheard by our panel of ten listeners. We chose to express the error rate per contrast in this way because there were not equal numbers of target-foil items representing each contrast. For example, the stop-nasal contrast was represented in the test by 18 target-foil items, whereas the /r/-/l/ contrast was represented by only 13 items.[7] It is possible, however, to quantify the error rate for each contrast as a proportion of *all* errors, in which case the proportions summed across contrasts would equal 1.00. Although it is not clear which approach to determining contrast error proportions is preferable, it could be argued that expressing the proportions relative to the entire set of errors, rather than on a contrast-by-contrast basis, is a more direct way to express the relationship between specific contrast errors and an overall intelligibility deficit *on this particular test*. The error proportions obtained on a contrast-by-contrast basis might be better suited to models that seek to generalize the influence of particular contrast deficits on a wide range of intelligibility measures (e.g., such as predicting intelligibility deficits on other word tests [e.g., the Yorkston-Beukelman test], or on tests of sentence intelligibility). These are issues that must be dealt with empirically, preferably by using both kinds of error proportion and comparing their performance in pilot models of intelligibility.

The representation of acoustic variables in a model of speech intelligibility is also open to some debate. At first glance, it might seem as if the ratio-scale measurements that could be derived from acoustic records would be ideal quantities for predictor variables. For example, various investigators (Monsen, 1974, 1978; Ansel, 1985; Metz et al., 1985) have used voice-onset time (VOT) measurements and differences in formant frequencies as *scalar* values in regression models of speech intelligibility, and Ansel (1985) has done the same for vowel durations. A potential problem with this approach is that equal increments along the acoustic scalar may be related to the speech perception event in a nonlinear way. In a sense, this is simply a restatement of the well-known phenomenon of categorical perception for certain acoustic-phonetic features, but the problem can be framed in a way that is more directly related to the development of a model of speech intelligibility. When Monsen (1978) and Metz et al. (1985) used VOT as a scalar in their regression analyses of acoustic variables and speech intelligibility, they made the implicit assumption, for example, that a 65ms VOT was 'more voiceless' than a 50ms VOT (or, that a -10ms VOT was 'more voiced' than a 10ms VOT). There is good reason to believe, however, that the VOT continuum should not be viewed this way, but rather should be conceptualized as a reflection of a more binary physiological phenomenon (see Weismer, 1980; Weismer and Cariski, 1984). Moreover, Repp (1979), following ideas developed by Winitz, LaRiviere, and Herriman (1975) and Abramson (1977), has shown that, even within the unrealistic setting of a categorical perception experiment,[8] a VOT boundary can be adjusted by manipulating the level of aspiration noise in the VOT interval. The point that we wish to emphasize here, using VOT as an example, is that the decision to represent the acoustic correlate of a contrast should be based on careful considerations regarding both the underlying physiological characteristics of the contrast, as well as perceptual correlates of the relevant acoustic continua, if they are known. There is, however, at least one argument for *always* using a scalar index of an acoustic contrast, regardless of how this index relates to normal speech physiology and perception. This argument holds that an optimal acoustic model of speech intelligibility would be one in which values of the index coefficients could be used as an objective metric of improvement or decline of a motor speech disorder (i.e., as a result of treatment, natural history, and so forth). The use of nominal indices in a clinically-useful model could be misleading, because certain 'real' changes in the coefficients might reflect adjustments that are not consistent with our current understanding of physiological phonetics, and/or may not have perceptual consequences. This line of thinking might suggest that the most conservative approach in the development of the model is to always use scalar measurements. As stated above, however, the danger of this approach is a possible misrepresentation of the contribution of certain variables to the overall intelligibility score. What is needed to understand the role of acoustic indices in a clinically useful model of speech intelligibility are studies that document specific changes as a function of behavioral or drug treatment, progression of degenerative diseases, and so forth. If these studies would show subtle acoustic changes that are tied consistently to aspects of service delivery or natural history, emphasis should be placed on the development of optimal scalar indices of the acoustic variables. There is certainly precedent in the articulation development and disorders literature to regard subtle acoustic effects, which could only be detected by scalar measures, as theoretically and clinically meaningful (see Macken and Barton, 1977; Weismer, 1984c).

The representation of obstruent acoustics in a model of speech intelligibility is difficult to discuss, because so little research attention has been devoted to the topic. In the case of stops, one might choose a categorical representation wherein each place of articulation would be associated with an operationally-defined acoustic characteristic, or range of characteristics. This approach would be consistent with the well-known template classifications of stop spectra reported by Blumstein and Stevens (1980) and Kewley-Port (1983; Kewley-Port and Luce, 1984). Moreover, a categorical representation of the acoustic correlates of stop place contrasts seems to be consistent with the largely categorical nature of stop place articulations as well as the perception of stop-burst spectra (Stevens & Blumstein, 1978; Kewley-Port, 1983). One possible difficulty with the categorical variable approach (e.g., where place could be coded 1=bilabial, 2=lingua-alveolar, 3=dorsal, 4=other [not fitting any of the operationalized spectral characteristics, see Shinn & Blumstein, 1983]) is that dysarthric speakers may not produce place contrasts in the categorical way expected of normal speakers. As a clinical observation, it is not uncommon to hear stops produced by dysarthric speakers at indeterminate, or multiple, places of articulation. Spectra associated with these kinds of stop could be classified in the 'other' category (see above), or the acoustic characteristics of stop bursts could be represented by a more fine-grained measure. Such a measure could be derived from spectral moments analysis, which has been shown to classify stop burst acoustics better than any published template system (Forrest, Weismer, Milenkovic, & Dougall, 1988). The measure could be in the form of the moments themselves, or the distance measure (Mahalanobis D^2) derived from the discriminant function analysis of the moment data. Unfortunately, there are no data on the relationship of either of these measures to perception of stops produced by disordered speakers.

Similar comments could be made about the representation of fricative acoustics in the model. Harmes, Daniloff, Hoffman, Lewis, Kramer, & Absher (1984) and Bladon and Seitz (1986) have described various spectral measures that might be used to describe fricatives; Harmes et al. found that the lower limit of relatively high energy frication noise was a good discriminator of fricatives produced by normal speakers and speakers with Broca's aphasia. The spectral moments approach can also be applied to fricatives (see Forrest et al., 1988), or for that matter to any spectrum of a speech event. One potential advantage of spectral moments is that they could provide a unified representation of several variables in an acoustic model of speech intelligibility. That is, the moments can be applied to any speech spectrum, and thus can serve as an index of any sound class. Whether or not this is preferable to acoustic measures that are specific to sound classes must be determined by the appropriate modelling work.

The representation of other contrasts that involve sonorants should be based on the same kinds of considerations about underlying physiology and perception that were discussed above in reference to the VOT problem. For example, we would guess that quantification of an acoustic dimensions underlying a contrast such as *stop-nasal* might best be accomplished using a nominal data approach, wherein nasalized stops (or fricatives) are coded '1' and non-nasalized stops are coded '0'. Because multiple regression techniques are available that permit a combination of interval- and nominal-data variables (Cohen and Cohen, 1975), it may be more prudent to categorize certain acoustic variables (such as nasality) in this way, than to attempt finer-grained measures that have questionable links to both production and perception. It is also possible that some of the semivowel contrasts (such as /r/-/w/) might be better captured with nominal-type indices than interval-type indices. Although there is some evidence that listeners hear a continuum of /r/-ness to /w/-ness when aspects of a synthetically-generated third formant are varied in discrete steps (Ohde and Sharf, 1987), the multiplicity of cues that contribute to most semivowel distinctions, and the high context sensitivity of these cues, may suggest that a reduction in the acoustic dimensionality of these contrasts is desirable. One approach to this problem would involve straightforward acoustic description of semivowel characteristics in a variety of phonetic contexts for both normal and dysarthric speakers.[9] This description could then point to the feasibility and form of a template system for indexing the acoustic characteristics of semivowels.

Finally, work must be done to determine if 'auditory-spectral' representations of acoustic events are more productive predictors of speech intelligibility deficits as compared to frequency representations. In recent years, there has been substantial interest in transforming frequency representations of speech events into spectra that more closely resemble the non-linear frequency resolution characteristics of the human auditory system. Syrdal and Gopal (1986), Kewley-Port and Luce (1984), and Forrest et al. (1988), among others, have shown that in certain cases 'auditory spectra' (such as Bark spectra: see Syrdal and Gopal, 1986) are better than frequency spectra for the classification of sound classes from acoustic data.

The implications for acoustic prediction of intelligibility deficits are obvious, and can be addressed by straightforward comparisons of the performance of frequency- and 'auditory-spectra' variables in the models.

Predicting intelligibility from the phonetic and acoustic characteristics of dysarthric speech

The central aim of an 'explanatory' intelligibility test, such as that proposed by Kent, et al. (1989), is to determine the phonetic, acoustic and, ultimately, the articulatory characteristics of dysarthric speech which result in reduced intelligibility. Using this information as a base, a further goal is to identify the means by which a dysarthric speaker's output should be modified in order to increase intelligibility. In this sense, the approach is not unlike that advocated by Nickerson and Stevens (1980) in relation to the speech of the deaf.

In this vein, Kent, et al. (in press) have reported phonetic 'error profiles' based on data derived from their intelligibility test. The error profile for 25 men with ALS presented in Figure 1 indicates that the phonetic contrasts with the greatest error proportions were, in decreasing order, stop versus nasal (0.18), initial /h/ versus null (0.15), initial consonant voicing (0.11), stop versus affricate (0.09) and alveolar versus palatal fricative (0.08).

In a further analysis of these data, the relationship between these top-ranked error proportions and the subjects' intelligibility scores was examined. In particular, we attempted to determine the extent to which the intelligibility of these dysarthric subjects could be predicted from their phonetic contrast errors. Error proportions from the phonetic contrasts yielding the five highest average error proportions were used as predictor variables in a multiple regression analysis of intelligibility. In addition, F2 slope values, obtained through spectrographic analysis, were included as a predictor variable, since previous analyses had suggested a moderately high correlation between this acoustic characteristic and the speech intelligibility of subjects with ALS (Kent. et al., 1989). Thus, a total of 6 predictor variables were selected for study, based on the results of previous phonetic and acoustic analyses.

As an initial step, Spearman rank order intercorrelations for all possible pairs of predictor variables were determined. Additionally, simple correlations between the 6 predictor variables and the subjects' intelligibility scores were calculated. These results are shown in Table 3.

GARY WEISMER AND RUTH E. MARTIN

Table 3. *Spearman rank order correlations among 6 predictor variables in stepwise regression analysis of intelligibility for 25 male ALS subjects*

	Phonetic contrasts						
	stop/ nasal	alveo/pal frictive	stop/ affricate	initial consonant voicing	initial /h/ null	F2 slope	intell. score
stop/ nasal		.816	.644	.599	.225	−.570	−.733
alveo./ palatal frictive			.634	.689	.426	−.719	−.785
stop/ affric.				.489	.477	−.431	−.639
init. C voicing					.702	−.743	−.687
init. /h/ null						−.504	−.641
F2 slope							−.843
intell. score							

At least moderate correlations were obtained between predictor variable pairs in most cases. One exception involved the initial /h/ versus null contrast which was moderately correlated with the initial consonant voicing variable (.702) but bore lower correlations with all other variables (.225, .426, .477, .504). In addition, the correlations between the stop versus affricate contrast and the initial consonant voicing (.489) and the F2 slope contrasts (-.431) were among the lowest values obtained.

In total, 7 correlations had absolute values that were less than .60. Of these, 6 correlations involved either the initial /h/ versus null or the initial consonant voicing contrast (both of which could be interpreted as reflecting laryngeal function) and one of the other variables. These results suggest that no clear relationship exists between the laryngeal and supralaryngeal aspects of the speech impairment in these male ALS speakers. It does not appear, for example, that the errors of the stop/nasal contrast, presumably reflecting velopharyngeal impairment, predict voicing errors very accurately.

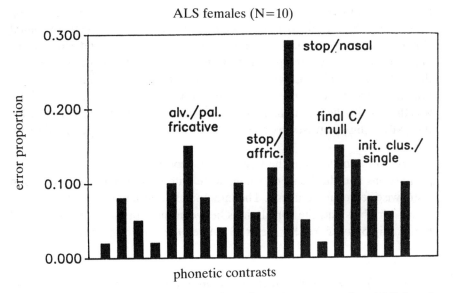

Figure 5. *Proportions of errors within phonetic contrasts for ALS females (N=10)*

Regarding the correlations between the 6 predictor variables and intelligibility, the F2 slope bore the highest simple correlation with intelligibility, followed by the alveolar versus palatal fricative contrast and the stop nasal contrast.

When these 6 variables were entered into a stepwise regression analysis, two variables accounted for 95.35% of the variance in the intelligibility scores. These were the stop versus nasal and the initial /h/ versus null contrasts. The stop versus nasal contrast alone accounted for 76.58% of the variance in the intelligibility scores. It is noteworthy that the two variables with the highest average error proportions also were the two that predicted intelligibility most reliably. Moreover, the set of intercorrelations in Table 3 suggests that these two variables are more independent than any of the other variable pairs. As noted above, this apparent statistical independence is consistent with the different subsystems of the speech mechanism represented by the stop-nasal (velopharyngeal) and initial /h/-null (laryngeal) contrasts.

A similar analysis was performed on data derived from the single word productions of 10 female subjects with ALS. As shown in Figure 5, the phonetic error profile for the female subjects indicated that the most involved contrasts were, in order of decreasing error poroportions, stop versus nasal (0.29), alveolar versus palatal fricative (0.15), final consonant versus null (0.15), initial cluster versus singleton (0.13) and stop versus affricate (0.12). Thus, the patterns of phonetic errors most characteristic of the male and female ALS groups were somewhat different. The most striking difference between the error profiles for the male and female subjects was that, while the initial /h/ versus null contrast frequently was in error for the males, this contrast was among the least involved for the female subjects.

As in the male data, the five phonetic contrasts with the highest error proportions and the F2 slope values were entered as predictor variables in a stepwise regression analysis. The intercorrelations among the pairs of predictor variables and the correlations between the 6 predictor variables and the intelligibility scores for the ALS women are shown in Table 4.

Table 4. Spearman rank order correlations among 6 predictor variables in stepwise regression analysis of intelligibility for 10 female ALS subjects

	Phonetic contrasts						
	stop/ nasal	alveo/pal frictive	stop/ affricate	initial consonant voicing	initial /h/ null	F2 slope	intell. score
stop/ nasal		.758	.767	.861	.382	−.636	−.782
alveo./ palatal frictive			.888	.724	.667	−.915	−.879
stop/ affric.				.706	.724	−.845	−.845
init. C voicing					.570	−.655	−.824
init. /h/ null						−.673	−.733
F2 slope							−.818
intell. score							

At least moderate correlations were obtained in most cases. Two relatively lower correlations, both below .60, were found between the initial cluster/singleton and stop/nasal contrasts, and the initial cluster/singleton and final consonant/null contrasts.

The simple correlations between the predictor variables and intelligibility indicated that the contrasts most strongly related to intelligibility were, in decreasing order, alveolar versus palatal fricative, stop versus affricate, and final consonant versus null. Interestingly, although the error proportion for the stop versus nasal contrast was substantially greater than any other contrast, the simple correlation between this contrast and intelligibility was less that those obtained for three other contrasts. Results of the stepwise regression analysis indicated that two variables, the alveolar versus palatal fricative and stop versus nasal, accounted for 91.09% of the variance in intelligibility scores. Further, 82.33% was accounted for by the alveolar versus palatal fricative contrast alone.

These preliminary analyses suggest that many of the variables that might be considered for a multivariate model of speech intelligibility tend to be at least modestly intercorrelated. Moreover, the stepwise multiple regression analyses point to the possibility that in some cases a single variable may account for a large amount of the variance in single word intelligibility scores. Because stepwise regression analyses are 'blind' discovery procedures that are highly sensitive to sampling error, it is imperative that models (equations) derived from one group of subjects be used to predict intelligibility scores for an independent group of subjects. We are hesitant to compare models across our two ALS groups, because we suspect that the response of the two sexes to neurological disease may be as different as the response of the sexes to normal aging (see Weismer & Fromm, 1983; Weismer & Liss, in press). In fact, the absence of contrasts that reflect laryngeal function in the top-ranked error proportions for the female ALS speakers, but their presence for the males, is curiously consistent with the well-known sex differences for the effects of aging on laryngeal functioning (Weismer & Liss, in press). Future work, then, should focus on validation of models within sex groups, as well as the application of models derived from our test (i.e., Kent et al., 1989) to the intelligibility scores derived from independent tests (such as Yorkston & Beukelman, 1981a). These studies are necessary to identify the *general principles* of intelligibility deficits, rather than isolated phenomena tied to a particular word list, response format, or other set of conditions specific to a particular test.

Influence of normal listening strategies on speech intelligibility

To this point in this chapter, we have focussed on considerations that bear primarily on single-word tests of intelligibility. We would not necessarily expect, however, the single-word intelligibility estimate from every dysarthric speaker to be a good predictor of sentence or connected discourse intelligibility. In fact, it seems reasonable to expect that two dysarthric speakers with the same single-word intelligibility might have significantly different sentence intelligibilities, for the following reasons. As noted above, when two dysarthric speakers have the same speech intelligibility score in a single-word test, a phonetic profile analysis may reveal strikingly different articulatory bases for the intelligibility deficits. These different articulatory deficits may not only be manifest at the single-word level, however, but also in the *manner of producing sequences of words*. The speaker with spastic dysarthria, for example, may produce a sequence of words in a scanning fashion, whereas the Parkinsonian speaker may have widely variable speaking rates and stress contrasts for the same utterance. The sentence intelligibilities of these two dysarthric speakers could be very different — even when the single-word intelligibilites are similar — because the listener's strategies for perceiving connected speech are better matched to one of these word sequencing styles. A better appreciation of this highly speculative argument may be gained by a brief discussion of modern work in the area of speech perception.

A very comprehensive discussion of the important issues in speech perception has been published by Pisoni and Luce (1986). These authors note that speech perception is a process involving the interaction of information derived from the acoustic signal and from higher level 'knowledge sources.' The knowledge described by Pisoni and Luce, as well as others (see for example, Marslen-Wilson, 1975; Cutler, 1976; Cutler & Foss, 1977; Nooteboom & van der Vlugt, 1988; Nooteboom, Brokx, & de Rooij, 1978), includes such things as notions about which parts of the speech signal are optimal for accurate perception ('islands of reliability,' including stressed words, onsets of words, regions of maximal spectral change), the effect of rate changes on low-level decisions about acoustic-phonetic structure, and the understanding of how sentence-level prosody focusses attention on 'high-content' regions of the speech signal. A key concept of this interactionist view of speech perception is that listeners employ strategies that optimize the process. The strategy of speech perception, then, is not simply to record a sequence of sounds as the speech signal enters the auditory system, but to attend preferentially to certain aspects of the signal, to make hypotheses regarding word identities before all the acoustic-phonetic information is available, and to have enough faith in the speed and experience of the process to delay certain decisions until the full range of knowledge sources can provide a high probability of perceptual success. In one sense, these considerations seem somewhat trite, because listening to and understanding connected speech is typically an effortless process. Conscious decisions regarding, for example, 'islands of reliability' are not typically made because the strategies are so well practiced and natural, having been shaped by the predictable structure of the incoming signal.

This situation changes dramatically when listening to a person with a motor speech disorder. Most people (certainly all speech-language pathologists who work in hospital settings) are quite familiar with the tremendous sense of effort that may be associated with understanding a patient with a neurogenic speech disorder. Much of this sense of effort is no doubt a function of the degraded sound structure of the patient's speech. As reviewed above, there is substantial evidence in the literature on intelligibility characteristics of the hearing impaired that segmental deficits do not always predict intelligibility deficits with a great degree of accuracy; we would expect the same thing in dysarthia, although the appropriate studies have not been done (see Platt et al., 1980). We would suggest, then, that an additional source of effortful listening and intelligibility deficit in dysarthria is our typical listening strategies, which may be poorly designed for understanding persons who produce connected speech in a way that is radically different from the normal speaker. Some years ago, Nash (1972) discussed this problem in the context of understanding a non-native speaker: "The crucial problem...is not the number and severity of distortions, but their effects upon the listener in the communication situation. This may or may not correspond to the actual amount of distortion" (1972: 570). And, she goes on to conclude that, "An inappropriate prosodic pattern...denies or contradicts the lexical message" (Nash, 1972: 571). Some speculative examples will illustrate how these considerations may bear on the intelligibility of dysarthric speech.

When listening to English, listeners expect certain stress contrasts to characterize words and sentences. Because stressed words serve as one of the 'islands of reliability', deviations from a normal stress pattern could disrupt the on-line processing of speech. Interestingly, there has been relatively little work done on the productive stress patterning of dysarthric utterances. Kent, Netsell, & Abbs (1979) have shown that persons with ataxic dysarthria reduce the temporal difference between stressed and unstressed syllables, a finding consistent with the perceptual impression of 'scanning speech' in this population (the same result has been demonstrated in the speech of the hearing impaired: see Stevens et al., 1983, and discussion above). Because the location of stressed words in normal speech appears to be anticipated by the listener (Cutler & Foss, 1977), and syllables carrying stress serve to organize lexical access strategies (Cutler & Norris, 1988), a deviant stress pattern should disrupt the normally efficient search for word identifications. Similarly, the fact that word onsets seem to be associated with greater intelligibility deficits than word offsets or word middles (Ziegler et al., 1988) may reflect the importance of word onsets in organizing lexical search strategies (Marslen-Wilson, 1987; Nooteboom & van der Vlugt, 1988). That is, the actual productive deficits of dysarthric speakers may not vary much across word position, but the weight of the word-initial deficit in understanding connected speech may be far greater than the weight in other word positions, as a result of normal listening strategies. The high quality synthetic speech that is currently available (Klatt, 1987), as well as LPC resynthesis techniques, makes the testing of these hypotheses fairly straightforward. For example, F0/stress characteristics of an utterance could be altered while maintaining the integrity of segmental contrasts. The prediction is that modifications of the F0/stress contour that made the location of stressed words less systematic or predictable would cause decrements in sentence intelligibility, even in the absence of variation in segmental integrity. Moreover, research on the intelligibility of synthetic speech (Slowiaczek & Nusbaum, 1985; Nusbaum & Pisoni, 1985) would suggest that as the segmental structure of an utterance is degraded, the 'focussing' aspect of stress prediction becomes more important. If the appropriate experiments would show these hypothesized effects in models of dysarthric speech (i.e., synthesized dysarthric speech), or in 'corrected' dysarthric speech, the results would have profound implications for the treatment of motor speech disorders.

Listening strategies associated with temporal cues to sound-identity may also be disrupted by dysarthric speech production. Nooteboom, Brokx, & de Rooij (1978) and Miller (1981) have reviewed the substantial evidence that overall speaking rate establishes boundary conditions for local segmental distinctions that depend on temporal cues. In other words, the local temporal boundaries are not fixed, but depend on the prevailing speaking rate. These rate-dependent changes in perceptual boundaries are mirrored by the adjustment in local temporal characteristics that occur when normal speakers voluntarily change their speaking rate. It is not known if the very slow, global speaking rates of some dysarthrics, or the very fast speaking rates among some hypokinetic dysarthrics, are accompanied by corresponding adjustments in local temporal cues to sound identity.[10] If they are not, the listener is faced with a mismatch between the two temporal characteristics. The consequence for processing the acoustic signal is obvious, and reveals another potential dimension of the influence of listener strategies on the intelligibility problem in dysarthria.

Clearly, the thoughts expressed in this section are prospective, because they apply to explanations of the intelligibility of connected speech, about which little is known both empirically and theoretically. For the reasons outlined here, there may not be good correspondence between the explanatory postulates we derive from single word tests, and those we may eventually formulate from the study of connected speech. This is really a general problem in speech perception, as summarized by Martin: "It is not clear that identification, discrimination and other methods found so useful in speech perception work up till now [that has used single syllables] will also be useful in the case of continuous speech" (1975: 173).

Summary

In this chapter we have tried to show how the standard use of speech intelligibility tests — that is, as severity metrics — can be expanded to include an explanatory component. A review of the literature on speech intelligibility in dysarthric and hearing-impaired persons suggests that limited attempts have been made to develop explanatory models of speech intelligibility. We have offered a fairly detailed discussion of our own explanatory test of intelligibility, and treated the issue of the selection and form of variables that would be appropriate in a model that incorporates both phonetic contrast variables and acoustic variables as predictors of overall speech intelligibility scores. In addition, a preliminary analysis of relationships between these variables suggested that the development of an explanatory model must proceed in the context of sets of variables that tend to be at least modestly intercorrelated. Finally, it is argued that the explanatory principles that are emerging from the study of single-word intelligibility are likely to be quite different than those that will be discovered in the study of sentence intelligibility.

Notes

1. Although Logemann and Fisher found voicing errors in their analysis of Parkinsonian dysarthria, we believe that had they run a control group of geriatric persons, similar kinds of voicing errors would have been recorded. This opinion is based on the fact that 'normal' geriatrics and Parkinson's patients had similar voicing control problems in the Weismer (1984) study, and that aging in general seems to be associated with loss of voicing control (Liss, Weismer, & Rosenbek, 1990), at least in the syllable-initial position.

2. Although it is beyond the scope of this chapter to treat this issue in depth, voicing status of stops may be cued by an unusually large variety of acoustic dimensions, which redundancy may explain why Miller and Nicely found this feature to be so resistant to various forms of distortion. Interestingly, there are no comprehensive investigations of the various acoustic counterparts of the voicing distinction in the literature on motor speech disorders.

3. Our experience suggests that spirantization of stop consonants is a common articulatory deficit in all motor speech disorders. Although Logemann and Fisher (1978) stated that their transcription analysis implicated spirantization as a hallmark of Parkinson's disease, our acoustic analyses have demonstrated the phenomenon to occur frequently in ALS (Weismer, Mulligan, and DePaul 1986) spastic dysarthria (Forrest and Weismer 1988) apraxia of speech (Weismer and Liss 1990) and ataxic dysarthria (unpublished observations). The phenomenon is also common in very old males (88-93 years old) who have not been diagnosed with a specific neurological disease (Liss, Weismer, and Rosenbek 1990).

4. The physiological correlate of the voiceless interval duration is the duration of the laryngeal devoicing gesture. See Hirose (1976), Weismer (1980) and Löfqvist (1980) for additional details.

5. Within certain theories of speech production, these two interpretations of stop-fricatives errors are associated with different notions of mechanism. Following the notions put forward by Öhman (1969), Perkell (1969), Fujimura and Kakita (1979), and refined by Fowler (1985), vocalic getures are largely controlled by extrinsic muscles, and consonant gestures by intrinsic muscles. Thus, a fricative-for-stop error resulting from the restricted/slow approach gestures during the vocalic gesture would reflect a different pathophysiology than the same error resulting from improper lingual adjustment at the point of articulatory contact.

6. As summarized in Weismer et al. (1988), the trajectories are first traced directly on the spectrograms, and then retraced on a graphics tablet that samples the tracings at 10Hz and stores the data in files for later analysis and plotting.

7. The number of items per contrast was based loosely on a notion of the frequency of occurrence — and thus, the potential importance to an intelligibility metric — of a particular contrast. In other words, the potential for stop-nasal errors, which involve segments having a fairly high frequency of occurence in English, was thought to be greater than the potential for /r/-/l/ errors, and was therefore implemented by a greater number of items.

8.   By 'unrealistic' we mean a setting that has minimal ecological validity.
9.   There is surprisingly little descriptive work on the acoustic characteristics of semivowels. Studies by Dalston (1975) and Lehiste and Peterson (1961) are available, but are based on a small number of speakers and limited range of phonetic contexts.
10. Our experience has been that neither the very slow or fast dysarthric speaker adjusts the local temporal characteristics (such as VOT, or vowel duration, or even formant transition durations) of segmental articulation in proportion to the overall speaking rate characteristics. This is an area that needs further investigation.

References

Abramson, A.S. 1977. "Laryngeal timing in consonant distinctions." *Phonetica* 34, 295-303.

Ansel, B.A. 1985. *Acoustic Predictors of Speech Intelligibility in Cerebral Palsied Dysarthric Adults.* Unpublished doctoral dissertation, University of Wisconsin-Madison, Madison, WI.

Bernstein, J. 1977. "Intelligibility and simulated deaf-like segmental and timing errors." *International Conference on Acoustics. Speech and Signal Processing* 25, 244-247.

Bladon, A., & Seitz, F. 1986. "Spectral edge orientation as a discriminator of fricatives." *Journal of the Acoustical Society of America* 80 (Suppl. 1), S18.

Blumstein, S.E., Stevens, K.N. 1980. "Perceptual invariance and onset spectra for stop consonants in various vowel environments." *Journal of the Acoustical Society of America* 67, 648-662.

Carrow, E., Rivera, V., Mauldin, M., & Shamblin, L. 1974. "Deviant speech characteristics in motor neuron disease." *Archives of Otolaryngology* 100, 212-218.

Caruso, A.J., & Burton, E.K. 1987. "Temporal acoustic measures of dysarthria associated with amyotrophic lateral sclerosis." *Journal of Speech and Hearing Research* 30, 80-87.

Cohen, J., & Cohen, P. 1975. *Applied Multiple Regression/Correlation Analysis for the Behavioral Sciences.* Hillsdale, NJ: Lawrence Erlbaum.

Crystal, T.H., House, A.S. 1988. "Segmental durations in connected speech signals: Current results." *Journal of the Acoustical Society of America* 83, 1553-1573.

Cutler, A. 1976. "Phoneme-monitoring reaction time as a function of preceding intonation contour." *Perception & Psychophysics* 20, 55-60.

Cutler, A., & Foss, D.J. 1977. "On the role of sentence stress in sentence processing." *Language and Speech* 20, 1-10.

Cutler, A., & Norris, D. 1988. "The role of strong syllables in segmentation for lexical access." *Journal of Experimental Psychology: Human Perception and Performance* 14, 113-121.

Dalston, R. 1975. "Acoustic characteristics of English /w,r,l/ spoken correctly by young children and adults." *Journal of the Acoustical Society of America* 57, 462-469.

Darkins, A.W., Fromkin, V.A., & Benson, D.F. 1988. "A characterization of the prosodic loss in Parkinson's disease." *Brain and Language* 34, 315-327.

Darley, F.L., Aronson, A.E., & Brown, J.R. 1975. *Motor Speech Disorders.* Philadelphia: W.B. Saunders.

Enderby, P.M. 1983. *Frenchay Dysarthria Assessment*. San Diego: College-Hill Press.

Farmer, A. 1980. "Voice onset time in cerebral palsied speakers." *Folia Phoniatrica* 32, 267-273.

Fletcher, S.G. 1971. *Diagnosing Speech Disorders from Cleft Palate*. New York: Grune and Straton.

Forrest, K., Weismer, G., Milenkovic, P., Dougall, R. 1988. "Statistical analysis of word-initial voiceless obstruents: Preliminary data." *Journal of the Acoustical Society of America* 84, 115-123.

Forrest, K., Weismer, G., & Turner, G.S. 1989. "Kinematic, acoustic, and perceptual analyses of connected speech produced by Parkinsonian and normal geriatric adults." *Journal of the Acoustical Society of America* 85, 2608-2622.

Fowler, C.A. 1985. "Current perspectives on language and speech production: A critical review." *Speech Science*, ed. by R.G. Daniloff, 193-301. San Diego: College-Hill Press.

Frearson, B. 1985. "A comparison of the AIDS sentence list and spontaneous speech intelligibility scores for dysarthric speech." *Australian Journal of Human Communication Disorders* 13, 5-21.

Fujimura, O., Kakita, Y. 1979. "Remarks on the quantitative description of lingual articulation." *Frontiers of Speech Communication Research*, ed. by B. Lindblom and S. Öhman, 17-24. London: Academic Press.

Gay, T. 1968. "Effect of speaking rate on diphthong formant movements." *Journal of the Acoustical Society of America* 44, 1570-1573.

Gay, T. 1970. "Effects of filtering and vowel environment on consonant perception." *Journal of the Acoustical Society of America* 48, 993-998.

Geers, A.E. 1978. "Intonation contour and syntactic structure as predictors of apparent segmentation." *Journal of Experimental Psychology: Human Perception and Performance* 4, 273-283.

Harmes, S., Daniloff, R.G., Hoffman, P.R., Lewis, J., Kramer, M.B., & Absher, R. 1984. "Temporal and articulatory control of fricative articulation by speakers with Broca's aphasia." *Journal of Phonetics* 12, 367-383.

Hirose, H. 1976. "Posterior cricoarytenoid as a speech muscle." *Annals of Otology, Rhinology and Laryngology* 85, 334-343.

Hirose, H., Kiritani, Sawashima, M. 1982. "Velocity of articulatory movements in normal and dysarthric subjects." *Folia Phoniatrica* 34, 210-215.

Hudgins, C.V., Numbers, F.C. 1942. "An investigation of the intelligibility of the speech of the deaf." *Genetic Psychology Monographs* 25, 289-392.

Huggins, A.W.F. 1977. "Speech timing and intelligibility." *Attention and Performance VII*, ed. by J. Requin, 279-298. Hillsdale, New Jersey: Lawrence Erlbaum.

Joanette, Y., Dudley, J.G. 1980. "Dysarthria symptomatology of Friedreich's ataxia." *Brain and Language* 10, 39-50.

John, J.E.J., Howarth, J.N. 1965. "The effect of time distortions on the intelligibility of deaf children's speech." *Language and Speech* 8, 127-134.

Kent, R.D. 1983. "The segmental organization of speech." *The Production of Speech*, ed. by P. MacNeilage, 57-89. New York: Springer-Verlag.

Kent, R.D., Kent, J.F., Weismer, G., Martin, R., Sufit, R.L., Brooks, B.R., & Rosenbek, J.C. 1989. "Relationships between speech intelligibility and the slope of second formant transitions in dysarthric subjects." *Clinical Linguistics and Phonetics* 3, 347-358.

Kent, R.D., Kent, J.F., Weismer, G., Sufit, R., Rosenbek, J.C., Martin, R.E., Brooks, B.R. (1990). "Impairment of speech intelligibility in men with amyotrophic lateral sclerosis." *Journal of Speech and Hearing Disorders*, 55, 721-728.

Kent, R.D., Moll, K.L. 1972. "Tongue body articulation during vowel and diphthong gestures." *Folia Phoniatrica* 24, 278-300.

Kent, R.D., Netsell, R. 1978. "Articulatory abnormalities in athetoid cerebral palsy." *Journal of Speech and Hearing Disorders* 43, 353-373.

Kent, R.D., Netsell, R., Abbs, J.W. 1979. "Acoustic characteristics of dysarthria associated with cerebellar disease." *Journal of Speech and Hearing Research* 22, 627-648.

Kent, R.D., Netsell, R., & Bauer, L.L. 1975. "Cineradiographic assessment of articulatory mobility in the dysarthrias." *Journal of Speech and Hearing Disorders* 40, 467-480.

Kent, R.D., Rosenbek, J.C. 1982. "Prosodic disturbances and neurologic lesion." *Brain and Language* 15, 259-291.

Kent, R.D., Weismer, G., Kent, J.F., & Rosenbek, J.C. 1989. "Toward explanatory intelligibility testing in dysarthria." *Journal of Speech and Hearing Disorders* 54, 482-499.

Kewley-Port, D. 1983. "Time-varying features as correlates of place of articulation in stop consonants." *Journal of the Acoustical Society of America* 73, 322-335.

Kewley-Port, D., & Luce, P.A. 1984. "Time-varying features of initial stop consonants in auditory running spectra: A first report." *Perception & Psychophysics* 35, 353-360.

Klatt, D.H. 1987. "Review of text-to-speech conversion in English." *Journal of the Acoustical Society of America* 82, 737-793.

Kreider, M.A. 1988. *The Effects of Context and Rate on the Intelligibility of the Conversational Speech of Moderately Disordered Speakers.* Unpublished M.S. thesis, University of Wisconsin-Madison.

Lehiste, I. 1965. "Some acoustic characteristics of dysarthric speech." *Bibliotheca Phonetica*, Fasc.2. Basel: Karger.

Lehiste, I., & Peterson, G.E. 1961. "Transitions, glides, and diphthongs." *Journal of the Acoustical Society of America* 33, 268-277.

Levitt,H., Stromberg, H. 1983. "Segmental characteristics of the speech of hearing-impaired children: Factors affecting intelligibility." *Speech of the Hearing-impaired: Research, Training and Personnel Preparation*, ed. by I. Hochberg, H. Levitt, M.J. Osberger, 53-73. Baltimore, MD: University Park.

Levitt, H., Stromberg, H., Smith, C.R., Gold, T. 1980. "The structure of segmental errors in the speech of deaf children." *Journal of Communication Disorders* 13, 419-442.

Licklider, J.C.R. 1951. "Basic correlates of the auditory stimulus." *Handbook of Experimental Psychology*, ed. by S.S. Stevens, 985-1039. New York: Wiley.

Liberman, A.M., Cooper, F.S., Shankweiler, D.P., Studdert-Kennedy, M. 1967. "Perception of the speech code." *Psychological Review* 74, 431-461.

Liss, J.M., Weismer, G., Rosenbek, J.C. (1990). "Selected acoustic characteristics of speech production in very old males." *Journal of Gerontology: Psychological Sciences*, 45, 35-45.

114   GARY WEISMER AND RUTH E. MARTIN

Löfqvist, A. 1980. "Interarticulator programming in stop production." *Journal of Phonetics* 8, 475-490.
Logemann, J.A., Fisher, H.B. 1978. "Vocal tract control in Parkinson's disease: Phonetic feature analysis of misarticulation." *Journal of Speech and Hearing Disorders* 46, 348-352.
Ludlow, C.L., Bassich, C.J. 1984. "The results of acoustic and perceptual assessments of two types of dysarthria." *Clinical Dysarthria*, ed. by W.R. Berry, 121-154. San Diego: College-Hill Press.
Ludlow, C.L., Connor, N.P., & Bassich, C.J. 1987. "Speech timing in Parkinson's and Huntington's disease." *Brain and Language* 32, 195-214.
Maassen, B. 1986. "Marking word boundaries to improve the intelligibility of the speech of the deaf." *Journal of Speech and Hearing Research* 29, 227-230.
Maassen, B., Povel, D. J. 1984a. "The effect of correcting temporal structure on the intelligibility of deaf speech." *Speech Communication* 3, 123-1350.
———. 1984b. "The effect of correcting fundamental frequency on the intelligibility of deaf speech and its interaction with temporal aspects." *Journal of the Acoustical Society of America* 76, 1673-1681.
———. 1985. "The effect of segmental and suprasegmental corrections on the intelligibility of deaf speech." *Journal of the Acoustical Society of America* 78, 877-886.
Macken, M.A., & Barton, D. 1977. "A longitudinal study of the acquisition of the voicing contrast in American-English word-initial stops, as measured by voice-onset time." *Journal of Child Language* 7, 41-74.
Marcus, S.M. 1984. "Recognizing speech: On the mapping from sound to word." *Attention and Performance X*, ed. by H. Bauma & D.G. Bouwhuis, 151-163. London: Lawrence Erlbaum.
Markides, A. 1970. "The speech of deaf and partially-hearing children with special reference to factors affecting intelligibility." *British Journal of Disorders of Communication* 5, 126-140.
Marslen-Wilson, W.D. 1975. "Sentence perception as an interactive parallel process." *Science* 189, 226-228.
———. 1980. "Speech understanding as a psychological process." *Spoken Language Generation and Understanding. Proceedings of the NATO Advanced Study Institute*, ed. by J.C. Simon, 39-67. Dordrecht, Holland: D. Reidel.
———. 1987. "Parallel processing in spoken word recognition." *Cognition* 25, 71-102.
Martin, J.G. 1975. "Rhythmic expectancy in continuous speech perception." *Structure and Process in Speech Perception*, ed. by A. Cohen and S.G. Nooteboom, 161-176. New York: Springer Verlag.
McGarr, N.S., & Osberger, M.J. 1978. "Pitch deviancy and intelligibility." *Journal of Communication Disorders* 11, 237-248.
Metz, D.E., Samar, V.J., Schiavetti, N., Sitler, R.W., & Whitehead, R.L. 1985. "Acoustic dimensions of hearing-impaired speakers' intelligibility." *Journal of Speech and Hearing Research* 28, 345-355.
Miller, 1981. "Effects of speaking rate on segmental distinctions." *Perspectives on the Study of Speech*, ed. by P.D. Eimas and J.L. Miller, 39-74. Hillsdale, New Jersey: Lawrence Erlbaum.

Miller, G.A., Nicely, P.E. 1955. "An analysis of perceptual confusions among some English consonants." *Journal of the Acoustical Society of America* 27, 338-352.

Monsen, R.B. 1974. "Durational aspects of vowel production in the speech of deaf children." *Journal of Speech and Hearing Research* 17, 386-398.

————. 1976a. "Normal and reduced phonological space: The production of English vowels by deaf adolescents." *Journal of Phonetics* 4, 189-198.

————. 1976b. "Second formant transitions of selected consonant-vowel combinations in the speech of deaf and normal-hearing children." *Journal of Speech and Hearing Research* 19, 267-278.

————. 1978. "Toward measuring how well hearing-impaired children speak." *Journal of Speech and Hearing Research* 21, 197-219.

Nash, R. 1972. "Phonemic and prosodic interference and intelligibility." *Proceedings of the Seventh International Congress of Phonetic Sciences*, ed. by A. Rigault and R. Charbonneau, 570-573. Paris: The Hague.

Netsell, R. 1969. "Evaluation of velopharyngeal function in dysarthria." *Journal of Speech and Hearing Disorders* 34, 113-122.

Nickerson, R.S., Stevens, K.N. 1980. "Approaches to the study of the relationship between intelligibility and physical properties of speech. *Speech Assessment and Improvement for the Hearing-Impaired*, ed. by J. Subtelny, 338-364. Washington, DC: A.G. Bell Assoc. for the Deaf.

Nooteboom, S.G., Brokx, J.P.L., & de Rooij, J.J. 1978. "Contributions of prosody to speech perception." *Studies in the Perception of Language*, ed. by W.J.M. Levelt and G.B. Flores d'Arcais, 75-107. New York: John Wiley.

Nooteboom, S.G., & van der Vlugt, M.J. 1988. "A search for a word-beginning superiority effect." *Journal of the Acoustical Society of America* 84, 2018-2032.

Nusbaum, H.C., & Pisoni, D.B. 1985. "Constraints on the perception of synthetic speech generated by rule." *Behavior Research Methods, Instruments, and Computers* 17, 235-242.

Ohde, R.N., Sharf, D.J. 1987. "Effect of formant transition rate on the differentiation of synthesized child and adult /w/ and /r/ sounds." *Journal of Speech and Hearing Research* 30, 215-222

Öhman, S.E.G. 1966. "Coarticulation in VCV utterances: Spectrographic measures." *Journal of the Acoustical Society of America* 39, 151-168.

Osberger, M.J., Levitt, H. 1979. "The effect of timing errors on the intelligibility of deaf children's speech." *Journal of the Acoustical Society of America* 66, 1316-1324.

Osberger, M.J., McGarr, N.S. 1982. "Speech production characteristics of the hearing-impaired." *Speech and Language: Advances in Basic Research and Practice* 18, 221-283.

Parkhurst, B.G., Levitt, H. 1978. "The effect of selected prosodic errors on the intelligibility of deaf speech." *Journal of Communication Disorders* 11, 249-256.

Perkell, J.S. 1969. *Physiology of Speech Production: Results and Implications of a Quantitative Study*. Cambridge: M.I.T. Press.

Pisoni, D.B., & Luce, P.A. 1986. "Speech perception: Research, theory and the principal issues." *Pattern Recognition by Humans and Machines: Speech Perception*, ed. by E.C. Schwab & H.C. Nusbaum, 1.1-50. New York: Academic Press.

Platt, L.J., Andrews, G., Young, M., Neilson, P.T. 1978. "The measurement of speech impairment of adults with cerebral palsy." *Folia Phonetica* 30, 50-58.
Platt, L.J., Andrews, G., Young, M., Quinn, P.T. 1980. "Dysarthria of adult cerebral palsy: I. Intelligibility and articulatory impairment." *Journal of Speech and Hearing Research* 23, 28-40.
Pollock, I., Pickett, J.M. 1963. "The intelligibility of excerpts from conversation." *Language and Speech* 6, 151-171.
Repp, B.H. 1979. "Relative amplitude of aspiration noise as a voicing cue for syllable-initial stop consonants." *Language and Speech* 22, 173-189.
———. 1982. "Phonetic trading relations and context effects: New experimental evidence for a speech mode of perception." *Psychological Bulletin* 92, 81-110.
Rose, P. 1987. "Considerations in the normalization of the fundamental frequency of linguistic tone." *Speech Communication* 6, 343-351.
Schiavetti, N., Metz, D.E., Sitler, R. 1981. "Construct validity of direct magnitude estimation and interval scaling of speech intelligibility: Evidence from a study of the hearing impaired." *Journal of Speech and Hearing Research* 24, 441-445.
Shinn, P., Blumstein, S.E. 1983. "Phonetic disintegration in aphasia: Acoustic analysis of spectral characteristics for place of articulation." *Brain and Language* 20, 90-114.
Slowiaczek, L.M., & Nusbaum, H.C. 1985. "Effects of speech rate and pitch contour on the perception of synthetic speech." *Human Factors* 27, 701-712.
Smith, C.R. 1975. "Residual hearing and speech production in deaf children." *Journal of Speech and Hearing Research* 18, 795-811.
Southwood, M.H. 1990. *A Term by Any Other Name: Bizarreness, Acceptability, Naturalness and Normalcy Judgements of the Speech of Speakers with Amyotrophic Lateral Sclerosis.* Unpublished doctoral dissertation, University of Wisconsin-Madison, Madison, WI.
Stevens, K.N., Blumstein, S.E. 1978. Invariant cues for place of articulation in stop consonants. *Journal of the Acoustical Society of America* 64, 1358-1368.
Stevens, K.N., Nickerson, R.S., & Rollins, A.M. 1983. "Suprasegmental and postural aspects of speech production and their effect on articulatory skills and intelligibility." *Speech of the Hearing-Impaired: Research, Training and Personnel Preparation*, ed. by I. Hochberg, H. Levitt & M.J. Osberger, 35-51. Baltimore, MD: University Park Press.
Syrdal, A.K., Gopal, H.S. 1986. "A perceptual model of vowel recognition based on the auditory representation of American English vowels." *Journal of the Acoustical Society of America* 79, 1086-1100.
Tikofsky, R.S. 1970. "A revised list for the estimation of dysarthric single word intelligibility." *Journal of Speech and Hearing Research* 13, 59-64.
Tikofsky, R.S., & Tikofsky, R.P. 1964. "Intelligibility measures of dysarthric speech." *Journal of Speech and Hearing Research* 7, 325-333.
Weismer, G. 1980. "Control of the voicing distinction for intervocalic stops and fricatives: Some data and theoretical considerations." *Journal of Phonetics* 8, 427-438.
———. 1984a. "Articulatory characteristics of Parkinsonian dysarthria." *The Dysarthrias: Physiology-acoustics-perception-management*, ed. by M.R. McNeil, J.C. Rosenbek, and A.E. Aronson, 101-130. San Diego: College-Hill.

———. 1984b. "Acoustic descriptions of dysarthric speech: Perceptual correlates and physiological inferences." *Seminars in Speech and Language*, ed. by J.C. Rosenbek. New York: Thieme-Stratton.

———. 1984c. "Acoustic analysis strategies for the refinement of phonological analyses." *Phonological Theory and the Misarticulating Child. ASHA Monographs* ed. by M. Elbert, D.A. Dinnsen & G. Weismer, 22.30-52.

Weismer, G., Cariski, D. 1984. "On speakers' abilities to control speech mechanism output: Theoretical and clinical implications." *Speech and Language: Advances in Basic Research and Practice*, 10, 185-241. ed. by N.J. Lass. New York: Academic Press.

Weismer, G., & Forrest, K. 1988. Acoustic characteristics of dysarthria associated with cerebral palsy. Paper presented at the annual convention of the American Speech-Language-Hearing Association, Boston, MA.

Weismer, G., & Fromm, D. 1983. "Acoustic analysis of geriatric utterances: Segmental and non-segmental characteristics which relate to laryngeal function." *Vocal Fold Physiology: Contemporary Research and Clinical Issues*, ed. by D.M. Bless and J.H. Abbs, 317-332. San Diego: College-Hill Press.

Weismer, G., Kent, R.D., Hodge, M., & Martin, R. 1988. "The acoustic signature for intelligibility test words." *Journal of the Acoustical Society of America* 84, 1281-1291.

Weismer, G., Kimelman, M.D.Z., & Gorman, S. 1985. "More on the speech production deficit associated with Parkinson's disease." *Journal of the Acoustical Society of America* 78(Suppl.1)S55.

Weismer, G., Liss, J.M. 1990. Acoustic/perceptual taxonomies of speech production deficits in motor speech disorders. Paper presented at the 5th Clinical Dysarthria Conference, San Antonio, TX.

Weismer, G., Liss, J.M. (in press). "Age and speech motor control." To appear in *Handbook of Aging and Communication*, ed. by D. Ripich. San Diego: College-Hill Press.

Weismer, G., Mulligan, M., & DePaul, R. 1986. "Selected acoustic characteristics of the dysarthria associated with amyotrophic lateral sclerosis." Paper presented at the 3rd Clinical Dysarthria Conference, Tucson, AZ.

Whitehead, R.L. 1986. "Consonantal influences on vowel duration as a function of speech intelligibility for hearing-impaired individuals." *Journal of the Acoustical Society of America* 79, 2084-2088.

Winitz, H., LaRiviere, C., & Herriman, E. 1975. "Variations in VOT for English initial stops." *Journal of Phonetics* 3, 41-52.

Wood, K.S. 1949. "Measures of progress in the correction of articulatory speech deficits." *Journal of Speech and Hearing Disorders* 14, 171-174.

Yorkston, K.M., & Beukleman, D.R. 1978. "A comparison of techniques for measuring intelligibility of dysarthric speech." *Journal of Communication Disorders* 11, 499-512.

———. 1981a. *Assessment of Intelligibility of Dysarthric Speech*. Tigard, Or: C.C. Publications.

———. 1981b. "Communication efficiency of dysarthric speakers as measured by sentence intelligibility and speaking rate." *Journal of Speech and Hearing Disorders* 46, 296-300.

Ziegler, W., & von Cramon, D.R. 1983a. "Vowel distortion in traumatic dysarthria."
   Phonetica 40, 63-78.
———. 1983b. "Vowel distortion in traumatic dysarthria: Lip rounding versus tongue
   advancement." *Phonetica* 40, 312-322.
———. 1986. "Spastic dysarthria after acquired brain damage: an acoustic study."
   British Journal of Disorders of Communication 21, 173-187.
Ziegler, W., Hartmann, E., & von Cramon, D. 1988. "Word identification testing in the
   diagnostic evaluation of dysarthric speech." *Clinical Linguistics and Phonetics* 2.291-
   308.

Chapter 4

The role of phonation in speech intelligibility:
A review and preliminary data from patients with Parkinson's disease

Lorraine Olson Ramig, Ph.D., CCC-SP
University of Colorado

Introduction

The role of phonation in the production of intelligible speech should be considered at various levels. The larynx should be studied for its role, in combination with the respiratory system, as the aerodynamic and acoustic *source* for speech production, as a generator of *suprasegmental features*, and as an *articulator*. Source characteristics of loudness and quality are dependent upon the respiratory system and vocal fold adductory and oscillatory systems. Suprasegmental features of pitch and prosody are dependent upon simultaneous modulations of source and articulatory characteristics. Laryngeal articulatory characteristics are dependent upon adductory gestures coordinated with sub- and supraglottal events to achieve segmental contrasts.

The vocal folds valve the respiratory air flow to generate the acoustic voice source. If vocal fold adduction (medial compression) or subglottal air pressure are insufficient, vocal loudness or intensity may be significantly reduced or intraoral air pressure may be inadequate for supraglottal valving. If the oscillations of the vocal folds are irregular or occur inconsistently, the voice source may be transient and voice quality may sound disordered. Respiratory, laryngeal and articulatory function must be coordinated to generate appropriate suprasegmental variations in pitch, loudness, duration and quality; disturbances of any of these variables may alter utterance meaning. If vocal fold adductory/abductory activity is inadequate, or not coordinated with sub and supraglottal events, the voice/voiceless articulatory contrast may be disturbed. All of these phonatory disruptions have the potential to reduce speech intelligibility.

A number of studies have reported a relationship between these phonatory disruptions and speech intelligibility (e.g. McGarr and Osberger, 1977; Parkhurst and Levitt, 1978; Monsen, 1983). The suprasegmental and laryngeal articulatory variables of pitch, prosody and voicing distinctions, together with their acoustic correlates, have been studied in individuals with hearing impairment, alaryngeal voice and motor speech disorders, and have been related to reductions in intelligibility in those populations (e.g., McGarr and Osberger, 1978; Yorkston and Beukelman, 1981). However, it is the relationship between segmental variables and speech intelligibility that has been given the greatest attention in the literature (e.g., Tikofsky, 1970; Tikofsky and Tikofsky, 1964; Darley, Aronson and Brown, 1969 a,b; Smith, 1972; Yorkston and Beukelman, 1981; Weismer, Kent, Hodge and Martin, 1988; Samar and Metz, 1988; Freyman and Nerbonne, 1989). In fact, one comes away from a review of the disordered speech literature with the impression that the role of phonatory characteristics in intelligible speech production is relatively limited when compared with segmental contributions. Freyman and Nerbonne (1989) recently concluded that a significant percentage of the information contributing to the intelligibility of speech is conveyed by consonants. Carney (1986) concluded that of three "speaker-oriented" variables (segmental production, suprasegmental production and hearing loss), segmental production appeared to correlate most strongly with speech intelligibility. Lessac (1967) stated that it is consonants that make the spoken word intelligible.

A closer look at this research reveals that in most of the studies of disordered speech and intelligibility, the significant support roles of the laryngeal and respiratory systems as the aerodynamic and acoustic source for speech production have been simply assumed. Generally, intelligibility has been evaluated from samples with reasonable audibility, suggesting that an adequate source was used for speech production. Furthermore, in a number of cases, samples have been equated for audibility (Freyman and Nerbonne, 1989) and consonant identification has been the only task for the listener (e.g., Owens and Schubert, 1977; Resnick, Dubno, Hoffnung and Levitt, 1975). In certain cases, the origin of segmental breakdowns may in fact be source-related (inadequate intraoral air pressure for supraglottal valving; Pickett,1956; Arkebauer, Hixon and Hardy, 1967), yet the primary focus has been on the segmental manifestation. This issue has been addressed in part when Stevens, Nickerson and Rollins (1983) suggested the need to consider the contribution of the 'postural aspects' of speech production to intelligibility. They suggest that certain aspects of segmental and suprasegmental characteristics depend upon the overall posture that is assumed by the laryngeal and respiratory structures in preparation for speech production. For example, they point out that breathy voice quality or reduced amplitude between syllables, such as observed in speech of the deaf, result from vocal fold positioning, i.e., too wide a glottal opening or the insertion of glottal closure between syllables (Hudgins, 1937; Bernstein, Rollins and Stevens, 1978). Stevens et al. (1983) assume that posture includes not only some static state of readiness for speaking, but also the range over which the configurations or states of various structures are allowed to vary. It should be noted that a consistent reduction in intelligibility has been observed in speakers with clearly inadequate source characteristics such as severely limited respiratory support or vocal fold adduction (hypoadduction or hyperadduction) accompanying, for example, neurological disease or alaryngeal voice (Kalb and Carpenter, 1981; Simpson, Till and Goff, 1988).

The critical role of source characteristics in intelligible speech production is highlighted further when one reviews the literature on speech enhancement. Various acoustic characteristics have been studied when normal and disordered speakers have attempted to improve their intelligibility or when instrumental methods have been used to enhance the understandibility of speech (Tolhurst, 1957; Pichney, 1981; Pichney, Durlach and Briada, 1985; 1986; Spector, Subtelny, Whitehead and Wirz, 1979). Speech enhancement may occur after treatment (Till and Toye, 1988), when speech is produced with background noise (Lane and Tranel, 1971; Summers, Pisoni, Bernacki, Pedlow and Stokes, 1988; Sundberg, Ternstrom, Perkins and Gramming, 1988) or in a performance mode (Ternstrom and Sundberg 1986), or when instrumental procedures are used to modify a signal to enhance its understandability (Lim, Oppenheim and Braida, 1978; Allen, Strong and Palmer, 1981; Montgomery and Edge, 1988). The speech enhancement literature suggests that the laryngeal source characteristics of intensity and spectral balance are among the phonatory variables that are consistently modified when a speaker attempts to improve intelligibility.

The following section will review phonatory source, suprasegmental and articulatory contributions to speech intelligibility as presented in the hearing impaired, alaryngeal, motor disorders and speech enhancement literature.

The relationship between intelligibility and phonatory characteristics in disordered and enhanced speech

It is the literature on hearing-impaired and deaf speakers that has addressed most explicitly the relationship between characteristics of phonation and speech intelligibility (e.g. McGarr and Osberger, 1978). The other primary sources for data on this issue come from the literature on alaryngeal voice, motor speech disorders, and speech enhancement. It is difficult to find any association between speech intelligibility and phonation in the laryngeal-based voice disorders literature, although the professional/performing voice literature suggests various modifications in voice characteristics for improvement in intelligibility (Berry, 1973; Turner,1977).

Contributions of the SOURCE functions of the larynx to speech intelligibility

Loudness

The role of loudness in speech intelligibility has been well established. The early work of Draegert (1951), Moore (1946), Curtis (1946) and Pickett (1956) concluded that greater intelligibility accompanies speech signals of greater intensity or force. Pickett (1956) reported drastic deterioration of intelligibility with low and high extremes of vocal effort . As loudness is raised in any voice, there is increased energy in the high part of the spectrum (spectral tilt decreases), which has been associated with improvements in the clarity of speech (Ternstrom and Sundberg, 1986). One technique used by performers which enables them to be heard over loud background noise is the "singer's formant". Performers use vocal tract modifications to shape the source characteristics for increased intensity which results in a spectrum envelop peak near 3KHz (Sundberg, 1977; Cleveland and Sundberg, 1983; Sundberg and Ternstrom, 1986).

A number of disorders of phonation result in the inability to generate adequate loudness. Breakdowns occur for functional reasons (e.g., voice disorders in the hearing impaired and deaf) and organic causes (e.g., laryngeal removal or neurolaryngeal disorders). The underlying physiologic basis may be that these individuals cannot create a sufficient air pressure difference to generate an acoustic signal of adequate amplitude due to insufficient respiratory support or inadequate or excessive adduction (hypoadduction or hyperadduction). For example, Bernstein, Rollins and Stevens (1978) reported that the tendency of deaf speakers to insert glottal closure between syllables and words creates a reduction in sound amplitude between two syllables and thus causes reduced amplitude and reduced intelligibility. Levitt, Smith and Stromberg (1974) reported intermittent phonation resulting in spasmodic and excess variation in loudness which correlated with reduced intelligibility. Smith (1975) found that errors involving poor phonatory control (intermittent phonation, spasmodic variations of pitch and loudness, and excessive variability of intonation) were highly correlated with reductions in intelligibility.

Reduced loudness has been well documented in alaryngeal speakers using esophageal speech (e.g. Drummond, 1965; Hyman, 1955; Diedrich, 1968) and has been associated with reductions in speech intelligibility observed in that patient population (Kalb and Carpenter, 1981). Recently, the tracheoesophageal shunt procedure has allowed these patients to use respiratory air rather than esophageal air to power voice production. Data support consistent increases in intensity as well as intelligibility with the use of this shunt (Robbins, 1984; Robbins, Fisher, Blom and Singer, 1984; Tardy-Mitzell, Andrews and Bowman, 1985; Pinzola and Cain, 1988; Doyle, Danhauer and Reed, 1988). These findings can be interpreted as support for the importance of the aerodynamic source in the intelligibility of tracheoesophageal voice production.

Reports indicate that reduced loudness is a deterrent to oral communication in patients with motor speech disorders (e.g. Rosenbek and LaPointe, 1985; Aronson, 1985; Simpson, Till and Goff, 1988). Respiratory as well as laryngeal adductory insufficiencies have been suggested as physiologic bases for these loudness reductions (Simpson, Till and Goff, 1988). For example, reduced intensity, monoloudness, weak overall effort and reduced intraoral pressures have been reported in parkinsonian speech (Canter, 1963, 1965; Mueller, 1971; Kent and Rosenbek, 1982; Ludlow and Bassich, 1983). Therapy techniques have focused on improving oral communication by enhancing respiratory support for speech and vocal fold adduction (Rosenbek and LaPointe, 1985; Ramig, Fazoli, Scherer and Bonitati, 1990). In addition, amplification systems are frequently recommended for motor disordered patients with significantly reduced loudness (Greene and Watson, 1968; Rubow and Strand, 1985) and have been associated with increases in intelligibility.

Increases in loudness or intensity are frequently reported when speakers attempt to improve their intelligibility in the presence of background noise (Hanley and Steer, 1949; Draegert, 1951; Tolhurst, 1954; 1955; Lane et al, 1970; Summers, Pisoni, Bernacki, Pedlow and Stokes,1988; Sundberg, Ternstrom, Perkins and Gramming, 1988), when asked to speak more clearly (Pichney, Durlach and Braida, 1986) when asked to stress or emphasize (Lieberman,1960; Klatt,1975; Cooper, Eady and Mueller,1985), or when asked to speak in low-redundancy contexts (Hunnicutt, 1985; 1987). For example, Garber, Siegel and Pick (1980) reported that in low-pass filtering conditions, subjects increased their intelligibility by increasing their vocal intensity rather than by any articulatory changes. Summers et al. (1988) reported that speakers modify both the prosodic and segmental acoustic-phonetic properties of their speech when they talk in noise. They speak louder and slower, raise pitch and introduce changes in the short-term power spectrum of voiced segments. Similar changes have been measured when subjects have been asked to stress or speak clearly. For example, Pichney, Durlach and Braida (1986) noted substantial differences (5-6 dB) in intensities of stop consonants and higher fundamental frequency values in acoustic analyses of "clear" versus conversational speech. In shouted speech, increases in fundamental frequency, vowel duration, the frequency of format one and a reduction in spectral tilt have been reported (Rostolland and Parant, 1974; Rostolland, 1982 a,b). However, because the magnitude of these changes is much greater in shouted speech and extreme articulations accompany shouting, speech is less intelligible. Thus, Rostolland (1982 a,b) concluded that clear speech cannot be obtained by merely boosting one's overall vocal output.

One classic feature associated with increased intelligibility in instrumental speech enhancement is the consonant to vowel (C/V) ratio, that is the ratio of the power of a consonant to that of the nearest vowel in the same syllable (Hecker, 1974; House, Williams, Hecker and Kryter, 1965; Montogomery and Edge,1988). For example, Hecker (1974) increased the C/V ratio of a low intelligibility talker and produced a 3.75% improvement in intelligibility. Ono, Okasaki, Nakai and Harasaki (1982) and Montogomery and Edge (1988) using hearing impaired listeners and Gordon-Salant (1986; 1987) with both normal and hearing impaired listeners reported improvements in intelligibility for monosyllables as a result of increases in C/V ratio. When Montogomery and Edge(1988) increased consonant intensity while holding the vowel constant at low presentation levels, they found that increasing amplitude produced significant improvements in intelligibility over unprocessed speech. He concluded that the 10% to 12% improvement produced by manipulating consonant amplitude was a demonstration of the influence that even modest increases in consonant intensity can exert on intelligibility and the importance of the C/V ratio in speech recognition. Recently, Freyman and Nerbonne (1989) reported that the degree to which variations in speech intelligibility could be explained by variations in C/V ratio was found to be quite different for different consonants. For example, for /s/, /ʃ/(sh), /tʃ/(ch)/ the C/V ratio accounted for a great deal of the variation in intelligibility; for voiceless stops, this was not the case. They suggested that this difference may be due to "the relative inaudibility of stops when speech-to-noise ratios are poor" (p.32) and support the recommendation by Turner and Robb (1987) that the audibility of consonants should be considered when analyzing speech recognition data. They concluded that when stimuli are calibrated according to vowel intensity, there is no evidence that the ratio between consonant and vowels is important for intelligibility.

In summary, it appears that generation of an adequate acoustic and aerodynamic source is a critical factor in intelligible speech production. Without sufficient vocal loudness or aerodynamic pressures, supraglottal valving for segmental production would be limited and intelligibility reduced.

Quality

Voice quality has been reported to be a source of information about physical, psychological and social characteristics of the speaker as well as playing a "vital semiotic role" in spoken interaction (Laver, 1968; Laver and Trudgill, 1979). Kohler and Dommelen (1987) suggested that the different overall human voice qualities "tense", "neutral" and "modal" may have prosodic effects on sound perception. Pittam (1987) reported that the voice qualities of "breathy", "creaky", nasal", "tense" and "whispery" all have been reported to function communicatively (Addington, 1968; Esling, 1978; Laver, 1980; Trudgill, 1974; Scherer, 1979).

Various approaches have been used to study vocal quality acoustically and perceptually. Numerous attempts have been made to relate qualities such as "hoarseness" and "harshness" to various short-term (cycle-to-cycle)

(Scherer et al, 1988) acoustic measures including jitter, shimmer and harmonics-to-noise ratio (e.g. Deal and Emanuel, 1978; Takahashi and Koike,
1975; Yumoto, Gould and Baer, 1982). In contrast, Laver (1980) and
Laver, Wirz, Mackenzie and Hiller (1981) applied principles of phonetic
analysis to vocal quality (similar to the concept of an articulatory setting)
and suggested that the vocal tract adopts long-term muscular adjustments
that underlie and act as contraints on short-term articulations. This idea
appears compatible with the 'postural aspects' concept of Stevens et al
(1983) discussed earlier. Based upon Laver's suggestion, Pittman (1987a,b)
emphasized that voice quality is a long-term phenomenon, present all the
time a person is talking and therefore should be studied as such with
techniques such as long-term spectral analysis. He used long-term spectral
analysis to discriminate among the voice qualities 'breathy', 'creaky',
'tense' and 'whispery'.

Disorders of voice quality have been reported in deaf and hard of hearing individuals. Spector, Subtelny, Whitehead and Wirz (1979) reported
that eleven percent of deaf individuals had voices that were harsh and
excessively tense. They associated this tension with an abrupt initiation of
voicing, faulty modulation of the air stream for consonant production and/
or inefficient control of air expenditure and suggested that these characteristics may adversely affect vocal pitch, pitch control, loudness and speech
intelligibility. McGarr and Osberger(1978) reported that children who
could not sustain phonation and whose speech contained numerous pitch
breaks were judged to have unintelligible speech. McGarr and Osberger
(1978) concluded that there is a relationship between poor phonatory control, on the one hand, and hearing level and intelligibility, on the other.
Monsen (1983) states that in the deaf, voice quality and speech intelligibility are intricately intertwined; with the relationship between voice quality
and intelligibility in the deaf being quite high.

When voice quality disorders are less severe, the effect on intelligibility
may be reduced. Samar and Metz (1988) reported that breathiness did not
degrade the message intelligibility of speech produced by hearing impaired
speakers under normal listening conditions. They interpreted this to be
related to a write down procedure of intelligibility assessment in which listeners report their linguistic perceptual experience, regardless of their perceptions of vocal aberrations such as breathiness. Monsen (1983) says rarely
is the voice quality of a normal hearing speaker deviant enough to impair
intelligibility under good listening conditions; he suggests that in a normal

hearing talker, peculiar voice quality may be considered apart from how well he is understood.

Disordered voice quality has been associated with reduced intelligibility and acceptability in alaryngeal speakers. Doyle, Danhauer and Reed (1988) associated low intelligibility in an esophageal speaker with rough voice quality. Niebor, Graaf and Schutte (1988) concluded that the quality of voice was better for patients with the tracheoesophageal puncture than esophageal speech. This improvement in quality has been associated with the addition of pulmonary air which improves listeners' perception of smoothness and acceptability (Pindzola and Cain, 1988). Relaxation of the pharyngoesophageal segment (pseudoglottis) by a myotomy has been associated with improved voice quality in tracheoesophageal speakers (Singer and Blom, 1981; Chodosh, Giancarlo and Goldstein, 1984). Weinberg and Bennett (1973) concluded that because of its more normal voice quality, the Toyko larynx was more "acceptable" than superior esophageal speech, Western Electric Reed and the Bell Electrolarynx.

Disordered voice quality has been reported in speakers with motor speech disorders such as flaccid dysarthria, pseudobulbar palsy and hypokinetic (Parkinsonian) dysarthria (Aronson, 1985). Breathiness, hoarseness, harshness, strained-strangled voice, wet and gurgly quality and tremor have been reported in these populations (Aronson, 1985; Boone and McFarland, 1988). Despite the clinical impression that these disordered qualities reduce speech intelligibility, this relationship has not been experimentally documented.

Disordered voice quality has been a focus of treatment techniques in the areas of deaf speech and motor speech disorders as well as the disordered voice literature. However, only in the area of deaf speech has an attempt been made to relate treatment related changes in voice quality to speech intelligibility. Spector et al. (1979) developed a program to reduce harsh/tense voice quality in adult deaf speakers. Perceptual judgments of pre- and post-training recordings revealed significant improvements in vocal tension, pitch register, pitch control, articulation and speech intelligibility. Boone and McFarland (1988) suggested that voice therapy can often improve the intelligibility of dysarthric speakers and various techniques for modification of disordered vocal quality in dysarthric speakers have been reviewed by Prater and Swift (1984) and Ramig and Scherer (1989). However it appears that few of these techniques have been studied explicitly for their effect on speech intelligibility.

In summary, it appears that vocal quality disorders reflecting a clear breakdown in phonatory source adequacy (such as excessive hypoadduction or hyperadduction) may have detrimental effects on speech intelligibility, such as the inability to produce voicing. The relationship between less severe disorders of voice quality and speech intelligibility is unclear at this time.

Contributions of SUPRASEGMENTAL *functions of the larynx to speech intelligibility*

Pitch

Vocal pitch has been defined as the perceptual correlate of the vibratory frequency of the vocal folds and has been studied perceptually and acoustically (fundamental frequency) in many populations. The relationship between pitch and speech intelligibility has been addressed primarily in the deaf and hard of hearing literature.

The overall pitch of the deaf and hard of hearing has been reported to be deviant (Green, 1956; Angelocci, Kopp and Holbrook, 1964; Martony, 1968; Bush, 1979; McGarr, Youdelman and Head, unpublished). Youdelman, MacEachron and McGarr (1989) report that inappropriate average pitch may sound unnatural and detract from the speaker's message and give conflicting cues about age and gender. Stevens et al (1983) suggested that improper adjustment of vocal fold posture can also result in a fundamental frequency contour that is overly sensitive to tongue position.

Monsen (1978), McGarr and Osberger (1978) and Samar and Metz (1988) conclude that there is no simple relationship between mean fundamental frequency and intelligibility in the deaf and hard of hearing. Sudden breaks in voicing and other evidences of inadequate control of phonation appear to be more highly correlated with poor intelligibility than inappropriate average pitch levels (McGarr, 1977; Levitt, et al., 1974).

The pitch of voice in esophageal speakers has been reported to be low (Weinberg and Bennett, 1972). Niebor et al. (1988) reported that the pitch of esophageal speakers plays an important role in assessment of voice quality. Shipp (1967) reported that one factor related to higher speech acceptability ratings was relatively higher mean fundamental frequency. The work of Robbins, et al. (1984a,b) suggested different fundamental frequencies for esophageal and tracheoesophageal speakers but did not address the relationship between fundamental frequency and intelligibility in these populations.

While disordered pitch has been reported in speakers with motor speech disorders (Aronson, 1985), its relationship with speech intelligibility in these populations has not been studied. For example, the pitch (fundamental frequency) of voices of patients with Parkinson's disease has been reported to be both excessively low (Darley, Aronson and Brown, 1975) and excessively high (Canter, 1963; Kammermeier,1969), but has not been identified as a factor which effects the intelligibility of these speakers.

Modification of pitch has been one goal of voice therapy throughout the years (Boone and McFarland, 1988). However, therapy-related pitch change has been associated with improvements in overall communication effectiveness rather than speech intelligibility. In relationship to speech enhancement, Pichnney, et al. (1986) found that a wider range of fundamental frequency is used in clear speech, with a slight bias toward higher fundamental frequencies.

In summary, it appears that the relationship between pitch or average speaking fundamental frequency and a speaker's intelligibility is unestablished at this time. The potentially distracting influence of a disordered pitch may be a contributing factor to intelligibility reductions.

Prosody-(stress and intonation)

Communicative functions of speech prosody include conveying emotional tone (e.g., Scherer, 1986), conveying linguistic distinctions (e.g., Cooper and Sorenson, 1981), signaling meaning (Yorkston, 1988), and assigning stress (e.g., Cooper, Eady and Mueller,1985). Price and Levitt (1983) suggest that listeners may use suprasegmental information to assign an initial syntactic structure before decoding the rest of the information. Weismer (1990) has recently suggested that if this prosodic information is deviant, it may affect the listener's strategy for decoding the message. Kent (1988) suggests the following "vocal control prerequisites" for prosody: loudness variation, adequate duration of phonation, appropriate pitch level, pitch variation and acceptable voice quality.

Prosodic disorders have been frequently reported in speech of the hard of hearing and deaf and related to reductions in speech intelligibility. Metz, Samar, Schiavetti, Sitler and Whitehead (1985) have suggested independent and primary roles for segmental and prosodic speech characteristics in determining intelligibility in severely to profoundly hearing impaired speakers; this has been supported by Parkhurst and Levitt (1978) and Stromberg and Levitt (1979). Stark and Levitt (1974), Gold (1975) and McGarr (1976) have shown that deaf children have difficulty in producing such features as stress, pausal juncture, and intonation. Flat monotonous speech, lacking in pitch contours has been reported in deaf speakers (Haycock,1933; Greene,1956; Hood,1966; Monsen, 1979). They suggest that the effect of these errors on speech intelligibility is significant. For example, if the speakers' voice is at the top of the frequency range, there are limitations for increases in pitch to indicate stress or to produce the rise in pitch required for some question forms (McGarr, Youldeman, Head, unpublished). Levitt, Smith and Stromberg (1974) reported that children with the same frequency of segmental errors had speech intelligibility scores differing by as much as 30%. Parkhurst and Levitt (1978) reported that excessive variations in pitch may reduce intelligibility. Breaks in pitch was one of the prosodic errors they reported to show a significant negative regression with intelligibility. McGarr and Osberger (1978) report that a grossly deviant pitch pattern may be sufficiently distracting in a communication situation to have indirect effects on intelligibility.

Prosodic features have been studied in alaryngeal speakers. Intonational contrast to signal phrase intent (Gandour and Weinberg, 1983), juncture in distinguishing ambiguous word pairs (Scarpino and Weinberg, 1981) and lexical stress to distinguish noun verb pairs (Gandour, Weinberg and Garzone, 1983) have been reported as normal or near normal in esophageal speakers. McHenry, Reich and Minifie (1982) reported that while the primary syllable stress to emphasize one word in a sentence was not within normal limits in esophageal speakers, it was high. Doyle, Danhauer and Reed (1988) and Pindzola and Cain (1988) report that the increased pulmonary support in tracheoesophageal speakers allows their prosodic feature production and intonation to closely resemble normal talkers (Robbins, 1984; Robbins et al., 1984; Shipp, 1967; Williams and Watson,1985). Weinberg (1986) reports that tracheoesophageal speakers could control fundamental frequency, duration, and intensity to mark suprasegmental (contrastive stress, intonation) contrasts. While these findings support near normal prosodic characteristics in esophageal and tracheoesophageal speakers, the relationship between these characteristics and speech intelligibility has not been investigated.

Breakdowns in prosodic characteristics have been reported in individuals with a variety of neurological disorders and have been associated with reductions in speech intelligibility (Ansel, 1987). Right brain damaged patients exhibit a disturbance of emotional and linguistic prosody (Shapiro and Danly, 1985). Left brain damaged patients demonstrate aprosodia (Ross, Anderson and Morgan-Fisher, 1989), involvement in the control of lexical and syntactic prosody (Behrens, 1985) and linguistic use of prosody in tones (Gandour and Dararananda, 1983). Ryalls (1986) and Ryalls, Joanette and Feldman (1987) suggest a whole brain basis for prosody and Kloude, Robin, Graff-Radford, Cooper (1988) observed prosodic impairment following callosal damage. Problems with prosody also have been observed to accompany Broca's aphasia (Danly and Shapiro, 1982), cerebellar ataxia (Kent and Rosenbek, 1982) and Parkinson's disease (Kent and Rosenbek, 1982; Blonder, Gur and Gur, 1989). Voices of Parkinson and ataxic patients have been described as having reduced pitch variability and monoloudness (Canter, 1963;1965; Kent and Rosenbek, 1982).

Prosody has often been a focus of treatment with motor disordered patients (Yorkston, Beukelman, Minifie and Sapir, 1984) and has been associated with changes in intelligibility in these patients. Yorkston and Beukelman (1981) suggest that in cases where prosodic patterns are often markedly abnormal and contribute to bizarreness of dysarthric speakers, forcing marginally intelligible speakers into specific stress patterns tends to increase intelligibility and reduce bizarreness. In contrast, Boothroyd et al. (1975) and Nickerson, Kalikow and Stevens (1976) reported improvement in suprasegmentals (lower fundamental frequency, consistent fundamental frequency contours and reduced pauses) post-treatment in deaf and hard of hearing children without corresponding improvement in intelligibility. They conclude that improvement in suprasegmental attributes alone is not sufficient to result in an immediate gain in intelligibility, although it may be accompanied by improvement in the naturalness or overall quality of the speech.

Hunicutt (1985, 1987) studied the prosodic correlates of peak dB level of word pairs, their durations, fundamental frequency maximum, range, excursion and contour complexity for words in high-redundancy versus low-redundancy contexts. The correlation between any one of these factors and intelligibility was low, however the differences were in the expected direction. She concluded "If prosody indeed correlates with intelligibility, it correlates as a whole, being expressed in various combinations of higher intensity, longer durations and more lively fundamental frequency contour."

In summary, it appears that disordered prosody can effect speech intelligibility. This may occur because the listener does not receive sufficent information to decode the message or because the disordered prosody prevents the listener from using her typical decoding strategy. Improved prosody may suggest that the speaker is better able to coordinate laryngeal and sub- and supraglottal events to generate the necessary variations in loudness, duration, pitch and quality which contribute to improved intelligibility.

Contributions of ARTICULATORY *functions of the larynx to speech intelligibility*

The voice-voiceless contrast is the primary articulatory function of the larynx that has been studied in relation to speech intelligibility (Smith, 1975; Yorkston and Beukelman, 1988) although recently, the initial glottal versus null (/hat/ versus /at/) contrast has been considered (Kent, Weismer and Kim, 1990; Kent, Weismer, Kent and Rosenbek,1990). Both contrasts require coordination of laryngeal adductory/abductory events together with sub- and supraglottal events in order to generate sufficient acoustic cues for the perception of the phonetic target. Breakdowns in production of the voice-voiceless contrast have been observed in the deaf and hearing impaired as well as in alaryngeal and motor disordered speakers.

One common error in deaf speech is confusion of the voiced-voiceless distinction (Smith, 1975; Mc Garr and Osberger, 1978). Observations have included voiced for voiceless errors (Smith, 1975) as well as voiceless for voiced errors (Markides, 1970). Metz et al. (1985) reported cognate pair voice onset time differences and mean sentence duration strongly predicted speech intelligibility based on readings of isolated word and contextual speech material. Monsen (1978) found that three speech characteristics: the voice onset time difference between /t/ and /d/, the second formant difference between /i/ and /o/ and a rating of the spectrographic quality of liquids and nasals emerged as the best predictors of speech intelligibility. He pointed out that correct production of these few phonemes per se is not the source of intelligibility but rather that the presence of these features suggests that a given speaker has achieved a certain level of articulatory skill. For example, he suggests that the speaker is able to coordinate the timing of the release of the plosive burst at the lips with the onset of glottal pulsation and to vary that timing for different target phonemes. He suggests that the inability to control the temporal coordination of laryngeal and supralaryngeal events may be responsible for problems with phonemic contrasts.

Alaryngeal speakers' most frequent perceptual confusion is the voice/ voiceless contrast (Doyle and Danhauer, 1986); voiceless stops are often perceived as voiced. This has been related to the non-adductor/abductor nature of the postlaryngectomy voicing mechanism and the reduced air supply available to the esophageal speaker. Weinberg, Horii, Blom and Singer (1982) have hypothesized that the esophageal voicing source is optimized using the trachesesophageal shunt. Doyle and Danhauer (1986) and Gomyo and Doyle, (in press) reported that tracheoesophageal speakers achieved the production of "voicing" cues with greater effectiveness than esophageal speakers and suggested that the addition of pulmonary air supply may result in changes in VOT and vowel duration and the generation of high pressures and flows needed for fricatives and plosives and may be related to improved speech intelligibility. Robbins, Christensen and Kempster (1986) suggest also that trachesophageal speakers' ability to generate greater and more sustained air pressures and flows likely results in slower pharyngoesophageal segment vibratory decay in contrast to the rapid decay in esophageal speech. They suggest that changes in the initiation or delay of phonation onset-offset as well as other temporal aspects such as vowel duration may result in perceptually salient changes in the speech signal.

Problems with laryngeal articulatory functions have been reported in the motor disordered population as well. In cases with inadequate vocal fold adduction (hypoadduction), voiced phonemes may be perceived as voiceless. This has been observed in cases of vocal fold paralysis. In other cases, extended consonantal voicing or continuous voicing (continuation of vocal fold vibration into voiceless stop closures) has been observed in Parkinson patients (Weismer, 1984) and patients with spastic dysarthria (Freeman, Cannito and Finitzo-Hieber, 1985). Farmer (1980) found frequent voiced for voiceless substitutions and VOTs which were longer and more variable in spastic and athetoid cerebral palsy speakers. She suggests that one important factor underlying the poor intelligibility of cerebral palsy speakers is the distortion caused by increased word and interword durations. Yorkston and Beukelman (1988) reported that imprecise phonatory control may prevent certain speakers from producing the voice/ voiceless distinctions that are important in intelligibility. Kent et al. (1990a,b) reported voiced-voiceless (e.g., bat-pat) as well as glottal and null (e.g., hat-at) confusions in patients with Parkinson's disease as well as amyotrophic lateral sclerosis and associated this with reduced intelligibility in these patient populations.

Articulatory contrasts have been the focus of therapy designed to improve speech intelligibility. Yorkston and Beukelman (1988) suggest contrastive drills marking voiced-voiceless consonant distinctions for dysarthric patients to improve intelligibility. Till and Toye (1988) reported that patient subjects modified their VOTs after specfic feedback of a voice/voiceless intelligibility confusion and not after general feedback of communication failure. In relation to enhanced speech, Pichney, et al. (1986) reported that VOT for unvoiced plosives increased substantially in clear speech. Chen (1980) observed this also in speech spoken clearly and conversationally in a carrier phrase.

In summary, it appears that there is a relationship between the articulatory functions of the larynx and speech intelligibility. Successful generation of the voice-voiceless contrast may offer the listener additional information to decode speech accurately. In addition, it may reflect the speaker's higher level of coordination of laryngeal events with sub- and supraglottal events which facilitate increased intelligibility across the board.

Summary

A common theme in the literature related to disordered phonation and speech enhancement seems to be that the disruption or the enhancement of the *source* aspects of laryngeal sound production underlie major changes in speech intelligibility. Once a speaker achieves a threshold of "adequacy of phonatory source" both acoustically and aerodynamically, the contribution of *suprasegmental or articulatory phonatory* characteristics to speech intelligibility may exist, but be less significant. Future research should assess the contribution of laryngeal function to intelligible speech production in an hierarchical way so that "phonatory source adequacy" is studied together with laryngeal contributions on suprasegmental and articulatory levels. It is critical to study systematically phonatory source contributions to intelligibility of segmental productions. One initial approach would be to employ speech synthesis to study the effects on speech intelligibility when the laryngeal and respiratory source characteristics are systematically varied while articulatory configurations remain constant.

Kent (1988; 120) has stated that "Because intelligibility is the essential feature of speech communication, the assessment of intelligibility is an issue of fundamental clinical importance." The virtual absence of the concept of speech intelligibility in the voice disorders literature together with the

limited discussion of the contribution of phonatory characteristics to intelligibility in all but the deaf and hearing impaired literature suggests that the
role of phonation has not been sufficiently studied for its role in clinical
assessment of speech intelligibility. The vast majority of the disordered
voice literature relates characteristics of phonation not to reduced intelligibility but to reduced "effectiveness", "acceptability" (Shipp, 1967; Weinberg and Bennett, 1973; Pindzola and Cain, 1988) or increased "distraction" or negative perception (Moran, LaBarge and Haynes,1988; Ruscello,
Lass and Podbesek, 1988). Speech intelligibility has been defined as "the
degree to which the speaker's intended message is recovered by the listener" (Kent, Weismer, Kent and Rosenbek, 1989: 483). At present, the
contribution of phonatory characteristics to that recovery is not established.
While the deaf and hearing impaired literature has begun to document the
role of disordered phonation in speech intelligibility reductions, it is critical
that disordered phonation of all etiologies be assessed for their impact on
speech intelligibility. Such information would allow a common metric for
determining the impact of speech breakdowns on communication functioning across client populations and offer a unifying perspective for the study
of phonation and speech intelligibility. Improvement following voice
therapy should be assessed for its impact on speech intelligibility as well;
unless treatment can be shown to positively impact an individual's overall
intelligibility, its social validity may be in question (Kent, 1988).

The following study makes an initial attempt to integrate ratings of
speech intelligibility with acoustic, kinematic and perceptual data on vocal
function before and after voice therapy for patients with Parkinson's disease. The study investigates the relationships among perceptual ratings and
acoustic and kinematic measures of source and suprasegmental characteristics such as loudness, quality and intonation and measures of vocal fold
adduction and oscillatory steadiness in patients whose vocal fold adduction
improved after voice therapy. The relationships among these variables and
perceptual ratings are studied to gain insight into which, if any, phonatory
variables were related to improvements in speech intelligibility after
therapy.

The relationship between improved vocal fold adduction and speech intelligibility in patients with Parkinson's disease

Disordered communication is a problem experienced frequently by patients with Parkinson's disease (e.g. Logemann, Fisher, Boshes and Blonsky, 1978). This problem primarily has been related to disorders of articulation (e.g. Weismer, 1984) and rate (e.g. Canter, 1969). Traditional speech therapy for these patients (e.g. overarticulate, increase articulatory precision, slow rate) generally has been unsuccessful (Allan, 1970; Green, 1980; Sarno, 1968). While disordered phonation has been reported in 89a of a group of patients with Parkinson's disease (Logeman, Fisher, Boshes and Blonsky, 1978), only recently have researchers and clinicians begun to focus treatment efforts on improving the phonatory abilities of these patients (Scott and Caird,1983; Robertson and Thompson, 1984; and Ramig, Mead, Scherer, Horii, Larson and Kohler, 1988a; Ramig, Fazoli, Scherer and Bonitati, 1990). Ramig et al. (1988a) identified a "phonatory inadequacy" in this patient population and designed a treatment program to focus on increasing basic respiratory/laryngeal source characteristics. They reported significantly improved vocal abilities in patients with Parkinson's disease following intensive voice therapy which focused primarily on increasing vocal fold adduction and improving use of respiratory support for speech. It has not been established however, whether these improvements in vocal function translated into improved perceptual characteristics of speech including increased speech intelligibility in this patient population. It was the purpose of the study reported here to investigate the relationship between vocal function and perceptual measures of speech including speech intelligibility in a group of patients with Parkinson's disease who experienced maximum improvement in vocal function following intensive voice therapy.

Methods

Subjects. Seven neuropharmacologically stable patients with idiopathic Parkinson's disease were selected from a group of two-hundred patients who participated in a four-week intensive program of speech therapy. All subjects were male, ranging in age from 63 to 77 years. Three were in Stage III and four were in Stage IV of Parkinson's disease (Hoehn and Yahr, 1969). These seven patients were selected for this study because they had attained maximum improvement in vocal function following therapy as defined by their acoustic, electroglottographic and videolaryngoscopic data (Ramig, Fazoli, Scherer and Bonitati, 1990). All seven patients demonstrated increased vocal fold adduction and phonatory stability as evidenced by a comparison of the pre- and post-treatment electroglottographic measures of the abduction quotient (Titze, 1984) and EGGW (Scherer and Vail, 1988), perceptual ratings of videolaryngoscopic examinations and acoustic measures of shimmer and the coefficient of variation of amplitude (Ramig, Fazoli, Scherer and Bonitati, 1990). All patients had participated in four-weeks of intensive (three to four times a week) voice therapy. This therapy was carried out in the context of a multidisciplinary treatment program which included physical therapy, occupational therapy, nutrition, counseling and exercise. Specific voice therapy procedures and underlying rationale have been discussed previously (Ramig, et al, 1988 a,b,c) and are summarized in Table 1.

Procedures. A variety of procedures were carried out to evaluate changes in patients' speech intelligibility following therapy. Each patient participated in a video taping session which sampled approximately five minutes of conversational speech before (pre) and after (post) therapy. All data were collected at the same time post- medication for each patient. Video tape recordings were made using a JVC Highband Saticon color video camera Model GX-S700 with a built in stereo microphone on to a JVC VHS video cassette recorder Model BR-1600U in a quiet environment. The microphone to patient distance was five feet and remained constant throughout all recordings. Given the well-established performance variability of Parkinson patients in a test situation (e.g. Weismer, 1984), conversational speech was selected inorder to maximize the likelihood of sampling functional communication abilities of these patients and minimize the effects of reading ability and visual acuity (Giolas and Epstein, 1963; Connolly, 1986). These pre- and post-video recordings were presented by a Panasonic NV8500 VHS recorder and two Panasonic CT110 nine inch color monitors in random order through earphones at constant and comfortable loudness to three speech pathologists familiar with rating the speech of Parkinson's disease patients. Netsell (1984) has suggested that perceptual ratings of speech should include at least three raters. These speech pathologists rated these samples on a visual analogue scale of speech characteristics (Schiffman, Reynolds and Young, 1981; Kempster, 1984) and on two scales of speech intelligibility: the Comunication Profile devel-

Table 1. *Framework and rationale for initial program of speech therapy administered to forty patients with idiopathic Parkinson's disease; treatmen philosophy is intensive therapy with a focus on phonation and immediate carryover into functional communication (Ramig et al. 1988a,b,c).*

Perceptual characteristics of speech	Hypothesized laryngeal and/or respiratory pathophysiology	Therapy goals and tasks	Acoustic, physiologic variables measured	Perceptual variables measured

"Reduced loudness, breathy, weak voice" (Logemann, et al. 1978, Aronson 1985)	Bowed vocal folds (Hansen, et al. 1984), rigidity, hypokinesia in laryngeal and/or respirtory muscles; reduced adduction; reduced inspiratory, expiratory volumes (Critchley 1981);	1. increase vocal fold adduction – isometric (pushing, lifting) with phonation
		
		increase maximum duration vowel phonation at increased intensity
		
		–think "shout"
		–speak over background noise
		
		2. increase respiratory support
		  –posture
		  –deep breath before speak
		  –frequent breaths
		  –phrasing of words in sentences
			Maximum duration of sustained vowel phonation (sec)
			
			vital capacity (L;%)
				loudness
				breathiness
				intelligibility

Table 1 continued

Perceptual characteristics of speech	Hypothesized laryngeal and/or respiratory pathophysiology	Therapy goals and tasks	Acoustic, physiologic variables measured	Perceptual variables measured
"Reduced pitch variability monopitch" (Logemann, et al. 1978,	Rigidity cricothyroid muscle (Aronson 1985)	1. increase maximum fundamental frequency range –high and low pitch scales –Sustain phonation at highest and lowest pitches	*maximum range of fundamental frequency (ST)*	
		2. increase fundamental frequency variation in connected speech –word emphasis –intonation in questions	*variability of fundamental frequency in connected speech (STSD)*	*monotone* *intelligibility*
Unsteady, hoarse, rough voice (Logemann, et al. 1978)	Rigidity, hypokinesia, tremor in laryngeal and respiratory muscles (Hansen, et al. 1984,	1. increase steadiness of phonation –maximum duration tasks with constant intensity –consistent, firm voice throughout sentence	*improved measures of phonatory stability* (coefficient of variation of frequency, coefficient of variation of amplitude, jitter, shimmer, harmonics to noise ratio)	*steadiness of voice* *hoarse* *tremorous* *intelligibility*

oped at the National Technical Institute for the Deaf (NTID) (Johnson,1975; McGarr and Osberger, 1978) and a modification of this profile. The following speech characteristics were rated on the visual analogue scale: loudness, shakiness of voice, scratchiness of voice, monotone, slurring, mumbling, speaking so that others can understand, participating in conversations and starting conversations. The visual analogue scale was designed to be a clinically feasible tool for both patients and professionals, which targets perceptual features related to treatment goals for these patients. Schiavetti, Metz and Sitler (1981) have demonstrated that because of nonlinearities, the NTID scale is not able to discriminate among individuals over the entire intelligibility range. We modified the NTID profile based on the findings of our pilot work which indicated that the scale in its original form was not sensitive to the type of improved communication our patients experienced after therapy. We presented both the original and modified version of this scale to listeners. Twenty percent of all ratings were repeated within task for an assessment of intratask reliability. In the clinical situation, visual analogue rating scales and NTID scales were completed by patients, caregivers, two speech pathologists and interdisciplinary team members pre- and post-treatment. The three scales are presented in Table 2.

Results

To assess intratask reliability, correlation coefficients were calculated for the within task repeated ratings of the perceptual variables on the visual analogue scale and the five and six point NTID scales by the three speech pathologists. For the visual analogue scale, these correlations ranged from .91 for loudness ratings to .98 for understandability or intelligibility ratings; coefficients for repeated ratings of the other perceptual variables fell between these two values. For the five and six point NTID scale of intelligibility, correlation coefficients were .92 and .97 respectively for repeated ratings. To assess the relationships among intelligibility assessed on the visual analogue scale and the NTID scales, correlation coefficients were calculated among these ratings. Intelligibility as assessed on the visual analogue scale correlated .69 and .70 with intelligibility ratings assigned on the five and six point NTID scales respectively. The relationship between pre- and post-therapy improvement in intelligibility (expressed in percent) as measured on the visual analogue scale and the five and six point NTID scales

Table 2 *Three perceptual scales used in this study*

---

a. 5 Point NTID Intelligibility Rating

---

1. Speech cannot be understood
2. Speech is very difficult to understand — only isolated words or phrases are intelligible
3. Speech is difficult to understand; however, the gist of the content can be understood
4. Speech is intelligible with the exception of a few words or phrases
5. Speech is completely intelligible

b. 6 Point Modification of NTID Intelligibility Rating

---

1. Speech cannot be understood
2. Speech is very difficult to understand — only isolated words or phrases are intelligible
3. Speech is difficult to understand; however, the gist of the content can be understood
4. Speech is intelligible with the exception of a few words or phrases
5. Speech is intelligible, but the listener must work hard
6. Speech is completely intelligible

c. Visual analogue scale

Always Loud Enough	Never Loud Enough
Never A Shaky Voice	Always A Shaky Voice
Never A Hoarse, "Scratchy" Voice	Always a Hoarse, "Scratchy" Voice
Never Monotone	Always Monotone
Never Slurs	Always Slurs
Never Mumbles	Always Mumbles
Always Speaks So Others Can Understand	Never Speaks So Others Can Understand
Always Participates In A Conversation	Never Participates In A Conversation
Always Starts A Conversation	Never Starts A Conversation

were reflected in correlation coefficients of .66 and .82 respectively. The average post-therapy intelligibility increase across all patients on the visual analogue scale was 21%. For the five and six point NTID scales it was 16% and 25.3% respectively.

To evaluate the impact of improved vocal function (increased adduction and stability) previously documented on perceptual measures, listener ratings were compared between the pre- and post-therapy conditions. There were statistically significant differences in listener ratings for all perceptual variables between the pre- and post-therapy conditions as assessed by paired t-tests; this included loudness, understandibility (intelligibility), scratchiness, shaky voice, monotone, mumbling and slurring from the visual analogue scale and intelligibility from the NTID scales. These data are summarized in Table 3.

Table 3   *Group means and standard deviations of perceptual ratings from the visual analogue scale and five and six point NTID intelligibility scales pre and post therapy for seven patients with Parkinson's disease. Increased rathings are associated with improvement.*

Perceptual variable		Therapy condition	
		Pre	Post
Loudness	m	53.3	87.4
	SD	19.1	9.4
Shakiness	m	71.3	85.0
	SD	9.2	7.6
Scratchines	m	59.4	87.1
	SD	25.4	8.9
Monotone	m	53.6	84.3
	SD	20.6	12.1
Slurring	m	62.1	86.6
	SD	17.7	8.7
Mumbling	m	57.9	85.7
	SD	20.7	9.6
Understandability	m	70.4	91.6
	SD	14.1	7.7
Intelligibility (NTID 5-point)	m	4.1	4.6
	SD	.4	.5
Intelligibility (NTID 6-point)	m	4.6	5.5
	SD	.7	.6

To evaluate the relationship between these perceptual ratings and kinematic (e.g., abduction quotient, eggw) and acoustic (coefficient of variation of amplitude, shimmer) data, Pearson product meoment correlation coefficients were calculated between changes in perceptual and kinematic and acoustic measures of vocal function from the pre- to post-treatment conditions. The only statistically significant relationships measured by the correlation coefficients were between the abduction quotient and ratings of both loudness and scratchiness; patients who increased vocal fold adduction most significantly were also rated as having the greatest increases in vocal loudness and reductions in scratchiness. There were no significant correlations with these measures and ratings of speech intelligibility.

To evaluate the impact of these perceptual changes on ratings of intelligibility pre- and post-therapy, correlation coefficients were calculated between changes in the perceptual measures and intelligibility as rated on the visual analogue scale. Ratings of monotone and shaky voice correlated with intelligibility .88 and .74 respectively; the other correlation coefficients ranged from .67 for loudness, .64 for slurs, .63 for mumbles and .32 for scratchiness. To evaluate the contribution of a combination of these various perceptual variables to overall ratings of intelligibility, a multiple regression analysis was carried out with intelligibility ratings as the criterion and the other perceptual variables as the predictors. The combination of monotone and shaky voice (intercorrelation of .53) resulted in a correlation coefficient of .94, suggesting that this combination of perceptual varaibles was able to account for 88% of the variance in speech intelligibility ratings for this group of speakers.

Discussion

These findings demonstrate that the improvement in vocal function documented by acoustic and kinematic measures in Parkinson's patients following intensive voice therapy translated to improvement in perceptual measures as well. These Parkinson's patients improved in perceptual measures of vocal function (loudness, monotone, shaky and scratchy voice) after intensive voice therapy. In addition, it appears that the increased vocal effort also positively affected articulatory variables as evidenced by improved ratings of slurring and mumbling. Overall, ratings of intelligibility were improved in the post-therapy condition and were most closely related to ratings of reduced monotony and shakiness of speech. The finding that monotony and shaky voice were related most closely to ratings of intelligibility supports the importance of phonatory characteristics in the intelligibility of these speakers. The patients' increased vocal effort appeared to improve overall communication performance because of improved acoustic and aerodynamic sources and perhaps because of generalization of this increased effort to articulatory performance as well.

It should be pointed out that the acoustic and kinematic data were analyzed from sustained vowel phonation and the perceptual ratings were made from conversational speech. Therefore direct relationships among acoustic, kinematic and perceptual variables can not be verified. However, these data support that the improvements measured from sustained vowels such as increased vocal fold adduction and amplitude steadiness appeared to be carried over into conversational speech and were reflected in ratings of increased loudness and reduced shakiness and scratchiness after therapy.

The relationship between improved ratings of monotony of speech and intelligibility can be interpreted in at least two ways. Perhaps the improved intonation provided the listeners with additional information to enhance speech intelligibility. On the other hand, perhaps as Price and Levitt (1983), Kent et al. (1989) and Weismer (1990) have suggested, the improved intonation patterns were consistent with listeners' perceptual set or tolerance to allow them to use familiar strategies to decode the message with greater ease and thus enhance intelligibility.

The patients in this study all had reduced vocal fold adduction associated with bowed vocal folds in the pre-therapy condition. While the voice-voiceless contrast is the primary measurement of adductory breakdown on segmental measures of speech intelligibility, our pilot work using voice-voiceless contrast word pairs with these patients suggests that most of them were able to make this contrast with ease. These same patients were rated as having reduced intelligibility and loudness and required additional effort on the part of the listener in order to be understood. One interpretation may be that in a particular contrastive word pair task the Parkinson's patients demonstrated their typical performance variablity by using maximum effort to achieve maximum performance which is not carried over to spontaneous speech. Another interpretation is that because of its segmental nature, the voice-voiceless contrast does not reflect overall breakdowns in adduction which reduce loudness across an entire utterance. Patients may be able to achieve sufficient respiratory, laryngeal and supraglottal coordination to generate the voicing contrast for a discrete unit of time, but are unable to achieve and maintain the adductory and respiratory forces necessary to generate adequate loudness across an entire utterance.

It should be noted that in many patients with Parkinson's disease, especially early in the disease process, reduced volume or loudness may be the primary complaint. While this loudness may not reduce intelligibility as documented by current procedures, it may require the "listener to work hard". The ability to document this additional effort on the part of the listener may prove to be very important. Our preliminary observations suggest that early intervention at this time with Parkinson's disease patients may be significant in terms of maintaining communication skills. If patients can learn techniques to maintain vocal function at this early point in the disease when their motivation and cognitive skills are frequently intact, it is likely that they will achieve greater success over time.

This study begins to address the interactions among acoustic, physiologic and perceptual measures of phonatory function and speech intelligibility. Future research should continue to address these relationships.

Acknowledgement

Preparation of this chapter was supported in part by NIH grants #8 RO1 DC00387-03 and RO1 DC01150-01 and NIDRR grant # H133 G00079. This research was supported in part by funds from the Lee Silverman Center for Parkinson's, Scottsdale, Arizona, the Axe-Houghton Foundation and the Parkinson's Association of the Rockies. Appreciation is expressed to Carolyn Mead Bonitati, Katy Fazoli, Ron Scherer, Roberta Borne, Carlos Fazoli and Ken Tagawa for assistance during various parts of this project.

References

Addington, D.W. 1968. "The relationship of selected vocal characteristics to personality perception." *Speech Monographs* 35, 492-503.
Allan, C.M. 1970. "Treatment of non-fluent speech resulting from neurological disease: treatment of dysarthria." *British Journal of Disorders of Communication* 5, 3-5.
Allen, D.R., Strong, W.T., and Palmer, E.P. 1981. "Experiments on the intelligibility of low frequency speech codes." *Journal of the Acoustical Society of America* 70, 1248-1255.
Andrews, G., Platt, L.J. and Young, M. 1977. "Factors affecting the intelligibility of cerebral plasied speech to the average listener." *Folia Phoniatrica* 29, 292-301.

Angelocci, A., Kopp. G., Holbrook, A. 1964. "The vowel formants of deaf and normal hearing eleven to fourteen year old boys." *Journal of Speech and Hearing Disorders* 29, 156-170.

Ansel, B.A. 1985. "Acoustic predictors of speech intelligibility in cerebral palsied dysarthric adults." Unpublished doctoral dissertation, University of Wisconsin-Madison, Madison, WI.

Aronson, A.E. 1985. *Clinical Voice Disorders.* New York:Thieme.

Arkebauer, H., Hixon, T. and Hardy, J. 1967. "Peak intraoral air pressures during speech." *Journal of Speech and Hearing Research* 10, 196-208.

Behrens, S.J. 1985. "The perception of stress and the lateralization of prosody." *Brain and Language* 26, 332-348.

Bellaire, K., Yorkston, K. and Beukelman, D. 1986. "Modification of breath patterning to increase naturalness of a mildly dysarthric speaker." *Journal of Communication Disorders* 19, 271-280.

Bennett, S. and Weinberg, B. 1973. "Acceptability ratings of normal, esophageal, and artificial larynx speech." *Journal of Speech and Hearing Research* 16, 608-615.

Bernstein, J., Rollins, A.M. and Stevens, K.N. 1978. "Word and syllable concatenation in the speech of the deaf." A paper presented at the meeting of the A.G. Bell Association for the Deaf, St.Louis, June.

Berry, C. 1973. *Voice and the Actor.* London: George G. Harrap and Company, Ltd.

Blonder, L.X., Gur, R and Gur, R. 1989. "The effects of right and left hemiparkinsonism on prosody." *Brain and Language.* 36, 193-207.

Boone, D.R. and McFarlane, S.C. 1988. *The Voice and Voice Therapy.* Englewood Cliffs:Prentice Hall.

Boothroyd, A., Archambault, P., Adams, R.E. and Storm, R.D. 1975. "Use of a computer- based system of speech analysis and display in a remedial speech program for deaf children." *The Volta Review* 77, 178-193.

Bush, M. 1979. "Articulatory proficiency and Fo control by profoundly deaf speakers." A paper presented at the meeting of the American Speech-Language-Hearing Association, November, Atlanta.

Canter, G. 1963. "Speech characteristics of patients with Parkinson's disease I. Intensity, pitch and duration." *Journal of Speech and Hearing Disorders* 28, 221-8.

————. 1965. "Speech characteristics of patients with Parkinson's disease: III. Articulation." *Journal of Speech and Hearing Disorders.* 30, 217-24.

Carney, A. E. 1986. "Understanding speech intelligibility in the hearing impaired." *Topics in Language Disorders* 6(3), 47-59.

Chodosh, P., Giancarlo, H., Goldstein, J. 1984. "Pharyngeal myotomy for voice rehabilitation post laryngectomee." *Laryngoscope* 94, 52.

Cleveland, T. and Sundberg, J. 1983. "Acoustic analysis of three male voices of different quality." *Proceedings of Stockholm Music Acoustics Conference,* ed. by A. Askenfelt, S. Felicetti, E. Jansson, and J. Sundberg, 143-156. Stockholm: The Royal Swedish Academy of Music.

Connolly, J.H. 1986. "Intelligibility: a linguistic view." *British Journal of Disorders of Communication* 21, 371-376.

Cooper, W.E., Eady, S.J.and Mueller, P.R. 1985. "Acoustical aspects of contrastive stress in question-answer contexts." *Journal of the Acoustical Society of America* 77, 2142-2156.

Cooper, W.E. and Sorenson, J.M. 1981. *Fundamental Frequency in Sentence Production*. New York:Springer-Verlag.

Critchley, E.M.R. 1981. "Speech disorders of parkinsonism: A review." *Journal of Neurology, Neurosurgery and Psychiatry*. 44, 751-758.

Curtis, J.F. 1946. "Intelligibility related to microphone position." *Speech Monographs* 13, 8-12.

Danly, M, and Shapiro, B. 1982. "Speech prosody in Broca's aphasia." *Brain and Language* 16, 171-190.

Darley, F., Aronson, A. and Brown, J. 1969a. "Clusters of deviant speech dimensions in the dysarthrias." *Journal of Speech and Hearing Research* 12, 462-469.

————. 1969b. "Differential diagnostic patterns of dysarthria." *Journal of Speech and Hearing Research* 12, 246-269.

————. 1975. *Motor Speech Disorders*. Philadelphia: W.B.Sanders.

Deal, R.E. and Emanuel, R.W. 1978. "Some waveform and spectral features of vowel roughness" *Journal of Speech and Hearing Research* 21, 250-264.

Diedrich, W.M. 1968. "The mechanism of esophageal speech." *Sound Production in Man*. Annals of the New York Academy of Sciences 155, 303-317.

Doyle, P.C. and Danhauer, J.L. 1986. "Consonant intelligibility of alaryngeal talkers: pilot data." *Human Communuication Canada* 10(4), 21-28.

Doyle, P.C., Danhauer, J.L. and Reed, C.G. 1988. "Listeners' perceptions of consonants produced by esophageal and tracheoesophageal talkers." *Journal of Speech and Hearing Disorders* 53, 400-407.

Draegert, G.L. (to appear). "Relationship between voice variables and speech intelligibility in high level noise." *Speech Monographs*.

Drummond, S. 1965. "The effects of environmental noise on pseudovoice after laryngectomee." *Journal of Laryngology* 79, 193-202.

Esling, J.H. 1978. "Voice quality in Edinburgh: a sociolinguistic and phonetic study." An unpublished doctoral dissertation. Edinburgh University.

Farmer, A. 1980. "Voice onset time production in cerebral palsied speakers." *Folia Phoniatrica* 32, 267-73.

Freeman,F. Cannito, M.P. and Finitzo-Heiber, T. 1985. "Classification of spasmodic dysphonia by perceptual-acoustic-visual means." *Spasmodic Dysphonia: The state of the art*, ed. by G. Gates, 5-18. New York: The Voice Foundation.

Freyman, R.L. and Nerbonne, G.P. 1989. "The importance of consonant-vowel intensity ratio in the intelligibility of voiceless consonants." *Journal of Speech and Hearing Research*. 32, 524-535.

Gandour, J. and Dararananda, R. 1983. "Identification of tonal contrasts in Thai aphasic patients." *Brain and Language* 18, 98-114.

Gandour, J. and Weinberg, B. 1983. "Perception of intonational contrasts in alaryngeal speech." *Journal of Speech and Hearing Research* 26, 142-148.

Gandour, J., Weinberg, B. and Garzone, B. 1983. "Perception of lexical stress in alaryngeal speech." *Journal of Speech and Hearing Research* 26, 418-424.

Garber, S.R., Siegel, G.M. and Pick, H.L. 1980. "The effects of feedback filtering on speaker intelligibility." *Journal of Communication Disorders* 13, 289-294.

Giolas, T.G. and Epstein, A. 1963. "Comparative intelligibility of word lists and continuous discourse." *Journal of Speech and Hearing Research* 6, 349-358.

Gold, T. 1975. "Perception and production of prosodic features by hearing impaired children." A paper presented at the Convention of the American Speech and Hearing Association, Washington, D.C., November.

Gomyo, Y. and Doyle, P.C. Forthcoming. "Perception of stop consonants produced by esophageal and tracheoesophageal speakers." *Journal of Otolaryngology.*

Gordon-Salant, S. 1986. "Recognition of natural and time-intensity altered CVs by young and elderly subjects with normal-hearing." *Journal of the Acoustical Society of America* 80, 1599-1607.

———. 1987. "Effects of acoustic modification on consonant recognition by elderly hearing-impaired subjects." *Journal of the Acoustical Society of America* 81, 1199-1202.

Greene, D.S. 1956. "Fundamental frequency of the speech of profoundly deaf individuals." An unpublished doctoral dissertation, Purdue University, West Lafayette, IN.

Greene, M.C.L. 1980. *The Voice and Its Disorders.* London: Pitman Medical.

Greene, M.C.L. and Watson, B.W. 1968. "The value of speech amplification in Parkinson's disease patients." *Folia Phoniatrica* 20, 250.

Hanley ,T.D. and Steer, M.D. 1949. "Effect of level of distracting noise upon speaking rate, duration and intensity." *Journal of Speech and Hearing Disorders* 14, 363-368.

Hansen, D.G., Gerratt, B.R. and Ward, P.H. 1984. "Cinegraphic observations of laryngeal function in Parkinson's disease." *Laryngoscope* 94, 348-353.

Haycock, G.S. 1933. *The Teaching of Speech.* Stoke-on-Trent: Hill and Ainsworth.

Hecker, M.H.L. 1974. "A study of the relationships between consonant and vowel ratios and speaker intelligibility." Unpublished doctoral dissertation, Stanford University, Stanford, CA.

Hoehn, M. and Yahr, M. 1969. "Parkinsonism onset, progression and mortality." *Neurology* 17, 427.

Hood, R.B. 1966. "Some physical concomitants of the perception of speech rhythm of the deaf." Unpublished doctoral dissertation, Stanford University, Stanford, CA.

House, A.S., Williams, C.E., Hecker, M.H.L. and Kryter, K. 1965. "Articulation testing methods:consonantal differentiation with a closed response set." *Journal of the Acoustical Society of America* 37, 158-166.

Hunnicut, S. 1985. "Intelligibility versus redundancy-conditions of dependency." *Language and Speech* 28, 47-56.

———. 1987. "Acoustic correlates of redundancy and intelligibility." *STL-QPSR* 2(3), 7-14.

Hyman, M., 1955. "An experimental study of artificial larynx and esophageal speech." *Journal of Speech and Hearing Disorders* 20, 291-299.

Johnson, D.D. 1975. "Communication characteristics of NTID students." *Journal of Academic Rehabilitative Audiology* 8(1/2), 17-32.

Kalb, M.B. and Carpenter, M.A. 1981. "Individual speaker influence on relative intelligibility of esophageal speech and artificial larynx speech." *Journal of Speech and Hearing Disorders* 46, 77-80.

Kammermeier, M.A. 1969. "A comparison of phonatory phenomena among groups of neurologically impaired speakers." An unpublished doctoral dissertation. University of Minnesota, Minneapolis.

Kempster, G.B., 1984. "A multidimensional analysis of vocal quality in two dysphonic groups." An unpublished doctoral dissertation. Northwestern University,Evanston.

Kent, R.D. 1988 "Speech intelligibility." *Decision Making in Speech-Language Pathology*, ed. by D.E. Yoder and R.D. Kent, 140-143. Philadelphia: Decker.

Kent, R.D. and Rosenbek, J. 1982. "Prosodic disturbance and neurologic lesion." *Brain and Language* 15, 259-291.

Kent, R.D., Weismer,G. Kent, J.F. and Rosenbek, J.C. 1990. "Toward phonetic intelligibility testing in dysarthria." *Journal of Speech and Hearing Disorders* 54(4), 482-499.

Kent, R.D., Weismer, G. and Kim, Hyang-Hee. 1990a. "Segmental and suprasegmental laryngeal dysfunction in neurological disease: amyotrophic lateral sclerosis, Parkinson's disease, stroke and cerebellar disease." A paper presented at the conference Neurological Disorders of Laryngeal Function. Los Angeles, CA.

Kent, R.D., Weismer, G. and Rosenbek, J.C. 1990b. "Acoustic-phonetic dimensions of intelligibility impairment in dysarthria." A paper presented at the conference Clinical Dysarthria. San Antonio, TX.

Klatt, D.H. 1975. "Vowel lengthening is syntactically determined in connected discourse." *Journal of Phonetics* 3, 129-140.

Klouda, G.V., Robin, D.A., Graff-Radford, N.R. and Cooper, W. 1988. "The role of callosal connections in speech prosody." *Brain and Language* 35, 154-171.

Kohler, K.J. and Dommelen, W.S. 1987. "The effect of voice quality on the perception of lentis-fortis stops." *Journal of Phonetics*, 15, 365-381.

Lane , H. and Tranel, B. 1970. "The Lombard signs and the role of hearing in speech." *Journal of Speech and Hearing Research* 14, 677-709.

Laver, J. 1980. *The phonetic description of voice quality*. Cambridge: Cambridge University Press.

Laver, J. 1968. "Voice quality and indexical information." *British Journal of Disorders of Communication* 3, 43-54.

Laver, J. and Trudgill, P. 1979. "Phonetic and linguistic markers in speech." *Social Markers in Speech*, ed. by K.R. Scherer and H. Giles, 1-32. Cambridge: Cambridge University Press.

Laver, J., Wirz, S., Mackenzie, J., and Hiller, S. 1981. A perceptual protocol for the analysis of vocal profiles. Work in Progress (University of Edinburgh, Department of Linguistics) 14, 139-155.

Lessac, A. 1967. *The Use and Training of the Human Voice*. New York; Drama Book Publishers.

Levitt, H., Smith, C.R., Stromberg, H. 1974. "Acoustic, articulatory and perceptual characteristics of the speech of deaf children." *Speech Communication Seminar*, Stockholm.

Lieberman, P. 1960. "Some acoustic correlates of word stress in American English." *Journal of the Acoustical Society of America* 32, 451-454.

Lim, J.S., Oppenheim, A.V., and Braida, L.D. 1978. "Evaluation of an adaptive comb filtering method for enhancing speech degraded by white noise addition." *IEEE Transactions on Acoustics, Speech and Signal Processing* 26, 354-358.

Logemann, J.A. Fisher,H.B., Boshes,B. and Blonsky, E.R. 1978. "Frequency and co-occurrence of vocal tract dysfunctions in the speech of a large sample of Parkinson patients." *Journal of Speech and Hearing Disorders* 43, 47-57.

Ludlow, C.L. and Bassich, C.J. 1983. "The results of acoustic and perceptual assessment of two types of dysarthria." *Clinical Dysarthria*, ed. W.R. Berry, 121-153. San Diego: College-Hill Press.

McGarr, N.S. 1976 "The production and reception of prosodic features." A paper presented at the annual meeting of the A.G. Bell Association, Boston, Mass, June.

———. 1978. "The differences between experienced and inexperienced listeners in understanding the speech of the deaf." Unpublished doctoral dissertation, City University of New York.

McGarr, N.S. and Osberger, M.J. 1978. "Pitch deviancy and intelligibility of deaf speech." *Journal of Communication Disorders* 11.

McGarr, N.S., Youdelman, K. and Head, J. (in press). Curriculum to remediate the monotone voice.

McHenry, M., Reich, A. and Minifie, F. 1982. "Acoustical characteristics of intended syllabic stress in excellent esophageal speakers." *Journal of Speech and Hearing Research* 25, 564-573.

Markides, A. 1970. "The speech of deaf and partially hearing children with special reference to factors affecting intelligibility." *British Journal of Disorders of Communication* 5, 126-140.

Martony, J. 1968. "On correction of voice pitch level for severely hard of hearing subjects." *American Annals of the Deaf* 113, 195-202.

Metz,D.E., Samar, V.J., Schiavetti,N., Sitler,R. and Whitehead, R.L. 1985. "Acoustic dimensions of hearing-impaired speakers' intelligibility." *Journal of Speech and Hearing Research* 28, 345-355.

Monsen, R.B. 1978. "Toward measuring how well hearing impaired children speak." *Journal of Speech and Hearing Research* 21, 197-219.

———. 1979. "Acoustic qualities of phonation in young hearing-impaired children." *Journal of Speech and Hearing Research* 22, 270-288.

———. 1983. "The oral speech intelligibility of hearing-impaired talkers." *Journal of Speech and Hearing Disorders* 48, 286-296.

Montgomery, A.A. and Edge, R.A. 1988. "Evaluation of two speech enhancement techniques to improve intelligibility for hearing-impaired adults." *Journal of Speech and Hearing Research* 31, 386-393.

Moore, P. 1946 "Intelligibility related to routinized messages." *Speech Monographs* 13, 46-49.

Moran, M.J., LaBarge, J.M. and Haynes, W.O. 19??. "Effect of voice quality on adult's perceptions of Down's syndrome children." *Folia Phoniatricia* 40, 157-161.

Mueller, P. 1971. "Parkinson's disease: Motor-speech behavior in a selected group of patients." *Folia Phoniatrica* 23, 333-346.

Netsell, R., Lotz, W. and Shaughnessy, A. 1984. "Laryngeal aerodynamics associated with selected voice disorders." *American Journal of Otolaryngology* 5(6), 397-403.

Nieboer, G.L.J., deGraaf, T. and Schutte, H.K. 1988. "Esophageal voice quality judgements by means of the semantic differential." *Journal of Phonetics* 16, 417-436.

Nickerson, R.S. 1975. "Characteristics of the speech of deaf persons." The Volta Review. 77.342-362.

Nickerson, R.S., Kalikow, D.N. and Stevens, K.N. 1976. "Computer-aided speech training for the deaf." *Journal of Speech and Hearing Disorders* 41, 120-132.

Ono, H., Okasaki, T., Naki, S., and Harasaki, H. 1982. "Identification of an emphasized consonant of a monosyllable in hearing-impaired subjects and its application to a hearing aid." *Journal of the Acoustical Society of America* 71, S58.

Osberberger, M.J. and McGarr, N.S. 19 "Speech Production Characteristics of the Hearing Impaired." *Speech and Language, Advances in Basic Research and Practice* 8, 221-283.

Owens, E. and Schubert, E.D. 1977. "Development of the California Consonant Test." *Journal of Speech and Hearing Research* 20, 463-474.

Parkhurst, B. and Levitt, H. 1978. "The effect of selected prosodic errors on the intelligibility of deaf speech." *Journal of Communication Disorders* 11, 249-256.

Pichney, M.A. 1981. "Speaking clearly for the hard of hearing." Unpublished doctoral dissertation, Massachusetts Institute of Technology, Cambridge, MA.

Pichney, M.A., Durlach, N.I. and Braida, L.D. 1985 "Speaking clearly for the hard of hearing: I:Intelligibility differences between clear and conversational speech." *Journal of Speech and Hearing Research* 28, 96-103.

————. 1986 "Speaking clearly for the hard of hearing II: Acoustic characteristics of clear and conversational speech." *Journal of Speech and Hearing Research* 29, 434-446.

Pickett, J.M. 1956. "Effects of vocal force on the intelligibility of speech sounds." *Journal of the Acoustical Society of America* 28(5), 902-905.

Pindzola, R.H. and Cain, B.H. 1988. "Acceptability ratings of tracheoesophageal speech." *Laryngoscope* 98, 394-397.

Pittman, J. 1987a. "Discrimination of five voice qualities and prediction to perceptual ratings." *Phonetica* 44, 38-49.

————. 1987b. "The long-term spectral measurement of voice quality as a social and personality marker: a review." *Language and Speech* 30 Part I, 1-12.

Prater, R.J. and Swift, R.W. 1984. *Manual of Voice Therapy*. Boston: Little, Brown Co.

Price, P.J. and Levitt, A.G. 1983. "The relative roles of syntax and prosody in the perception of the /s/-/c/ distinction." *Language and Speech* 26, 3.

Ramig, L.A., Mead, C.L., Scherer, R.C., Horii, Y., Larson, K. and Kohler, D. 1988a. "Voice therapy and Parkinson's disease:a longitudinal study of efficacy." A paper presented at the Clinical Dysarthria Conference, San Diego.

Ramig, L.A., Mead. C.L. and DeSanto, L. 1988b. "Voice therapy and Parkinson's disease. *American Speech and Hearing Association* 30(109), 128.

Ramig, L.A., Mead, C.L. and Winholtz, W. 1988c. "Speech therapy:Parkinson's disease." Produced by the Recording and Research Center of the Denver Center for the Performing Arts.

Ramig, L.A., Fazoli, K., Scherer R. and Bonitati, C. 1990. "Changes in phonation of Parkinson's disease patients following voice therapy." A paper presented at The Clinical Dysarthria Conference. San Antonio, TX.

Ramig, L.A. and Scherer, R. 1989. "Speech therapy for neurological disorders of the larynx." *Neurological Disorders of the Larynx*, ed. by A. Blitzer, C.Sasaki, S. Fahn, M.Brin and K.Harris New York:Thieme.

Resnick,S.B., Dubno, J.R., Huffnung, S. and Levitt, H. 1975. "Phoneme errors on a nonsense syllable test." *Journal of the Acoustical Society of America* 58, S114.

Robbins, J. 1984. "Acoustic differentiation of laryngeal, esophageal, and tracheoesophageal speech." *Journal of Speech and Hearing Research* 27, 577-585.

Robbins, J., Christensen, J. and Kempster, G. 1986. "Characteristics of speech production after tracheoesophageal puncture: voice onset time and vowel duration." *Journal of Speech and Hearing Research* 29, 499-504.

Robbins, J.,Fisher, H.B., Blom, E.D., and Singer, M.I. 1984. "A comparative acoustic study of normal, esophageal, and tracheoesophageal speech production." *Journal of Speech and Hearing Disorders* 49, 202-210.

Robertson, S. and Thompson, F. 1984. "Speech therapy in Parkinson's disease: a study of the efficacy and long-term effect of intensive treatment." *British Journal of Disorders of Communication* 19, 213-224.

Rosenbek, J.C. and LaPointe, L.L. 1985. "The Dysarthrias: description, diagnosis and treatment." *Clinical Management of Neurogenic Communicative Disorders*. ed. by D. Johns, 97-152. Boston: Little, Brown and Co.

Ross, E.D., Anderson, B. and Morgan-Fisher, A. 1989 "Crossed aprosodia in strongly dextral patients." *Archives of Neurology* 46 (2), 206-209.

Rostolland, D. 1982a. "Acoustic features and shouted voice." *Acustica* 50, 118-125.

Rostolland, D. 1982b. "Phonetic structure of shouted voice." Acustica 51, 80-89.

Rostolland, D. and Parant, C. 1974. "Physical analysis of shouted voice." A paper presented at the Eighth International Congress on Acoustics, London.

Rubow, R.T. and Swift, E. 1985. "Microcomputer-based wearable biofeedback device to improve treatment carry-over in parkinsonian dysarthria." *Journal of Speech and Hearing Disorders* 50, 178-185.

Ruscello, D.M., Lass, N.J. and Podbesek, J. 1988. "Listeners' perceptions of normal and voice-disordered children." *Folia Phoniatrica* 40, 290-296.

Ryalls, John. 1986. "What constitutes a primary disturbance of speech prosody? A reply to Shapiro and Danly." *Brain and Language* 29, 183-187

Ryalls, J., Joanette, Y. and Feldman, L. 1987. "An acoustic comparison of normal and right-hemisphere-damaged speech prosody." *Cortex* 23, 685-694.

Samar, V.J. and Metz, D.E. 1988. "Criterion validity of speech intelligibility rating-scale procedure for the hearing-impaired population." *Journal of Speech and Hearing Research* 31, 307-316.

Sarno, M. 1968. "Speech impairment in Parkinson's disease." *Archives of Physical Medicine and Rehabilitation* 49, 269-275.

Scarpino, J. and Weinberg, B. 1981. "Junctural contrasts in esophageal and normal speech." *Journal of Speech and Hearing Research* 24, 120-126.

Scherer, K.R. 1986. "Vocal affect expression: a review and a model for future research." *Psychological Bulletin* 99, 143-165.

————. 1979. "Personality markers in speech." *Social Markers in Speech*, ed. by K.R. Scherer and Giles, Cambridge: Cambridge University Press.

Scherer, R.C., Gould, W.J., Titze, I.R., Meyers, A. and Sataloff, R. 1988. "Preliminary evaluation of selected acoustic and glottographic measures for clinical phonatory function analysis." *Journal of Voice* 2, 230-244.

Scherer, R.C. and Vail, V.J. 1988. "Measures of laryngeal adduction." *Journal of the
Acoustical Society of America* 84 (S1), S81(A).

Schiavetti, N., Metz, D.E. and Sitler, R.W. 1981. "Construct validity of direct magnitude estimation and interval scaling of speech intelligibility: evidence from a study
of the hearing impaired." *Journal of Speech and Hearing Research* 24, 441-445.

Scott, S. and Caird, F. 1983. "Speech therapy for Parkinson's disease." *Journal of
Neurology, Neurosurgery and Psychiatry* 46, 140-144.

Schiffman, S., Reynolds, M.L. and Young, F.W. 1981. *Introduction to Multidimensional Scaling: Theory, Methods and Applications.* New York: Academic Press.

Scuri, D. 1935. "Restirazione e fonazione nei sordomute", In Nickerson, R.S. 1975.
"Characteristics of the speech of deaf persons." *The Volta Review*, 342-362.

Shapiro, B. and Danly, M. 1985. "The role of the right hemisphere in the control of
speech prosody in propositional and affective contexts." *Brain and Language* 25, 19-
36.

Shipp, T. 1967. "Frequency, duration, and perceptual measures in relation to, judgments of alaryngeal speech acceptability." *Journal of Speech and Hearing Research*
10, 417-427.

Simpson, M.B., Till, J.A. and Goff, A.M. 1988. "Long-term treatment of severe dysarthria: a case study." *Journal of Speech and Hearing Disorders 53, 433-440* .

*Singer, M.I. and Blom E.D. 1981. "Selective myotomy for voice restoration after total
laryngectomee." Archives of Otolaryngology 107, 670.*

Smith, C.R. 1972. "Residual hearing and speech production in deaf children." Unpublished doctoral dissertation, City University of New York.

Smith, C.R. 1975. "Residual hearing and speech production in deaf children." *Journal
of Speech and Hearing Research* 18, 795-811.

Spector, P.B., Subtelney, J.D., Whitehead,R.L. and Wirz, S.L. 1979. "Description and
evaluation of a training program to reduce vocal tension in adult deaf speakers." *The
Volta Review* 81(2), 81-90.

Stark, R.E. and Levitt, H. 1974. "Prosodic feature perception and production in deaf
children." *Journal of the Acoustical Society of America* 55, A.

Stevens, K.N., R.S. Nickerson, and A.M. Rollins. 1978. "On describing the suprasegmental properties of the speech of deaf children." In Bolt, Beranek and Newman
Report No. 3955, November.

―――. 1983. "Suprasegmental and postural aspects of speech production and their
effect on articulatory skills and intelligibility." *Speech of the Hearing Impaired:Re-
search, Training and Personnel Preparation*, ed. by I. Hochberg, H.Levitt, M.J.
Osberger, M.J., 35-51. Baltimore:University Park Press.

Summers, W.V., Pisoni, D.B., Bernacki, R.H., Pedlow, R.I. and Stokes, M.A. 1988.
"Effects of noise on speech production: acoustic and perceptual analyses." *Journal
of the Acoustical Society of America* 84(3), 917-928.

Stromberg, H. and Levitt, H. 1979. "Multiple linear regression analysis of errors of deaf
speeech." A paper presented at the Acoustical Society of America, Cambridge, MA.

Sundberg, J. 1977. "The acoustics of the singing voice." *Scientific American* 234, 82-91.

Sundberg, J., Ternstrom, S., Perkins, W. and Gramming, P. 1988. "Long-term average spectrum analysis of phonatory effects of noise and filtered auditory feedback." *Journal of Phonetics* 16, 203-219.

Takahashi, H. and Koike, Y. 1975. "Some perceptual dimensions and acoustic correlates of pathologic voices." *Acta Oto-Laryngologica Supplement* 338, 1-24.

Tardy-Mitzell, S., Andrews, M.L., and Bowman, S. 1985. "Acceptability and intelligibility of tracheoesophageal speech." *Archives of Otolaryngology* 111, 213-215.

Ternstrom, S. and Sundberg, J. 1984. Acoustical aspects of choir singing. *Acoustics for Choir and Orchestra*, ed. by S. Ternstrom, 12-22. Stockholm:Royal Swedish Academy of Music.

Tikofsky, R.S. 1970. "A revised list for the estimation of dysarthric single word intelligibility." *Journal of Speech and Hearing Research* 13, 59-64.

Tikofsky, R.S. and Tikofsky, R.P. 1964. "Intelligibility measures of dysarthric speech." *Journal of Speech and Hearing Research* 7, 325-333.

Till, J.A. and Toye, A.R. 1988. "Acoustic phonetic effects of two types of verbal feedback in dysarthric subjects." *Journal of Speech and Hearing Disorders* 53, 449-458.

Titze, I.R. 1984. "Parameterization of glottal area, glottal flow, and vocal fold contact area." *Journal of the Acoustical Society of America* 75, 570-580.

Tolhurst, G.C. 1949 "Audibility of the voiceless consonants as a function of intensity." *Journal of Speech and Hearing Disorders* 14, 210-215.

————. 1955. "The effect on intelligibility scores of specific instructions regarding talking" (USAM Report #NM001 064 01 35). Pensacola, FL: Naval Air Station.

————. 1957. "Effects of duration and articulation changes on intelligibility, word reception, and listener preference." *Journal of Speech and Hearing Disorders* 22, 328.

Trudgill, P. 1974. *The Social Differentiation of English in Norwich*. Cambridge: Cambridge University Press.

Trudeau, M.D. , Fox, R.A. and Fornataro, L.M. 1988. "Use of the tracheostoma valve in the marking of contrastive stress and sentence intonation." *Journal of Communication Disorders* 21, 21-31.

Turner, James Clifford. 1977. *Voice and Speech in the Theatre*. (3rd revised ed. by Malcolm Morrison. London: Pittman, Ltd.

Turner, C.W. and Robb, M.P. 1987. "Audibility and recognition of stop consonants in normal and hearing-impaired subjects." *Journal of the Acoustical Society of America* 81, 1566-1573.

Voelker, C. 1938. "An experimental study of the comparative rate of utterance of deaf and normal hearing speakers." *American Annals of the Deaf* 83, 274-284.

Voiers, W.D. 1964. "Perceptual bases of speaker identity." *Journal of the Acoustical Society of America* 36, 1065-1073.

Weinberg, B. 1988. "Speech management in the alaryngeal patient." *Decision Making in Speech-Language Pathology*, ed. by D.E. Yoder and R.D. Kent, 148-149. Philadelphia: Decker.

Weinberg. B. and Bennett, S. 1973. "Acceptability ratings of normal, esophageal, and artificial larynx speech." *Journal of Speech and Hearing Research* 16, 608-615.

Weinberg, B., Horii, Y., Blom, E. and Singer, M. 1982. "Airway resistance during esophageal phonation." *Journal of Speech and Hearing Disorders* 47, 194-199.

Weismer, G. 1984. "Articulatory characteristics of Parkinsonian dysarthria." *The Dysarthrias: Physiology-Acoustic-Perception-Management.* ed. by M.R. McNeil, J.C. Rosenbek and A. Aronson, 101-130. San Diego: College Hill Press.

———. 1990. "Keynote Address" A paper presented at the Clinical Dysarthria Conference. January, San Antonio.

Weismer, G., Kent, R., Hodge, M. and Martin, R. 1989. "The acoustic signature for intelligibility test words." *Journal of the Acoustical Society of America.*

Williams, S.E. and Watson, J.B. 1985. "Differences in speaking proficiencies in three laryngectomee groups." *Archives of Otolaryngology* 111, 216-219.

Yorkston, K. 1988. "Prosody in the adult." *Decision Making in Speech-Language Pathology*, ed. by D.E. Yoder and R.D. Kent, 140-143. Philadelphia: Decker.

Yorkston, K.M. and Beukelman, D.R. 1978. "A comparison of techniques for measuring intelligibility of dysarthric speech." *Journal of Communication Disorders* 11, 499-512.

———. 1981a. "Ataxic dysarthria: treatment sequences based on intelligibility and prosodic considerations" *Journal of Speech and Hearing Disorders* 46, 398-404.

———. 1981b. *Assessment of Intelligibility of Dysarthric Speech* C.C. Publications: Tigard, OR.

Yorkston. K.M., Beukelman, D.R. and Bell, K.R. 1988. *Clinical Management of Dysarthric Speakers.* Boston: Little, Brown and Company.

Yorkston, K, Beukelman, D., Minifie, F. and Sapir, S. 1984. "Assessment of stress patterning." *The Dysarthrias:physiology, Acoustics, Perception, Management*, ed. by M. McNeil, J. Rosenbek and A. Aronson, 131-162. San Diego: College-Hill Press.

Yumoto, E., Gould, W. and Baer, T. 1982. "Harmonics-to-noise ratio as an index of the degree of hoarseness." *Journal of Acoustical Society of America* 71, 1544-1550.

Youdelman,K., MacEachron, M. and McGarr, N.S. 1989. "Using visual and tactile sensory aids to remediate monotone voices in hearing-impaired speakers." *The Volta Review* 91(4), 197-208.

Chapter 5

The intelligibility of English vowels spoken by British and Dutch talkers

James Emil Flege
University of Alabama at Birmingham

1. Introduction

Intelligibility testing first began as a means for evaluating the effectiveness of communication devices such as telephones (Fletcher and Steinberg 1929). It was later used as a way to assess the articulatory effectiveness of talkers (Black, 1976) and speech synthesizers (Green, Logan, and Pisoni, 1986; Logan, Green and Pisoni, 1989). In more recent years, the role of the listener in assuring the effective transmission of messages via speech has been recognized (e.g. Rubin, 1983; Pisoni, Nusbaum and Green, 1985). The chapter presents a model of second language (hereafter, L2) speech learning. The intelligibility of vowels spoken in a second (foreign) language is then examined. The results show that the phonetic relationship between vowels in the L2 and in the native language (L1) is an important determinant of the intelligibility of L2 vowels. It is also shown that vowels differ inherently in intelligibility, and that the native dialect of the listener plays a role in determining the intelligibility of vowels spoken in an L2.

1.1 *Establishing a phonetic inventory*

Young children just beginning to learn speech must discover which classes of phones (hereafter, *sounds*) in their L1 are contrastive. They must also learn how to articulate sounds according to the phonetic norms of their L1. For example, a native French child must learn to produce /t/ as a voiceless unaspirated stop with a dental place of tongue contact ([t̪]) whereas a native English child must learn to produce /t/ as a voiceless *aspirated* stop with an alveolar place of constriction ([tʰ]).

Mastery of many sounds requires a period of skill acquisition. Although children may misarticulate certain L1 sounds for a time, most sounds are eventually mastered once learning has run its full course. One important characteristic of L1 acquisition is so obvious that it is seldom noticed: although they may misarticulate their L1, children never seem to speak it with a foreign accent. This is because foreign accent does not derive primarily from insufficient learning, but from the inappropriate use of sounds developed for one language in speaking another.

When attempting a sound that does not occur in the L1, L2 learners — at least relatively inexperienced ones — often substitute the nearest L1 sound. For example, a Spanish speaker is likely to produce the English word *beat* with a Spanish /i/. Spanish and English both have an /i/, but Spanish /i/ is produced with a slightly lower tongue position than English /i/ (Flege, 1989b). Many Spanish speakers of English, even those who are highly experienced in English, seem to use a Spanish /i/ in English words (Flege, 1991b). To take another example, a German may produce English *bat* with an [ɛ]-quality vowel because German has no /æ/ (Bohn and Flege, 1991).

Nearly all L2 speech errors involve sounds which either do not exist in the L1, or differ from their L1 counterpart (James, 1984, 1985a). For example, Flege and Hillenbrand (1984) found that adult native French speakers of English produced English /t/ with voice onset time (VOT) values that were intermediate to the phonetic norms of French and English for voiceless stops, defined in part by the mean short-lag VOT values measured in /t/s produced by French monolinguals and the long-lag VOT values observed for English monolinguals. Stops with "compromise" VOT values were also observed in L2 stops produced by adult native speakers of English who had learned French.

The nonauthentic production of L2 /t/s by the French and English subjects in the Flege and Hillenbrand (1984) study was probably *not* the result of an inability to detect auditorily the phonetic difference in how /t/ is implemented in French and English (Flege, 1984; see also Flege and Hammond, 1982). The L2 learners' ability to note at least some of the acoustic differences that distinguish the /t/s of French and English was demonstrated by the fact that both French and English subjects were able to modify /t/

partially when speaking their L2. This raises the question: Why did the L2 learners not modify their production sufficiently to permit an *authentic* production of the L2 /t/?

1.2 *The Sensitive period Hypothesis*

One explanation offered frequently for the unmodified substitution of L1 for L2 sounds, or for the partial modification just mentioned, is that a "sensitive period" exists for speech learning (see Snow, 1988 and Flege, 1987b). In a recent cross-sectional study examining the effect of age on L2 learning, Johnson and Newport (1989) found that second language learners' ability to learn L2 syntax begins to diminish gradually (or is used less) long before puberty. If the same phenomenon applies to speech learning, then one might suppose that young children learn to pronounce their L1 without accent because L1 learning occurs during early childhood, a time when speech learning ability is presumably at its height. By hypothesis, learning the sound system of an L2 after the sensitive period has passed will be less rapid and/or complete because speech learning ability has diminished or for some reason is only partially exploited.

The French and English subjects examined by Flege and Hillenbrand (1984) were living in an environment where L2 was the predominant language. They had used the L2 as their primary language for an average of 12 years, and appeared to be highly motivated to pronounce the L2 authentically. It is therefore unlikely that these subjects would ever approximate the phonetic norms of their L2 for /t/ more closely than they already had. This suggests that an upward limit exists for the learning of certain L2 sounds, and leads to the following sensitive period hypothesis:

> H1:   Adult L2 learners are less able than child L2 learners to translate into gesture, via the establishment of central sensorimotor representations, the auditory and visual stimulation that accompanies the production of L2 sounds not found in the L1.

By hypothesis, the French subjects examined by Flege and Hillenbrand (1984) were less able than young children learning English as an L1 to learn the pattern of glottal-supraglottal timing needed to implement /t/ as $[t^h]$. If one assumes that producing stops with short-lag VOT is somehow basic or unlearned (e.g., Kewley-Port and Preston, 1974) and thet all new learning is mediated by previous learning, then hypothesis could be reformulated as follows:

H2:   Adult L2 learners are less able than young children to *modify*
       existing (L1) pattern of speech production in order to produce
       L2 sounds authentically.

A sensitive period hypothesis is consistent with the belief that individuals who learn an L2 as young children often speak both of their languages without a foreign accent, whereas those who learn an L2 later in life typically speak it with a foreign accent (see Tahta, Wood and Loewenthal, 1981). For example, Flege (1988a) found that native English-speaking listeners gave significantly lower (i.e., more foreign accented) scores to English sentences spoken by Chinese subjects who learned English as adults than to sentences spoken by native speakers of English. Many have supposed that the offset of a sensitive period for speech occurs around the time of puberty, but another finding of the Flege (1988a) study suggested an earlier offset: Chinese subjects who began learning English L2 at an average age of eight years also produced English sentences with a detectable foreign accent.

The perception of foreign accent is based on many aspects of segmental and suprasegmental articulation. Acoustic analyses of speech sound production have also been consistent with a sensitive period hypothesis. Flege (1991) found that native Spanish children who began learning English as an L2 in a Texas school at about the age of 5-6 years of age were able to produce both English and Spanish /t/s authentically. These "Early L2 Learners" produced Spanish /t/ with appropriate short-lag VOT values, and English /t/ with appropriate long-lag VOT values. "Late L2 Learners" who began learning English L2 in adulthood, on the other hand, were unable to differentiate fully Spanish and English /t/. As in many previous L2 production studies, the Late L2 Learners produced English /t/ with "compromise" VOT values that were intermediate to the phonetic norms of Spanish and English.

2.   Purpose of the chapter

A sensitive period hypothesis seems to account for the well-known phenomenon of foreign accent, but there are several problems with it, at least as just formulated. For example, a sensitive period hypothesis provides no explanation for why the French speakers of English examined by Flege and Hillenbrand (1984) only *partially* approximated the English phonetic norm for /t/. Why should it be any easier to modify laryngeal timing to give the approximately 20-ms increase in VOT that was observed than to learn a modification that would give the approximately 40-ms increase needed to achieve the long-lag phonetic norm of English? The same thing can be asked of the native English learners, whose learning task was to shorten VOT, that is, to produce French /t/ with short-lag VOT rather then the accustomed long-lag VOT values.[1] Nor does a sensitive period hypothesis offer any insight into what specific speech learning mechanisms or processes are changed or attenuated as humans mature physiologically and develop cognitively.

The speech production data now available make it appear likely that previous L1 learning affects subsequent L2 learning through the intermediary of central cognitive-linguistic and phonetic structures more abstract than the sensorimotor level implied by a sensitive period hypothesis. Therefore, the present chapter has two major purposes: (1) to definiate a speech learning model (henceforth SLM) that attempts to describe the mechanisms and processes by which L1 phonetic interference affects the production of L2 vowels and consonants and account for age-related differences in the learning of sounds in an L2; and (2) to present the results of a vowel production study that provided a preliminary test of the model.

Most empirical L2 research has focussed on consonants, especially the VOT dimension in word-initial stops. The study presented in this chapter will test the SLM by examining the production of six English vowels (/i,æ,ɑ,u,I,ʌ/) spoken by 50 Dutch university students who began learning English in school at about the age of 12 years. Flege and Eefting (1987) previously obtained assessments of the degree of foreign accent in English sentences spoken by the Dutch subjects. As predicted by a sensitive period hypothesis, all 50 had detectable foreign accents even though many were majoring in English and had frequent access to native speakers of English at school or during trips to England. The Dutch subjects' success in learning English vowels was assessed by determining how often each of the six vowels was identified by native English-speaking listeners.

As noted by Leather (1983: 210), one general problem in testing speech learning hypotheses is that auditory perceptual judgments, even those of trained observers, are likely to be unacceptably inconsistent unless measures are taken to reduce measurement error. Thus some of the many factors (other than articulation) that can influence vowel intelligibility will be considered briefly below before turning to specific predictions of the SLM.

Development of the SLM was initially prompted by the observation that, in general, sensorimotor skills increase through childhood and the adolescent years. A number of studies have shown that the ability to imitate sounds not found in the L1 increases with age (Politzer and Weiss, 1969; Olson and Samuels, 1973; Snow and Hoefnagel-Höhle, 1982a; Ekstrand 1982). Why then, should speech learning ability decline with age? The SLM attempts to account for the psycholinguistic and phonetic processes that underlie speech learning. The SLM is in accord with the general principle that sensitive periods are generally centered around the period when learning takes place most rapidly, and that stable systems are less susceptible to change than rapidly evolving ones (Bornstein, 1987).[2]

One important hypothesis generated by the SLM is that the phonetic categories needed to produce and perceive L2 sounds rapidly and accurately in conversational speech can be established readily until about the age of 5-6 years, when the phonetic system begins to stabilize. After that age, additional categories can be established for "new" but not "similar" L2 sounds. Although both new and similar (but not "identical") L2 sounds differ acoustically from sounds in the L2, there is thought to be a qualitative as well as a quantitative difference in the degree of phonetic dissimilarity between new and similar sounds and sounds found in the L1. A new L2 sound is defined as an L2 sound that differs sufficiently from any sound in L1 that it evades the effects of equivalence classification, a basic cognitive mechanism thought to shape both L1 and L2 speech learning. The distinction between new and similar sounds, which remains elusive, will be described further below.

The SLM assumes a continuity in the mechanisms used to acquire the L1 and to learn an L2 later in life. It posits that speech learning does not necessarily end when the L1 has been "mastered" because humans continues to learn phonetically whenever they are required to communicate via a phonetic system that differs systemmatically from the one(s) they have used previously. More specifically, the SLM hypothesizes that the phonetic system may evolve over the lifespan to permit the addition of phonetic categories for new L2 sounds that occupy a portion of the phonetic space that has not been exploited previously; and the model posits the updating of any existing phonetic category so that it may better reflect the acoustic substance of the wide array of phones in L1 and L2 that have been identified as

realizations of it. The SLM also hypothesizes that changes in motoric processes are possible following perceptual modifications: additional phonetic
realization rules may be developed to output new and modified phonetic
categories.

The SLM, as formulated below, leads to the prediction that the Dutch
subjects would be more successful in learning new than similar English
vowels. However, before predictions generated by the SLM are discussed,
assumptions about the nature of vowel production and perception will first
be presented and the current procedures used to classify L2 vowels as similar and new (or as "identical") described.

2.1 Speech production and perception

Williams and Nottebohm (1985) identified direct links between motor output and auditory input for male zebra finches, an avian species which com-
pletes song learning about 90 days after hatching and shows no changes in
song thereafter, even after deafening. Echoing the "motor theory" of
speech perception, the authors concluded that conspecific sounds may be
decoded "by reference to the vocal gestures used to produce them" (p.
279). Unfortunately, the linkage between vocal production and perception
in less well understood in humans than in birds. It is uncertain how best to
account for the observation that, in infancy, the effect of the surrounding
linguistic environment begins to influence perception before it influences
production (Jusczyk, 1989), or why young children are often able to comprehend words more accurately than they can produce them. Divergences
in productive and perceptual abilities has suggested to some the existence
of separate lexicons for production and perception (Menn, 1982), and to
others (e.g., Matthei, 1989) a single lexicon with separate productive and
perceptual access routes to abstract linguistic information.

The SLM hypothesizes that speech production and perception are both
organized at three sequential levels. A consideration of the speech of adult
monolinguals suggests that a broad correspondence exists between production and perception at the three levels, especially at the most abstract,
phonemic, level. However, the structures that regulate the encoding and
decoding of the phonic elements needed for aural-oral communication may
not be isomorphic in adult L2 learners. This was shown recently by the finding that Chinese speakers who themselves produced English with a foreign
accent were as able as native English speakers to differentiate native from

Chinese-produced sentences (Flege, 1988a). The assumption is made, as is common in both L1 and L2 research (e.g., Gottfried and Beddor, 1988: 72), that changes in perception are generally a necessary but not a sufficient condition for corresponding changes in speech production.

2.1.1 *Speech production*

Speech production is conceptualized as being organized at three levels: a phonemic level, a somewhat less abstract phonetic category level, and a sensorimotor level. As described by Keating (1984), phonemes are implemented by a finite set of universal phonetic categories which, in turn, are physically output through learned language-specific realization rules. Relatively little empirical research has focussed on the process of phonetic category formation or the evolution of phonetic categories. This is surprising because phonetic categories represent an essential interface between the abstract phonemic level, at which words are specified in the mental lexicon, and the sensorimotor representations used to articulate speech.

Results obtained by Flege and Eefting (1988) suggested that Spanish-English bilinguals may have two phonetic categories for implementing the phoneme /t/, one for producing voiceless unaspirated stop [t̪]s in Spanish and one for producing voiceless aspirated [tʰ]s in English. The subjects imitated a VOT continuum ranging from /da/ to /ta/ that contained stops with lead, short-lag, and long-lag VOT values. The Spanish and English monolingual subjects produced stops with VOT values in only two of the three modal VOT ranges whereas native Spanish subjects who had learned English by the age of 5-6 years (Early L2 Learners) produced stops with VOT values in *all three* modal ranges.

In a previous study (Flege and Eefting, 1987b) these same subjects had identified the members of the VOT continuum in a two-alternative forced-choice test. The phoneme boundaries derived from that study coincided with the location along the continuum where VOT values in the vocal imitation responses shifted between modal VOT categories (i.e., from lead to short-lag, and from short-lag to long-lag). The identification data suggested that both the monolingual and bilingual subjects possessed two phonological categories (viz. /t/ and /d/), whereas the imitation data suggested that the bilinguals had *three* phonetic categories. One might conclude from these results that Early L2 Learners possess an enriched phonetic system containing phonetic categories from both the L1 and the L2, which may explain why early childhood bilinguals seem to produce both of their languages without a detectable accent rather than manifesting an accent in the less dominant language (McLaughlin, 1978, 1984; Mack, 1989).

Studies examining the L2 production of Late L2 Learners have shown that they may produce /p,t,k/ in the L2 with "compromise" VOT values. Flege (1991a) found, for example, that Spanish Late L2 Learners produced /t/ with significantly longer VOT values in English than Spanish, but nevertheless differed significantly from native English speakers. By hypothesis (see below), the Late L2 Learners had not established a phonetic category for English /t/; they succeeded in partially differentiating /t/ in Spanish and English through the use of a phonetic realization rule.

Realization rules specify the timing, amplitude, and duration of muscle contractions that position the speech articulators in space and time (e.g. Chomsky and Halle, 1968; Lieberman, 1970; Ladefoged, 1975, 1980, 1983). The need for realization rules in a model of speech production is suggested by the existence of small but systematic acoustic differences that may distinguish corresponding sounds in two languages. For example, both Danish and English have phonemes implemented as voiceless aspirated stops. By hypothesis, the slightly longer VOT values observed for Danish than English /p,t,k/ (Christensen, 1984) result from the application of different language-specific realization rules of course, such differences might be accounted for by the existence of different language-specific (rather than universal) phonetic categories. However, an independent justification for realization rules is the need to account for differences in segmental articulation that result from rate changes, requests for clarification, or for changes in interlocutor. For example, Labov (1981) noted that monolingual native speakers of English systematically altered their production of English /u/ by fronting this vowel in certain speaking situations.

An important determinant of intelligibility for speech produced by text-to-speech systems is the number and sophistication of realization rules which specify the parametric input to synthesis rules (Logan et al., 1989). In a way that parallels the development of speech perception and the refinement of text-to-speech systems, there is evidence that children learning their L1 add and/or refine realization rules gradually after discovering more basic means for implementing stop phonemes (e.g., Macken and Barton, 1980; Mack and Lieberman, 1985).

Within several years after the appearance of language, children can usually produce most sounds of their L1 recognizably. This implies that they have established phonetic categories with which to implement the

phonemes of their L1. Studies have shown that speech motor control continues to be refined for several years (e.g., Eguchi and Hirsh, 1969; Smith
1977). Other studies have shown that children's production changes gradually so that their speech conforms ever more closely to the phonetic norms
of their L1 (e.g., Zlatin and Koenigsknecht, 1976; Mack and Lieberman,
1985; Flege, McCutcheon, and Smith, 1987; Flege, 1988c), probably as the
result of changes in realization rules. It is assumed here that adults remain
able to add or refine phonetic realization rules.

2.1.2 *Speech perception*

The perceptual processing of speech is conceptualized as occurring at three
levels of organization: phonemic, phonetic, and auditory.

The auditory level of analysis is earliest both in terms of ontogeny and
on-line processing. Infants are able to discriminate most, if not all, of the
phonetic contrasts exploited by human languages. They do so on the basis
of innate auditory abilities in much the same way that macaques, for example, can discriminate between stops differing in place of articulation (Kuhl
and Paden, 1983) or vervets can discriminate vowels (Sinnott, 1989).

Most but not all (e.g. Klatt, 1979) models of speech perception posit
that words are recognized through the intermediary of phonetic and/or
phonemic category representations. It appears that infants' early sensory-
based ability to discriminate speech sounds is modified once they begin to
process speech sounds phonetically. For example, Werker and Tees (1982,
1983, 1984a,b) found that 6 to 8-month-old infants being raised in an English-speaking environment could discriminate a phonetic contrast that
occurs in Hindi but not English (viz. a contrast between dental and retro-
flex /t/) whereas infants aged 10 to 12 months could not.[3]

The maintenance of an ability to discriminate some but not all of a
"universal" set of potential phonetic contrasts (Werker, 1986; see also
Jusczyk, 1986) suggests that infants soon acquire at least some knowledge
of the segmental phonetic inventory of the language spoken around them.
A recent study using a headturn preference procedure (Jusczyk, Friederici
and Wessels, 1989) supports this view. Nine-month old infants from an
English environment looked longer at a loudspeaker emitting English
words than at another loudspeaker emitting Dutch words. The preference
for words from the ambient language was not evident in six month-old
infants, nor was it evident in the nine-month-old infants when the segmental information was removed by low-pass filtering.

Werker (1986) suggested that infants will remain sensitive only to those phonetic differences that have "phonemic significance" in the ambient language after their auditory processing of speech is "reorganized" at around 12 months of age. This reorganization, which Werker and others regard as stemming from reversible attentional processes, depends on infants' ability to note the phonetic similarity present in a class of acoustically different phones. Kuhl (1979) found that infants could ignore nondistinctive acoustic differences in vowels such as pitch contour and information pertaining to the talker's gender. Hillenbrand (1983, 1984) showed that infants could "sort" consonants into phonetically relevant categories.

Near the end of the first year of life, then, it appears that infants begin to organize disparate sound elements found in the ambient language into what might be termed phonetically-relevant categories. Data reported by Greiser (1984; Greiser and Kuhl, 1989) suggested that infants and native-English adults may possess similar prototypes for /i/. This raises the possibility that certain early-appearing phonetic categories may be "natural" categories, like focal colors (Rosch, 1975; Bornstein, 1975). However, given the wide range of sounds that occur in human languages, at least some phonetic categories are likely to be influenced by experience with specific varieties of speech.

Aslin and Pisoni (1980) hypothesized that children may "tune" innate auditory processes as the result of language-specific experience. Jusczyk (1989) suggested that attentional allocation is modified by learning, which may alter the weight given to various acoustic properties in the speech signal. The resulting "interpretative schemes", which may develop through "innately guided" learning processes, are optimally suited for the rapid processing of phones found in the L1.

In most instances, listeners consciously perceive phones in terms of *phonemic* categories established as the result of previous perceptual learning (Gibson, 1969). English-speaking listeners, for example, ordinarily disregard the acoustic difference between the realizations of /t/ in words like *tab* and *bat* because they have learned that the audible acoustic differences between /t/s that are released and aspirated as opposed to those which are unaspirated and (often) unreleased are not used to signal differences in meaning in English. Although the [tʰ] and [t] allophones of /t/ are phonetically different, they are perceived to be the "same" at the most abstract — and conscious — level of categorization. Another way of stating this is to say that native speakers of English possess phonological knowledge that English words cannot be distinguished by a [tʰ] vs. [t] difference.

Even though [tʰ] and [t] phones are phonologically the same for native speakers of English, they may be processed perceptually using different phonetic categories. A recent study (Flege, 1989a; Flege and Wang, 1990) examined the identification of the contrast between English word-final /d/ and /t/ by Chinese subjects. The L1s of these subjects possess a contrast between a voiceless unaspirated /d/ and a voiceless aspirated /t/ in word-initial position, but no Chinese languages has a stop voicing contrast in the final position of words. Both Chinese and native English listeners identified word-final English /t/ and /d/ tokens at high rates. However, when release bursts were removed, only the Chinese listeners showed a significant decrease in performance. This suggested that the Chinese but not the native English subjects were using phonetic categories established for word-initial /t/s and /d/s to identify stops in word-*final* position. This strategy worked well for word-final stops with bursts but not for those without bursts, which had to be identified on the basis of cues not used to distinguish voiced from voiceless stops in word-initial position e.g., preceding vowel duration.

2.1.3 *Phonetic perception*

Werker and her colleagues have provided experimental evidence for an optional phonetic level of processing that is distinct from either a phonemic or auditory level (Werker and Logan, 1985; see also Repp, 1981). Other indirect evidence exists for a phonetic level. For example, Koreans who learn English are much more sensitive than native English speakers to the phonetic difference between released and unreleased tokens of word-final /p,t,k/ in English because the presence versus absence of release bursts underlies a phonemic contrast in their L1 (Robson, 1982). However, it is quite easy to make this phonetic difference accessible to English speakers. One has only to direct their attention to it. If listeners did not have access to a phonetic level of representation under certain circumstances it would be difficult to understand how, for example, native speakers of English can detect the subphonemic difference between [tʰ] and [t] realizations of /t/ in standard and Spanish-accented English (Flege and Hammond, 1982). It would also be difficult to explain how adult listeners learn to discriminate certain nonnative phonetic contrasts, such as the contrast between Hindi unvoiced and breathy voiced dental stops (Werker and Tees, 1983), or how listeners may detect socially or stylistically conditioned variations in the realization of an L1 phoneme.

As noted earlier, listeners' conscious perception of sounds normally occurs at a phonemic rather than a phonetic level. However, it does not appear that phonemic-level processing is obligatory, or takes precedence over phonetic processing in the same way that phonetic-level processing takes precedence over auditory processing of speech (Repp, Healy, and Crowder, 1979). The nature of the processing task is likely to influence whether a phonemic or phonetic mode is engaged. For example, even though consonant perception is often described as "categorical", within-category discrimination can occur, especially when inter-stimulus intervals are short and the testing paradigm employed minimizes response uncertainty (Carney, Widin, and Viemeister, 1977).

The instructions given to listeners in a speech perception experiment may determine whether they engage an auditory or a phonetic mode of processing (e.g. Repp, 1981; Remez, Rubin, Pisoni, and Carrell, 1981). So too, listeners can be induced to process stimuli in a phonetic rather than *phonemic* mode. Native speakers of English are accustomed to hearing only voiced and voiceless stop phonemes because English possesses only two phonemic stop series. A study by Pisoni, Aslin, Perey and Hennessey (1982) showed, however, that native English subjects could be trained to partition into three categories the members of a synthetic continuum encompassing stops with lead, short-lag, and long-lag VOT values that would normally be divided into voiced vs. voiceless phonemic categories. The conditions under which access to a phonetic level of representation occurs may vary from listener to listener. They may also vary according to the nature of the listening task, the nature of the stimuli (Logan, Lively, and Pisoni, 1989), and the nature of the phonetic contrast. "Robust" phonetic contrasts that are not found in the listener's L1 but that occur in many other human languages may be more easily accessible than "fragile" ones (Burnham, 1986).

According to the SLM, phonetic-level perception is mediated by phonetic category "prototypes" which specify the ideal weighting of a set of independent and continuously varying properties that define each phonetic category (e.g. Repp, 1976; Oden and Massaro, 1978; Massaro and Oden, 1980; Massaro and Cohen, 1983, 1984; Samuel, 1977, 1982).[4] Phonetic categories for vowels may specify duration and the patterns of movements to and from "target" formant frequencies. The prototype may be defined as possessing all of the properties associated with a category, each to the largest degree possible. To be identified correctly, an individual token need not possess all properties, nor must the properties represented be present to the maximum degree possible. For example, a prototypical /i/ may be longer than a prototypical /I/ (Bennett, 1968), but a relatively short [i]-quality vowel may nevertheless be identified as an instance of /i/.

Phonetic category prototypes may evolve so as enable the litener to process the phones of a particular language effectively. By hypothesis, it is with reference to a prototype that listeners determine how a vowel "ought" to sound in a particular context (see Linell, 1982). Also by hypothesis, it is the existence of a tolerance region around each prototype which enables the listener to detect divergences from phonetic norms either as "distortions" (for children or adults with speech defects) or as "foreignness" (in nonnative speakers).

The tolerance region may be greater around vowel than consonant prototypes (Hudgins and Numbers, 1942), perhaps because vowels can vary continuously. However, relatively little work has focussed on defining the range of auditorily acceptable variants for either vowels or consonants.

Phonetic category prototypes seem to evolve as a function of phonetic input even after they have been established and tuned during L1 acquisition (see, e.g., Flege and Eefting, 1986). It appears that the ability to detect foreign accent increases with age (Scovel, 1981). Perhaps listeners become better able to gauge the degree of divergence of particular phones from prototypes as the prototypes defining the "center" of phonetic categories become better defined as the result of experience with an increasingly wide range of variants. Although little work has focussed on second dialect learning, it is my impression that vowels in another dialect of one's native language sound less accented as a function of experience with the new dialect.

2.2 Perceiving L2 sounds

A large cognitive learning task still awaits the child acquiring L1 phonology after phonetic categories are established and methodsare found for-implementing them. Children must discern what are the *phonemic* categories of their L1 (Ferguson, 1986). In keeping with a linguistic approach to speech analysis, Jusczyk (1989) noted that even after children have arrived at a correct description of the phonetic categories in their L1, they still face an additional "mapping problem" that involves relating phonetic categories to the phonological categories of the L1. For native English children this involves, among other things, learning that [tʰ] and [t] are context-conditioned allophonic variants of /t/ that occur in initial pre-stressed and final post-stressed positions, respectively. Another part of the process of phonological learning is acquiring systematic knowledge of what pattern of sound *sequences* are permissible in the L1.

Oller and Eilers (1983) found that children just beginning to acquire the phonology of their L1 appear to be better able to discriminate phones that are phonemically contrastive in their L1 than phones which are not. However, the phoneme learning task may be complicated in instances where a phonemic category is implemented by more than one phonetic category. For example, the phoneme /t/ may be implemented as an unaspirated stop or flap in post-stressed intervocalic position. It may be implemented as a lingual stop (usually unreleased) in word-final position, or as a glottal stop. Jusczyk (1985) suggested that variants in complementary distribution (e.g., initial [tʰ] and final [t]) will not be associated in a single phonemic unit until children learn to read.

The learned strategy of focussing attention only on those aspects of sounds needed for phonemic contrasts also seems to characterize the perception of L2 sounds by adults. Most researchers who have examined the production of L2 sounds have recognized the fundamental importance of the L2 learner's attempt to match or find correspondences between phonic elements in L1 and L2 (e.g., Weinreich, 1953; Briere, 1966; Wode, 1977, 1978; see also Best et al., 1988). Trubetzkoy (1939/1969) hypothesized that the phonology of L1 causes L2 learners to "filter out" acoustic differences that are not phonemically relevant in L1. This view has been restated over the years by many students of L2 learning (e.g., Borden, Gerber, and Millsark, 1983). For example, it is widely agreed that Japanese speakers confuse English /r/ and /l/ perceptually because the phones used to realize these phonemes are not contrastive in Japanese. Logan et al. (1989) observed that learning such a nonnative contrast may be difficult because children's perceptual sensitivity to speech changes as the result of experience so that only those phonetic contrasts that "denote differences in meaning remain distinctive" (p. 3). This suggests filtering at a phonemic level, whereas the view taken here is that such filtering actually takes place at a *phonetic* level of processing.

A classic view of perceptual development is that children become increasingly less reliant on sensory information as they develop cognitively (Gibson, 1969). Bruner (1964) suggested three major stages: an enactive stage, with its reliance on motoric codes; an iconic stage, where reliance shifts to sensory or perceptual codes; and finally a symbolic stage. Bruner (see also Inhelder and Piaget, 1969) suggested that, as children mature, they rely less on the common features which identify specific exemplars as belonging to a category and more on higher order, superordinate, categories in the hierarchy. In keeping with this, the SLM posits that the difficulty adults may have in producing similar L2 sounds authentically is the result of the general cognitive mechanism of equivalence classification.

When asked to imitate an ensemble of familiar and "alien" (i.e., non-L1) synthetic vowels, both children and adults tend to respond with familiar, L1 vowels (Kent and Forner, 1979). Moreover, token-to-token variability in F_2 frequency is less for L1 than non-L1 vowels (but cf. Kent, 1974). These imitation data point to the common tendency of listeners to identify vowels in terms of previously established (i.e. L1) categories. Not surprising, researchers have noted that during L2 learning there is a tendency for sounds in the L1 to exert a "gravitational attraction" (Schouten, 1975) or "assimilatory" pull (Best et al., 1988) on L2 sounds. This phenomenon is referred to here as equivalence classification.

Equivalence classification is important for speech learning because it permits listeners to make perceptual groupings of a wide variety of disparate phones with a common communicative function. This basic mechanism, which is evident even in prelinguistic infants (e.g., Kuhl, 1979; Hillenbrand, 1983, 1984), permits humans to perceive constant categories in the face of variability found in the many physical exemplars which may instantiate a category. Without equivalence classification it would be impossible, for example, for talkers to use the word *chair* correctly in identifying the many physical exemplars of this furniture type.

The role of equivalence classification in speech development seems to find a broad parallel in cognitive development. Children and adults use somewhat different strategies to categorize word, picture, or object arrays (e.g., Anglin, 1977; Bruner et al., 1966; Nelson, 1974). If the development of phonetic category prototypes follows the same general course as concept formation, we would also expect to see an evolution in phonetic perception as children develop. Equivalence classification may underlie the child's ability to produce L1 phones authentically, but it may also be responsible for L2 learners' foreign accent.

The SLM predicts that Late L2 Learners will be less successful in learning similar L2 sounds than Early L2 Learners because they equate similar

L2 sounds with sounds in the L1. This may happen even though similar L2 sounds differ acoustically — and audibly in some testing circumstances — from the corresponding L1 sound.

Although it is uncertain why young children should treat similar L2 sounds differently than older L2 learners, one potential basis for the hypothesized difference is that adults and older children may make greater use of higher-order syntactic and semantic information than young children. Auditory-acoustic processing of the speech signal might be terminated prematurely in adults and older children as the result of the relatively rapid recognition of words brought about by greater (or earlier) use of higher order information in parallel with bottom-up phonetic information.

Another possibility is that a difference between young and older L2 learners occurs because of the *state of development* of phonetic categories at the time L2 learning commences. As children encounter an increasingly wide range of phonetic category realizations, they may become increasingly better able to identify sounds in non-ideal listening conditions because the tolerance limits of the category expand. Although such a development could be regarded as highly adaptive as far as processing of the L1 is concerned, it would make it harder to note phonetic differences between similar L1 and L2 sounds. For example, a native Spanish 5-year-old may be better able to note the acoustic phonetic difference between [t̪] and [tʰ] phones used to realize /t/ in Spanish and English than a native Spanish adult. At the same time, the center of each category center may become better defined. This may make it easier for children as they grow older to detect distortions and to gauge degree of foreign accent (see Flege, 1988a).

Jusczyk (1989) noted that trying to assign meaning is an important factor in encouraging a child to attend to "similarities and differences that exist in the acoustic attributes" of the speech signal. As children's lexicons expand to include an ever larger number of minimally paired items, they may performer deeper and more abstract analyses of the acoustic signal, which may influence their readiness to recognize the existence of new phonetic groupings of sounds. For example, Burnham (1986) found that children with good comprehension abilities for their age were more likely to identify sounds in accordance with the phonemic categories of their L1, and to ignore phonetic contrasts that were not phonemically relevant in L1, than were children with relatively poor comprehension abilities.

An increasing tendency to equate similar L2 sounds with sounds in the L1 might be encouraged by greater phonemic awareness, which seems to increase at about the time children learn to read (Liberman, Shankweiler, Fisher, and Carter, 1974; Bradley and Bryant, 1983). It is still a matter of controversy as to whether an explicit awareness of phonemes arises from learning to read (Morais, Cary, Alegria, and Bertelson, 1979; Mann, 1986) or simply as the result of maturation (Kirtley, Bryant, MacLean, and Bradley, 1989). It is clear, however, that good readers have greater phonemic awareness than poor readers. That is, good readers generally have a greater (and earlier appearing) ability to segment sounds and syllables than poor readers (e.g., Liberman, Shankweiler, Fisher, Liberman, Shankweiler, Fisher, and Carter, 1974; Bradley and Bryant, 1983).

Mann (1984) noted a number of differences between good and poor readers that suggest differences in phonetic processing which, in turn, may be related to a propensity for equivalence classification. She noted that poor readers were less able to remember strings of nonsense words (but not faces or drawings) than good readers. Although both good and poor readers were less able to remember strings of letters that rhymed (e.g., "B", "D", "E") than strings that did not rhyme, the deleterious effect of rhyming was much smaller for poor than good readers in a recall experiment, and also in a study examining the vocal repetitions of sentences consisting of rhyming or non-rhyming words.

Mann (1984) noted that the segmental substitution errors made by poor readers when repeating word strings showed that they, like good readers, code speech phonetically. She was therefore led to conclude that poors readers' phonetic representations "decay more rapidly" or are "less well formed" (p. 8) than the phonetic representations of good readers. This was supported by a study examining the effect of noise on speech perception (Brady, Shankweiler, and Mann, 1983). High- and low-frequency words were equally intelligible for good and poor readers in ideal listening conditions, whereas poor readers made significantly more identification errors than good readers for words presented in noise. Mann (1984) concluded that good and poor readers differ in terms of how effectively they use phonetic representations to process speech.

The possibility exists that the just-noted reading ability differences between children are analogous to speech processing changes that occur in the ontogenetic development of all individuals; and that differences in phonetic categorization might distinguish individuals, although to a lesser degree, throughout their lifespans. van Balen (1980) found that high school students who received relatively high scores on a test of English listening proficiency tended also to receive high scores on a comparable test in Dutch. Greenberg and Roscoe (1988) used a list recall task to examine the phonetic coding of speech by students in first-year college foreign-language classes who differed in terms of L2 comprehension ability. A tone or word "suffix" was appended to a list of digits to be recalled. It was assumed that the presence of a word (but not tone) suffix would decrease ability to recall list-final digits more if recall was based more on "vulnerable" sensory information in echoic memory than on "stable, higher-order" phonetic codes. Students who were poor L2 comprehenders showed a significantly greater suffix effect than students with good comprehension ability, suggesting that the good comprehenders were more efficient in their phonetic coding.

Nonnatives comprehend speech more poorly in noise than native speakers (Florentine, 1985). This appears to be due at least in part to the fact that nonnatives' phonetic representations are less well suited for processing incoming L2 phones than native speakers'. Individuals who rapidly code L2 sounds in terms of existing categories, even if they differ substantially from L1 sounds, may succeed well in comprehending the L2, but at the cost of failing to recognize the phonetic differences that may distinguish sounds in L1 and L2.

Paradoxically, individuals who are skilled in comprehending L2 speech in noise, which has been regarded as a suitable index of overall proficiency in the L2 (e.g., Spolsky, Sigurd, Sako, Walker, and Atterbrun, 1968), may experience relatively great difficulty in learning L2 pronunciation because they rapidly and reliably code L2 sounds in terms of existing L1 categories. Lambert (1977) suggested that some L2 Learners ("code users") are likely to perceive an L2 sound which differs auditorily from sounds in the L1 in terms of L1 categories, whereas others ("code formers") tend to develop new central representations in such instances. Such differences might ultimately be used to account for why some adults profit more from auditory perceptual training on a novel phonetic contrast than others (e.g., Flege, 1989a; Flege and Wang, 1990).

The SLM differs from previous approaches in not regarding equivalence classification as performing a kind of affective, auditory, or phonological "filtering" of subphonemic acoustic differences between L1 and L2 sounds. By hypothesis, all audible acoustic differences between similar L1 and L2 sounds may influence the phonetic system, even those that are not accessible perceptually (that is, those that cannot be heard consciously because of previous perceptual learning). This can be illustrated by considering English voiceless stops from the standpoint of native speakers of French. Flege (1984) found that native French adults who were highly experienced in English produced English /t/ with significantly longer VOT values in English than in French, but with significantly *shorter* VOT values than native speakers of English. By hypothesis, they were prevented from producing English /t/ authentically because they had not established a long-lag stop category for English /t/. Their phonetic category prototype for /t/ had probably changed, however, because of the many English [tʰ] phones they had identified as /t/.

The hypothesis that already-established (L1) categories may evolve as a function of L2 experience in the direction of L2 sounds agrees with the observation by Obler and Albert (1978: 159) that bilinguals identify phonemes "without regard for language specific (acoustic) information" because their perceptual processing is "intermediate to that of...monolinguals". This may not be true for all L1 categories and all L2 sounds, however. An hypothesis of the SLM is that L1 categories will not be modified in an attempt to accommodate the learners need for producing and perceiving L2 sounds referred to as "new".

2.3 *The new vs. similar distinction*

The distinction between new and similar L2 sounds has been made before. For example, Delattre (1964, 1969) noted that some sounds in an L2 differ "radically" from any sound in the L1 and should be regarded as "new" from the standpoint of the L2 learner. Wode (1978: 114) noted that a major difference between child and adult learners of an L2 is "the state of development" of their phonological systems. In his view, both children and adults match phonic elements of the L2 to their L1 "grid". As the L2 is processed, the acoustic input is "scanned" and phones falling within some "crucial similarity range" are judged to be equivalent to an element of L1, and therefore substituted by it. Other phones falling outside a crucial (but undefined) range are judged to be non-equivalent, and will undergo "other developments" than simple substitution, according to Wode.

The SLM posits that the basis for a sensitive period is the increasing tendency by older children and adults to classify as similar sounds in the L2 that would be classified as *new* by young children. One might characterize L1 learning by young children as a "bottom-up" process of learning, whereas L2 learning by older children and adults might better be characterized as a "top-down" process (Mack, 1989). For children learning their L1, *all* sounds are new. The number of phonetic categories they will establish depends on the number of sounds (i.e. phone classes) encountered in the L1. For example, English-learning children will establish many more vowel categories than Spanish-learning children. Older children and adults who are learning an L2, on the other hand, have already established a phonetic system suitable for distinguishing a large and ever growing number of lexical items. The number of additional categories they establish will be limited by their previous phonetic learning via the mechanism of equivalence classification.

2.4 *Phonetic norm*

Many studies of L1 speech learning, both those comparing groups in cross-sectional designs (e.g. Smith, 1977) or examining single subjects in detail in longitudinal designs (Mack and Lieberman, 1985), have assumed that children's speech evolves towards something referred to as a "phonetic norm". The L1 norm, which should probably be regarded as a heuristic for research rather than a reality, is typically defined as monolingual adults' mean values for various phonetic parameters of interest. The adults chosen to represent the norm that children are said to be approximating are typically drawn from the same community as the children being studied.

The concept of phonetic norm is also used frequently in studies of L2 speech learning as a benchmark for assessing the extent to which L2 learners have succeeded in producing L2 sounds, and as a starting point for assessing the phonetic distance between sounds in L1 and L2. Defining the L2 phonetic norm can be problematical. For example, Holden and Nearey (1986) raised the issue of how one is to chose among the "widely divergent dialects" of an L2 in defining the L2 phonetic norm.

If one is interested primarily in determining how successful learning has been, the L2 norm should probably be based on *all L2 speech* that has been processed meaningfully. For many L2 learners, this would include the speech of other nonnative speakers who speak the L2 with a foreign accent, and native speakers who are representative of various regional and social dialects in addition to those who use the standard or prestige dialect. The norm should also reflect the variations in L2 speech typical of varying levels of formality.

For a variety of practical and methodological reasons, the L2 norm has seldom if ever been defined in an ideal fashion. An additional methodological problem is the need to relate an *individual* L2 Learner's performance to that of a group of speakers of the L2 (i.e., the L2 norm). For example, a Spanish speaker whose typical realization of /i/ is an [I]-like vowel might have greater difficulty in learning English /I/ than a Spanish speaker who typically realizes /i/ as an [i]-quality phone. Holden and Nearey (1986) showed that which Russian vowel was identified with English /ʌ/ varied according to the dialect of the native Russian listener.

A particular listener's prototype for a vowel might be estimated by presenting a wide range of synthetic variants differing according to the acoustic features that distinguish adjacent vowel categories (see Holden and Nearey, 1986). The phonetic norm for a language could then be based on data obtained for representative native speakers of that language. However, this would be an enormous undertaking, even for a single subject, because of the number of combinatorial possibilities for the relevant acoustic parameters in vowels (e.g., duration, F_0, F_1-F_3 "target" frequencies and movement patterns).

Speech production and perception are related to one another, at least for individuals with stable phonetic systems. Because of this, the prototypes of a language might be estimated indirectly, through an examination of speech production. A simple (but not necessarily optimal) way of doing so is by plotting target formant frequency values at a single measurement point for individual tokens (or means for individual talkers) in an F_1-F_2 space (see e.g., Holtse, 1972). Motivation for this is provided by multidimensional scaling experiments which have shown that F_1 and F_2 are independent dimensions that account for most of the variance in spectral quality ratings for vowels in a relatively large vowel inventory (Pols, van der Kamp, and Plomp, 1969). The perceptual prototype can be estimated as the value found at the center of the area thus delimited.

When plotted in this way, the realizations of vowels adjacent to one another in the phonetic space often overlap (Peterson and Barney, 1952) suggesting that vowels may be confused perceptually if represented only by F_1 and F_2 (Carlson, Granström, and Fant, 1970; DiBenedetto, 1989). The majority of vowel tokens can nevertheless be classified correctly on the basis of the F_1 and F_2 frequency values by statistical procedures. The rate of correct classification can be increased by normalization, and increased further still by taking into account vowel duration and the pattern of dynamic formant movements in the first two formants (Assman et al, 1982; DiBenedetto, 1989; see also Miller, 1989 for three-dimensional plots).[6]

For the purposes of L2 research, a perceptual "tolerance region" for vowels in the L2 can be defined as some portion of the space defined by the vowels producted of native speakers, for example, a space encompassing a 95% confidence interval along the principal components of variation of F_1 and F_2. Other, correctly identifiable, tokens produced by nonnative talkers that are foreign-accented may fall outside the tolerance region defining a vowel category.

Practical considerations dictate that only a small number of native speakers can be examined to estimate the phonetic norms of the L1 and a target L2 being learned. This raises the important issue of deciding *which* native speakers (and which speaking style) should represent the phonetic norm. In most previous studies, the talkers chosen to represent L2 have been drawn from the community in which the L2 learners reside. The L1 norm has often been based on L2 learners' productions of their own native language, a practice that may bias results if learning the L2 has affected L1 production. The style examined in most L2 research is usually the maximally careful style elicited in formal production experiments, which may limit the generalizability of findings.

2.5 *The relationship of L2 and L1 sounds*

A useful method for characterizing the relationship between phonetic categories in L1 and L2 is to classify the L2 sounds as "new", "similar", or "identical". A three-way classification of L2 sounds is implicit or explicit in much L2 research (e.g., Brière, 1966). No universally-accepted method now exists for differentially classifying L2 sounds as new or similar. In attempting to operationalize the distinction, the most important question to consider is: When does an L1 versus L2 acoustic difference make a *phonetically relevant* difference?

To determine this, the SLM employs three criteria for classification. A preliminary step is to consider the IPA symbols used to represent the L1 and L2 sounds. This is followed by acoustic measurements and listeners' perceptual judgments of sounds in L1 and L2. The SLM posits that interlingual identification occurs at a phonetic rather than a phonemic level, so the procedures operate on sounds (that is, phonetically-relevant phone classes).

An *identical* L2 sound is a sound represented by the same IPA symbols used to represent a sound in the L1. When acoustic analyses are performed for representative native speakers, there is not a significant acoustic difference between corresponding L1 and L2 sounds. When a detailed perceptual analysis is performed, listeners cannot detect a difference between the L1 and L2 sounds. An identical L2 sound is usually produced authentically as the result of a process referred to as "positive transfer" (Weinreich, 1953). Identical sounds have therefore received little attention because most L2 speech errors involve similar and new sounds (James, 1984, 1985a). However, for consonants at least, positive transfer may not extend to new syllable positions. Recent research has shown that Chinese subjects have difficulty producing and perceiving a contrast between /t/ and /d/ in the final position of English words even though an English-like /t/-/d/ contrast occurs in the initial position of words in their L1 (Flege and Davidian, 1985; Flege et al, 1987; Flege, 1988c).

To be classified as either similar or new, some acoustic difference(s) between pairs of L1 and L2 sounds must exist, and there must be evidence that the sounds are auditorily discriminable. A "phonetic symbol" criterion might be used as a provisional measure because, at present, no well-accepted, objective metric exists for measuring the phonetic distance between sounds in two language. An L2 sound that is *similar* to a sound in L1 is represented by the same IPA symbol as the L1 sound, even though statistical analyses reveal significant — and audible — acoustic differences between the two.

For example, Flege (1987a) examined formant frequency values in French /i/ and English /i/, and also between the /u/s of French and English. Significant acoustic differences were obtained for both pairs of French-English vowels; and native English listeners were able to identify French vowels at significantly above-chance rates when asked to determine which member of a vowel pair had been spoken by a native French speaker. Both the acoustic and perceptual tests conformed to traditional phonetic descriptions of French /i/ and /u/ being more "peripheral" than their English counterparts.

An L2 sound that is *new* differs acoustically and perceptually from the sound(s) in L1 that most closely resembles it. But, unlike a similar sound, it is represented by an IPA symbol that is not used for any L1 sound. An example of a new sound from the standpoint of English is French /y/. This vowel sound differs acoustically and perceptually from the nearest possible vowels of English (/i/, /I/, and /u/), and is represented by a symbol not used traditionally in describing the vowels of English.

The phonetic symbol criterion has the advantage of making use of the expert phonetic classifications of researchers who have worked with the languages under consideration, but it is not without problems. The most obvious problem is that many phonetic transcription systems are now in use; and even seasoned researchers who are using the nominally same system don't always agree. For example, the distinction between the vowels in English words like *beat* and *bit* is sometimes represented as a distinction between /i/ and /I/, and sometimes as one between /i:/ and /i/. The latter symbolization, which emphasizes the duration difference that accompanies the spectral distinction between this tense-lax vowel pair, seems to be favored by analysts whose L1 makes important use of duration for phonemic distinctions.[7]

Thus it appears necessary to supplement the phonetic symbol test with additional acoustical criteria. Bohn and Flege (1991) suggested that an L2 vowel should be considered new only if most of its realizations occupy a portion of the acoustic phonetic vowel space that is unoccupied by the realizations of any L1 vowel. This implies that few of the vowels in an L2 will be new for learners whose L1 has a large vowel inventory. Perceptual tests might also be used to differentiate new and similar vowels.[8] Other behavioral measures of speech processing might also furnish a useful metric.[9]

2.6 *Applying the classification scheme*

Application of the criteria is illustrated in Figure 1(a-d) for four hypothetical languages. In these illustrations, the simplifying assumption is made that the languages possess only the small number of vowels shown, and that non-spectral dimensions such as duration, diphthongization or nasalization are not used contrastively.

Figure 1(a) represents an L1 with three vowel phonemes (/i/, /u/, /a/) and an L2 with four (/i/, /u/, /a/, /ɛ/). The vowel /i/ occupies approximately the same portion of the acoustic vowel space in L1 and L2; the L2 /i/ is classified as identical because the small and nonsignificant acoustic differences between it and the L1 /i/ are inaudible. The L2 /a/ is classified as identical for the same reasons. The L2 /u/, on the other hand, is classified as similar because it is realized as a slightly lower [u]-quality vowel (viz. [u$_T$]) than the L1 /u/, even though its major (and only) allophone is represented by the same symbol used for the major allophone of L1 /u/ (viz., /u/). The L2 /ɛ/

is classified as new because, in addition to differing acoustically and auditorily from adjacent L1 vowels, it is represented by a symbol not used for a major allophone for any of the L1 vowels.

Figure 1(b) illustrates how allophonic variation is to be handled. Once again, the L1 has three vowel phonemes (/i/, /u/, /a/) and the L2 has four (/i/, /u/, /a/, /ɛ/). However, in this instance one of the L1 vowel phonemes, /a/, has two allophonic variants ([ɛ], [a]) that are acoustically and auditorily indistinguishable from the major allophones used to implement the /ɛ/ and /a/ phonemes of L2. Since interlingual identification is hypothesized to occur at a phonetic category level, the L2 /ɛ/ and /a/ are classified as identical vowels.

As noted earlier, conscious speech perception normally occurs at a phonemic level, so the identity of the L1 and L2 vowels might not be apparent immediately. If so, a learner might produce an L2 word like /ba/ as [bɛ] in early stages of learning because /a/ is realized as [ɛ] in open syllables. The SLM predicts, however, that this phonemically-motivated substitution pattern will not persist because interlingual identification occurs at a phonetic category level. This leads to the expectation that learners will eventually use their [ɛ] and [a] phonetic categories to implement the L2 /ɛ/ and /a/ phonemes.

The allophonic relationship between the [ɛ] and [a] phones in the example just given can be regarded as learned "phonological" knowledge. Steensland (1981) found that, when Swedes were asked to identify Russian /e/ in terms of Swedish vowel categories, the Russian /e/ more closely approximated Swedish /ɛ/ than Swedish /e/ when it was produced in the context of palatal than plain consonants in Russian. These phonetically-conditioned differences in vowel height would presumably have been less obvious to native speakers of Russian had some means been found to test their perception. For example, Jaeger (1986) used the concept formation paradigm to show that native speakers of English group [kʰ] and [k] phones into a single /k/ phonemic category despite the fact that they differ audibly.

The claim that such phonological knowledge will not affect L2 production after an initial stage of learning may need to be restricted to vowels; Benson (1988) found that Vietnamese subjects had no difficulty producing consonants such as /p,t,k/ in the final position of English words except those containing the diphthong /aⁱ/. In this context final stops are not permitted in Vietnamese. The fact that the subjects honored L1 phonotactic constraints in English L2 suggests, indirectly, that they perceived the vowel in English

Figure 1(a-d). *Illustration of how vowels in four hypothetical L1-L2 pairs are classified using procedures outlined in the text.*

Figure 1a   F$_2$ Frequency in Mels

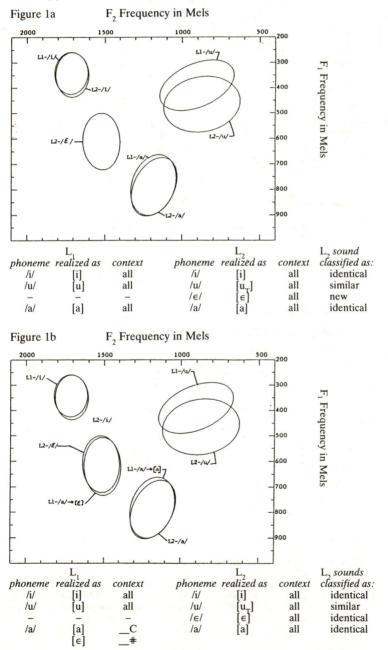

phoneme	L$_1$ realized as	context	phoneme	L$_2$ realized as	context	L$_2$ sound classified as:
/i/	[i]	all	/i/	[i]	all	identical
/u/	[u]	all	/u/	[u$_T$]	all	similar
–	–	–	/ɛ/	[ɛ]	all	new
/a/	[a]	all	/a/	[a]	all	identical

Figure 1b   F$_2$ Frequency in Mels

phoneme	L$_1$ realized as	context	phoneme	L$_2$ realized as	context	L$_2$ sounds classified as:
/i/	[i]	all	/i/	[i]	all	identical
/u/	[u]	all	/u/	[u$_T$]	all	similar
–	–	–	/ɛ/	[ɛ]	all	identical
/a/	[a]	_C	/a/	[a]	all	identical
	[ɛ]	_#				

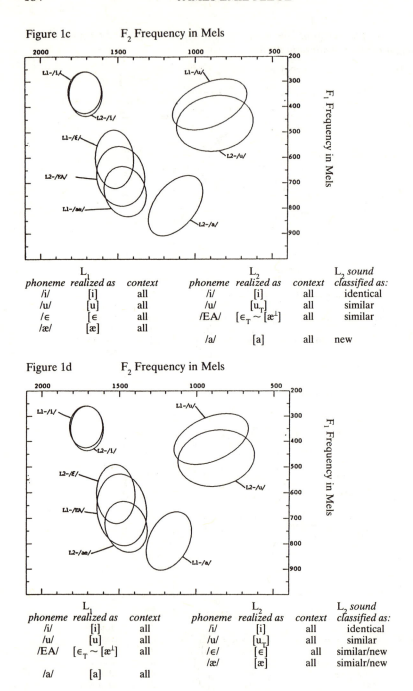

Figure 1c   F₂ Frequency in Mels

	L₁			L₂		L₂ sound
phoneme	realized as	context	phoneme	realized as	context	classified as:
/i/	[i]	all	/i/	[i]	all	identical
/u/	[u]	all	/u/	[u_T]	all	similar
/ɛ/	[ɛ]	all	/EA/	[ɛ_T ~ [æ⊥]	all	similar
/æ/	[æ]	all	/a/	[a]	all	new

Figure 1d   F₂ Frequency in Mels

	L₁			L₂		L₂ sound
phoneme	realized as	context	phoneme	realized as	context	classified as:
/i/	[i]	all	/i/	[i]	all	identical
/u/	[u]	all	/u/	[u_T]	all	similar
/EA/	[ɛ_T ~ [æ⊥]	all	/ɛ/	[ɛ]	all	similar/new
/a/	[a]	all	/æ/	[æ]	all	simialr/new

words such as *bite* as [aɪ], not as a related Vietnamese vowel that might have occurred in a consonant-final word (e.g. /ʌ/).

Figure 1(c) represents a kind of phonemic merger, that is, an instance in which the L1 has a phonemic contrast not found in the L2. The L2 phoneme is represented here as /EA/ because the wide range of phones used to realize it have (hypothetically) lead researchers to transcribe it as either /ɛ/ and /æ/. The simple substitution of an L1 /ɛ/ for the L2 /EA/ will sometimes result in correct identification by a native L2 listener, but sometimes it will not. Whether or not correct identification occurs will depend upon the nature of L2 listeners' prototypes for /EA/. So too, the simple substitution of an L1 /æ/ for /EA/ will sometimes but not always result in correct identification. The L2 /EA/ is classified as similar, but it is not obvious here whether it is similar to L1 /ɛ/ or to L1 /æ/. A post-hoc analysis of L2 production data could reveal this: A learner who substitutes L1 /ɛ/ is likely to have identified the L2 /EA/ with L1 /ɛ/, whereas the learner who substitutes L1 /æ/ probably identified /EA/ with L1 /æ/.

Finally, Figure 1(d) illustrates a kind of phonemic split, that is, an instance in which the L2 has a phonemic contrast not found in the L1. It underscores the point that the classification of L2 sounds must be made with reference to the individual speaker-hearer. The /ɛ/ and /æ/ phonemes of L2 are realized with phones that might be used to realize a single phoneme in L1, represented here as /EA/. The hypothetical L1 /EA/ is realized by a wide range of variants, [æ]-quality vowels by older talkers and [ɛ]-quality vowels by young talkers. A young native speaker of L1 who realizes /EA/ as [ɛ] and uses the L1 [ɛ] category to produce L2 /ɛ/ should be understood. For such an individual, the L2 /ɛ/ can be classified as an identical vowel if the learner's L1 [ɛ] realizations are judged to be "good" exemplars of L2 /ɛ/. The L2 /æ/ would necessarily be regarded as a new vowel. Just the opposite set of L1-L2 relationships would hold true for a hypothetical older talker who realized the L1 /EA/ as an [æ]-quality vowel.

3.   Predictions of the model

Early L2 learners are tentatively defined as individuals who begin learning the L2 by the age of 5-6 years; Late L2 learners are defined as those who begin learning their L2 later in life. The SLM posits that phonetic categories are needed for the authentic production of L2 sounds. By hypothesis, Early L2 Learners are able to establish phonetic categories for all L2 sounds not found in the L1, and so possess an enriched phonetic system which includes the phonetic categories possessed by monolingual speakers of both the L1 and the L2. This leads to the hypothesis that:

> H3: Early L2 learners will produce identical, similar, and new L2 sounds authentically if they have received sufficiant phonetic imput.

The SLM posits that Late L2 learners will differ from Early L2 Learners with respect to similar sounds but not identical or new sounds. This position diverges from the one taken by some (but not all) previous investigators. Stockwell and Bowen (1965) felt that the absence of an L2 sound in the L1 was the source of the greatest learning difficulty (see also Olson and Samuels, 1973), whereas the partial resemblance of an L2 sound to a sound in the L1 generally facilitates learning. Based on the results of a short-term training experiment, Brière (1966: 795) concluded that L2 sounds which are "close equivalents" of L1 sounds at either a phonemic or a phonetic (i.e., "allophonic") level will be "easier to learn" than L2 sounds without such equivalents. The position taken by Oller and Ziahosseiny (1970), on the other hand, was that L2 sounds that differ only minimally from sounds in the L1 are the most difficult to master.

There may be an element of truth to both positions. Snow and Hoefnagel-Höhle (1982) report that those Dutch sounds that showed relatively little improvement over 20 trials in a laboratory study evaluating imitation by native English adults and children showed a relatively great amount of improvement during a one-year period of naturalistic acquisition of Dutch in the Netherlands. L2 sounds with close equivalents in the L1 may be relatively easy to produce in the earliest stages of L2 learning whereas L2 sounds which are more dissimilar are relatively difficult because they require new gestures to be produced in an acceptable — or even an identifiable — fashion. Relatively greater success for similar than new sounds is what the SLM predicts for students in classroom learning situations where native speaker input is unavailable or limited; it might also be seen in early stages of naturalistic acquisition for learners who have native-speaker input. However, the SLM proposes that the reverse is true for later stages of naturalistic L2 learning.

The SLM posits that Late L2 Learners can establish phonetic categories for new L2 sounds whereas they can not do so for similar L2 sounds. Thus the SLM leads to a prediction that L2 learners will ultimately be more successful in producing L2 sounds authentically if they differ *substantially* from L1 sounds than if they differ *just a little.*

By hypothesis, Late L2 learners may at first identify new sounds with some sound(s) in the L1, but this will not persist because the new L2 sound will not be equated with an L1 sound. It is predicted that Late L2 learners will, given sufficient phonetic input, note the phonetic difference between the new L2 sound and any sound in L1, and that this will precipitate the establishment of a phonetic category for the new L2 sound. Once a realization rule has been developed with which to output the newly established L2 category, production of the L2 sound will be authentic.

In regards to the experiment to be presented below, experienced speakers of Dutch were expected to produce new English vowels more authentically than inexperienced ones. Equivalence classification is hypothesized to be the primary obstacle to effective speech learning beyond early childhood for similar sounds, but no such barrier should exist for new vowels. Thus the intelligibility of new vowels produced by experienced Dutch subjects should be as great as that for native speakers of English. This can be formalized as:

H4:   In early stages of learning, Late L2 learners may fail to produce a new L2 sound authentically, substituting one or more L1 sounds for it. However, experienced Late L2 learners will eventually develop phonetic categories for new L2 sounds and produce them authentically.

The SLM leads to a radically different expectation concerning Late L2 learners' production of *similar* L2 sounds. The SLM posits that Late L2 Learners continue to equate similar L2 sounds with a sound(s) in the L1 no matter *how long* they have spoken the L2 and now matter *how good* they are at learning languages:

By hypothesis, equivalence classification places an upper limit on the extent to which L2 learners can approximate the phonetic norms of L2 for similar vowels (Flege, 1981, 1984, 1988b; Flege and Hillenbrand, 1984) by preventing them from establishing a phonetic category for the similar L2 sound. So, for example, French ten-year-olds but not five-year-olds are expected to equate English [tʰ] and French [t] realizations of /t/. If so, then ten-year-old learners should at best phonetically approximate the VOT norm for English /t/ even though they are able to detect auditorily the acoustic difference between English and French /t/ realizations. They are expected to realize /t/ with longer VOT values in English than French, but this would result from the use of different realization rules, not from implementing the phoneme /t/ using two different phonetic categories.[10] This leads to the formalization of two additional hypotheses:

H5:   Late L2 learners will not produce similar L2 sounds authentically, no matter how experienced they are, because category formation is blocked by equivalence classification.

H6:   Experienced Late L2 learners will differ from inexperienced Late L2 learners to a greater extent for new L2 sounds (for which categories can be established) than for similar L2 sounds.

These hypotheses generate the prediction that Dutch subjects, even those with an excellent overall pronunciation of English, will continue to show phonetic interference in producing similar L2 sounds.

Determining the exact age at which L2 Learners are no longer likely to establish an additional phonetic categories for similar L2 sounds (i.e., the age of demarcation between Early vs. Late L2 Learners) will require additional research. It should be noted that the age proposed here, 5-6 years of age, differs greatly from the age proposed by Best et al., (1988). The authors suggested that by the age of 10-12 mos, infants begin categorizing sounds phonemically. As a result, they may lose the ability to discriminate two novel but phonetically distinct sounds classified as allophonic variants of an L1 phoneme. Two phonetically distinct sounds which are not "assimilated" to an L1 phoneme will remain discriminable even though neither occurs in the L1. This was the explanation given for why children being reared in an English-speaking environment, and English-speaking adults, remained able beyond the age of 10-12 months to discriminate Zulu clicks. According to Best et al., such non-assimilating (i.e., new) sounds may continue to be perceived in an auditory or phonetic (articulatory) mode.

4.   Vowel production data

Relatively few previous studies of L2 learning have provided data suitable for evaluating the SLM's predictions concerning vowel production. An /ɛ/-for-/æ/ substitution reported for Bulgarian-accented English by Danchev (1987) at first seems to contradict the SLM's predictions. Bulgarian is analyzed as having /ɛ/ and /ɑ/ phonemes but no /æ/ (Maddieson, 1984), leading one to think that /æ/ is a new vowel and will therefore be produced authenticaly by Bulgarians who are experienced in English. Danchev (1986) reported, however, that Bulgarians substitute their /ɛ/ (and, less frequently /ɑ/) for English /æ/. He noted that an /ɛ/-for-/æ/ substitution may be "consciously or unconsciously accepted" by native English listeners and Bulgarian teachers of English because of the acoustic overlap seen between /ɛ/ and /æ/ in British English (henceforth, BE).

The substitutions in Bulgarian-accented English probably do not represent a disproof of the prediction about new vowels, however. First, Danchev's (1986) observations were based on several sources of data which included spelling errors and loanword phonology as well as actual pronunciations by L2 learners. The L2 learners were high school and university students and individuals enrolled in intensive English classes who may not have fulfilled the condition of "sufficient native speaker input". English-learning children must receive several years of input before they succeed in producing /æ/ (Amastae, 1978; Mack and Lieberman, 1985; Pollock and Keiser, 1990), so there is no reason to expect Bularian adults to do so on the basis of less imput.

The predictions regarding L2 vowel production generated by the SLM received some support from two instrumental studies of vowel production. One (Flege, 1987a) measured formant frequencies to test the difference between similar and new vowels in French, viz. /u/ and /y/. Previous research had suggested that English speakers substitute English /u/ for the new French vowel /y/ in early stages of L2 learning, but little was known concerning how experienced English speakers of French would perform. The most experienced of the three native English groups examined did not differ from French monolinguals in producing the new vowel /y/, whereas all three groups differed from French monolinguals in producing the similar vowel /u/.[11]

Perceptually-based results obtained by Major (1987) suggested that new vowels may be learned more successfully than similar vowels. That study examined the production of English /æ/ and /ɛ/ by 50 Brazilian subjects. From the standpoint of Portuguese, English /æ/ is apparently a new vowel and English /ɛ/ is a similar vowel.[12] Accordingly, the SLM predicts that Portuguese learners of English will establish a phonetic category for English /æ/, and eventually produce that vowel authentically, whereas they will be unable to establish an /ɛ/ category and thus will continue to produce that vowel nonauthentically.

Native speakers of English in the Major (1987) identified /æ/ (in *sat*) and /ɛ/ (in *bet*) in a two-alternative forced-choice test. The percentage of correct identifications was calculated for two groups of Brazilian subjects differing in overall degree of foreign accent. The relatively non-proficient subjects' /ɛ/ was more intelligible than their /æ/ (87% vs. 26% correct identifications), whereas the reverse was true for the proficient subjects (50% vs. 68% correct). These differences led to a significant Group x Vowel interaction in an ANOVA examining the percent correct scores (p < .01).[13] It appeared that as the Brazilians were learning English /æ/ their production of English /ɛ/ somehow deteriorated, perhaps because they over-generalized their solution for a known pronunciation problem. A definite conclusion cannot be reached, however, because the listeners were offered only two choices, which means that results for one vowel necessarily affected results for the other vowel.

The study presented below also used a perceptual method to assess the authenticity of L2 vowel production, but it made use of 14 rather than just two response choices. The number of response categories is just one of many factors that may influence how well vowels are identified in an identification experiment. Some of these factors will be discussed before the English vowels examined in the present study are classified (as identical, similar, or new) and predictions generated concerning Dutch subjects' ability to produce them.

5.   Factors affecting vowel intelligibility

Intelligibility is determined by how a talker articulates and also by the interlocuter's listening skill. For example, the English spoken by deaf talkers is more intelligible for listeners familiar with deaf individuals, such as teachers of the deaf, than it is for listeners who are not familiar with deaf speech (McGarr, 1978). The effect of listener experience appears to be greater for isolated words than sentences, and greater in testing paradigms with high than low uncertainty (see Rubin, 1983). One study (Rubin, 1983) did not show the expected advantage of previous deaf listening experience, but this was probably because the deaf talkers were presented in a variable-talker rather than a constant-talker format (see below).

Generally speaking, the greater the use of higher order information in reaching phonetic decisions, the more intelligible vowels will be (Miller,

Heise, and Lichten, 1951). Kalikow, Stevens, and Elliot (1977) showed that words presented in noise were identified better when they occurred in a semantically constraining context than at the end of sentences like *John was discussing the___*. Varonis and Gass (1982) had native English listeners rate sentences produced by non-native speakers. Both grammatical errors and non-authentic pronunciation affected judgments of comprehensibility. Gass and Varonis (1984) found that familiarity with the topic of conversation had an important effect on listeners' comprehension; familiarity with particular talkers and foreign accents were also important.

Not all of the English vowels spoken by native English talkers are identified correctly by native English listeners, so one would not expect perfect intelligibility for nonnative talkers, even if they produced English vowel in a completely native-like way. Table 1 summarizes the results of several previous studies that have assessed the intelligibility of the six English vowels examined in the present study. The overall rate of correct identifications was greater for high vowels (/i/, /I/, /u/), which were identified at near-perfect rates, than for non-high vowels (/æ/, /ɑ/, /ʌ/), which were not. The misidentifications of the non-high vowels occurred even in studies employing

Table 1. *Percent correct identification by native English listeners of vowels spoken in CVC words by American and Canadian talkers. The vowels in each of six previous studies (A-F) were identified in fixed-talker conditions using a variable number of response categories (keywords).*

A	B	C	D	E	F	Average							
/I/ (100)	/i/ (99+)	/i/ (99)	/u/ (100)	/i/ (99+)	/I/ (100)	/i/ (98.8)
/i/ (100)	/ɑ/ (99+)	/I/ (99)	/i/ (99)	/u/ (99+)	/i/ (97)	/I/ (98.7)
/u/ (100)	/I/ (99)	/ɑ/ (96)	/ɑ/ (99)	/æ/ (98)	/u/ (97)	/u/ (98.2)
/æ/ (100)	/u/ (97)	/u/ (96)	/I/ (98)	/I/ (96)	/ɑ/ (96)	/ɑ/ (95.8)
/ʌ/ (93)	/ʌ/ (96)	/ʌ/ (96)	/æ/ (97)	/ɑ/ (96)	/æ/ (90)	/æ/ (95.2)
/ɑ/ (89)	/æ/ (94)	/æ/ (92)	/ʌ/ (87)	/ʌ/ (92)	/ʌ/ (78)	/ʌ/ (90.3)

A. Macchi (1980): 11 vowels in a /t_t/ context, 15 talkers, 96 listeners
B. Strange (1989): 11 vowels in /b_b/, /d_d/ and /d_t/ contexts, 1 talker, 36 listeners
C. Strange (1989): 10 vowels in six CVC contexts, one talker, 112 listeners
D. Assman et al. (1982): 10 vowels in a /p_p/ context, 10 talkers, 14 listeners
E. Strange et al. (1976): 9 vowels in a /p_p/ context, 15 talkers, 11 listeners
F. Strange and Gottfried (1980): 10 vowels in a /k_k/ context, 6 talkers, 20 listeners

listeners who had been carefully screened and/or trained. When misidentifications occurred, /æ/ was typically heard as /ɛ/ or /ʌ/, /ɑ/ was heard as /ʌ/, and /ʌ/ was heard as /ɑ/ or /æ/.

The misidentifications of /æ/, /ɑ/, and /ʌ/ probably derived from the relative lack of peripheral auditory discriminability. Sinnott (1989) found that although human subjects discriminated perfectly pairs drawn from a synthetic set of 10 English vowels based on Peterson and Barney (1952) values, they were relatively slow in doing so for /ɑ/-/ʌ/, /æ/-/ɛ/, and /ɛ/-/I/. Non-human primates were slow for the same pairs. In addition, the animals showed errors in discriminating /ɑ/-/ʌ/, /ɛ/-/I/, and /æ/-/ɛ/. It is notable that the macaques made far more discrimination errors for /ɑ/-/ʌ/ (20.5%) and /æ/-/ɛ/ (12.0%) than for /i/-/I/ (0.5%).[14]

The importance of vowel identity on intelligibility can be illustrated by considering the results obtained by Eguchi and Hirsh (1969). The /i/, /ɛ/, and /æ/ stimuli in that study had been edited from the sentence *He has a blue pen* as spoken by 84 adults and children. As shown in Figure 2, the correct identification rates were far from perfect for any group, but they were higher for adults and older children than for children aged 3-5 years. The relatively low intelligibility of the young children's vowels was probably due to their vowel articulation rather than to the (adult) listeners' inability to normalize for formant frequency differences between adult- and child-produced vowels, for token-to-token variability in F_1 and F_2 frequencies decreased steadily with age.

The Eguchi and Hirsch (1969) data in Figure 2 show that /i/ and /ɛ/ were identified more often than /æ/ (just 9% correct), which was often heard as /ɛ/ because of allophonic, style-conditioned variation.[15] Increases in speaking rate are well known to decrease the rate of information transmission in many communication systems, including fingerspelling (Reed, Delhorn, and Durlach, 1987). The temporal and spectral contrasts between vowels are reduced as speech rate is increased (Koopmans van Beinum, 1980), leading to decreased intelligibility. It appears that a relatively slow speaking rate may facilitate the comprehension of an L2 by nonnatives (Koster, 1987).

Most studies of L2 production have examined isolated words that have been read from a list. This virtually assures that fast-rate effects will not lessen intelligibility. However, speaking rate may influence the intelligibility of English vowels spoken by some nonnative speakers in real-life situations. Anderson-Hsieh and Koehler (1989) found that English passages produced

6 Response category test

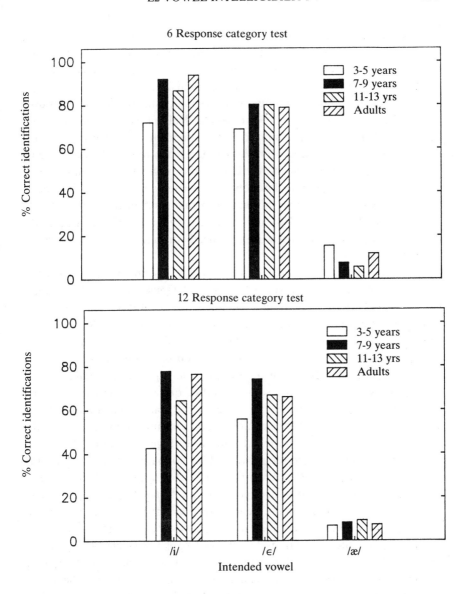

12 Response category test

Figure 2. *The intelligibility of the vowels /i/, /ɛ/, and /æ/* edited from an English sentence spoken by child and adult native speakers of English. One group of listeners (top) used six response categories and another group of listeners (bottom) used 12 response categories. The data are from Eguchi and Hirsh (1969).

at a fast rate by native Chinese subjects with poor English pronunciation were much less comprehensible than their normal-rate sentences. The fast-rate decrement noted for a subject with good English pronunciation was much smaller, resembling that of a native English speaker.

Including the phonetic context that originally surrounded a vowel usually makes it easier to identify. For example, Rubin (1983) found that vowels in /bVb/ words were identified 3% more often when the words were presented at the end of their carrier phrase than when removed from the carrier phrase, and about 7% more often in the original /b_b/ context than when presented in isolation. Phonetic context may also aid the listener in identifying vowels spoken by nonnative speakers. Amastae (1978) transcribed English vowels read by nine native speakers of Mexican Spanish. More vowels from a word list were produced correctly than vowels read in a text (95% vs. 89%).

Consonantal context has been described as a factor which "perturbs" the acoustic structure of vowels (Stevens and House, 1963). This implies that vowels might have invariant acoustic properties if it were not for coarticulation; and that coarticulation impedes identification. More recent studies examining vowels in CVC syllables have shown that consonant context may actually *aid* vowel recognition. When presented in isolation, the "target" portion of vowels can be identified at high rates (Assman et al, 1982). However, vowels may also be identified quite well on the basis of the transitions leading to and from the target (see Rubin, 1983; Strange, 1989) because acoustic effects of the gestures used in forming a vowel may be distributed over the entire periodic (transitions + target) portion of CVCs.

Much the same pattern seems to hold for nonnative speakers. Miranda and Strange (1989) presented words formed by inserting 10 native-produced English vowels into a /d_d/ context in a "full syllable" and a "silent center" condition, in which the center (target) portion of the vowel was removed. The rate of correct identifications was the same in the full-syllable and silent-center conditions for native English subjects (99%); it was slightly higher in the full-syllable than silent-center condition for nonnative subjects (63% vs. 58%). In a "center-only" condition, where the target remained and the transitions were removed, native speakers correctly identified 95% of vowels and nonnatives identified 74% of vowels.

Generally speaking, the fewer the response categories available to listeners, the higher will be the rate of correct identifications. As was shown earlier in Figure 2, listeners in the Eguchi and Hirsh (1969) study achieved a higher correct identification rate with six than 12 response alternatives (71% vs. 46% correct). Verbrugge, Strange, and Shankweiler (1976) obtained a slightly lower correct identification rate for vowels in an /h_d/ context than did Peterson and Barney (1952). The difference (90% vs. 94%) may have been due to the fact that listeners in the Verbrugge et al (1976) study had 15 response alternatives (keywords such as *heed*, *hid*, *hoed*) whereas those in the Peterson and Barney study had just 10.[16] Identification rates are generally lower when multiple talkers are presented than when the vowels of a single talker are presented in a constant-talker condition (Macchi, 1980; Strange et al, 1976). Thus another factor that may have contributed to the difference between the Verbrugge et al (1976) and Peterson and Barney (1952) studies was that a larger number of talkers were presented in each block in the former than the latter study (30 versus 10). Verbrugge et al (1976) presented /p_p/ words spoken by 15 talkers in two conditions to test whether listeners "calibrate" on the vowels spoken by a talker in a constant-talker condition. The overall rate of correct identifications was higher in a constant-talker than variable-talker condition (94% vs. 87%); the greatest improvement noted for any of the nine monophthongal vowels examined was for /æ/ (17%).

Other studies have shown that the time needed to recognize words increases, and the rate of correct identifications decreases (especially for words degraded by digital techniques), in a variable-talker compared to a constant-talker condition (Mullinex, Pisoni, and Martin, 1989; see also Assman et al, 1982). Recent results pertaining to /r/-/l/ identification by Japanese subjects suggest that the cognitive "cost" associated with processing different talkers in a variable-talker conditions, including a lower rate of correct identifications, may be greater for nonnative than native listeners (Logan et al, 1989).

Finally, nonnative talkers' vowels may suffer more from non-ideal listening conditions than native speakers' vowels if they are more distant from a native listener's prototype than native speakers' vowels. Nabèleck and Donahue (1984) found that the English spoken by 20 non-native speakers was as intelligible as that of 20 native speakers of English under normal listening conditions, but significantly less intelligible in reverberant conditions.

6. Dutch vs. English vowels

The present study examined Dutch subjects' production of six English vowels which, from the standpoint of Dutch, included vowels classifiable as identical, similar, or new. Four of the vowels defined the corners of the vowel quadrilateral (/i,æ,ɑ,u/), one was a high front lax vowel (/I/), and the remaining vowel was a short, central vowel (/ʌ/).

Dutch is usually analyzed as having three diphthongs (/ɑu/, /ʌ/, /ɛi/) and 12 monophthongs, which Moulton (1962) divided into two classes based primarily on phonological considerations: short (/ɔ/, /ɑ/, /æ/, /I/, /ɛ/) or long (/i/, /u/, /y/, /o/, /a/, /ø/, /e/). Duration measurements have shown, however, that except before /r/, three of the supposedly long vowels (/i/, /y/, /u/) are short (Nooteboom, 1972; Nooteboom and Slis, 1972). In addition, Dutch has three long vowels that occur in foreign loanwords (/ɔ:/, /æ:/, /ɛ:/) and a schwa (/ə/) in unstressed syllables.

Figure 3 shows the acoustic relationship between the six English vowels examined in the present study and the 12 Dutch monophthongs that occur in stressed syllables. The ellipses for English /i/, /I/, /æ/, /ʌ/, /ɑ/, and /u/ represent 95% confidence intervals drawn around the F1-F2 values reported by Peterson and Barney (1952) for American English (henceforth AE) vowels as spoken by 33 adult male native speakers.[17] The phonetic symbols indicating the mean F_1-F_2 values for Dutch vowels are based on values reported for 50 adult male native speakers of Dutch by Pols et al (1973). Figure 4 shows the relationship between the Pols et al. (1973) Dutch vowel data and and the mean values reported by Holtse (1972) for English vowels as spoken by six male native speakers of British English (henceforth BE). The BE males were speakers of general Received Pronunciation.

6.1 *An identical vowel*

English /I/ was classified as an identical vowel because, as seen in Figures 3 and 4, the mean values for Dutch /I/ are very similar to those reported for the /I/ of AE and BE. An ANOVA carried out by Disner (1983) showed that the F_1-F_3 values for Dutch /I/ (Pols et al, 1973) and AE /I/ (Peterson and Barney, 1952) did not differ significantly. It appears that the /I/s of Dutch and BE do not differ auditorily, for Collins and Mees (1984: 86) stated that Dutch /I/ can "pass straight into (British) English without being modified" and should thus pose "no problem" for pronunciation.[18]

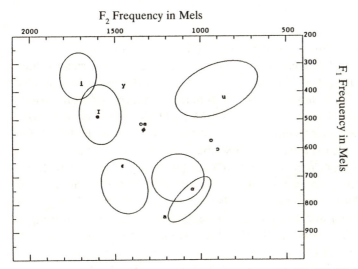

Figure 3. *The acoustic relationship between American English /i/, /I/, /u/, /ɑ/, /æ/, /ʌ/* and Dutch vowels. The ellipses for the English vowels surround approximately 95% of the F_1 and F_2 values reported by Peterson and Barney (1952) for 33 male English speakers. The phonetic symbols represent the mean F_1-F_2 values reported by Pols, Tromp, and Plomp (1973) for 12 monophthongal Dutch vowels spoken by 50 native Dutch men.

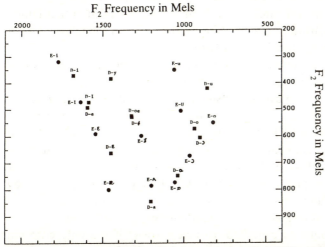

Figure 4. *The mean values for Dutch vowels (marked "D") reported for Dutch men by Pols et al (1969) and for English vowels (marked "E") reported for six British male speakers of RP by Holtse (1972).*

6.3   *A new vowel*

English /æ/ was classified as new because Dutch has no vowel phoneme represented phonetically as /æ/. As can be seen in Figure 3, the mean values
for Dutch /ɛ/ fall just within the upper boundary of the space occupied by
English /æ/. Figure 4 shows that BE /æ/ is more distant from a Dutch vowel
than any other BE vowel. Collins and Mees (1984) observed that both
beginning and advanced Dutch learners of English substitute Dutch /ɛ/ for
English /æ/ (see also van Heuven, 1986) but did not quantify their observation. Perceptual data reported by Schouten (1975) are consistent with the
belief that Dutch learners of English will eventually recognize that English
/æ/ is a new, non-Dutch vowel. Results were obtained from both advanced
(3rd and 4th year) and beginning (1st year) Dutch students majoring in
English at the University of Utrecht. The advanced students identified /æ/
more often than the beginning ones (93% vs. 57% correct). Not surprisingly, the only consistent error was /ɛ/ (12% of responses).

6.2   *Similar vowels*

English /i/ was classified as similar because Dutch /i/ is lower in the acoustic
space than either the /i/ of AE (Figure 3) or BE (see Figures 3 and 4). Disner (1983) found that the F_1-F_3 values of Dutch /i/ and AE /i/ differed significantly. Consistent with this, Collins and Mees (1984) stated that Dutch
learners typically substitute Dutch /i/ for English /i/ even though the Dutch
vowel is "less fronted" than its English counterpart.
   English /u/ was also classified as a similar vowel, but it may pose more
of a learning problem for Dutch L2 learners than English /i/. Dutch /u/ differs acoustically from English /u/ (Disner, 1983) and has been described as
intermediate to the /u/ and /U/ of English (van Heuven, 1986). Dutch learners may at first substitute Dutch /u/ for English /u/. More advanced Dutch
learners are said to substitute the vowel "sequence" /yu/ for English /u/
(Collins and Mees, 1984), perhaps because /u/ is fronted so much in BE that
some investigators regard it as a front vowel (Bauer, 1985). In a study by
Schouten (1975), Dutch students identified synthetic English /u/ tokens correctly in only 60% of instances; most misidentifications of /u/ were as /U/.
   English /ʌ/ would be classified as a new vowel if the only criterion
applied was a consideration of phonetic symbols, for Dutch has no vowel
phoneme represented as /ʌ/. However, several considerations led to /ʌ/'s

classification as similar. First, acoustic data suggest that English /ʌ/ occupies a portion of the acoustic phonetic vowel space that goes unused in Dutch. As seen in Figure 3, the mean values for Dutch /ɑ/ fall within the area occupied by AE /ʌ/; and the same appears to be true for BE vowels. As seen in Figure 4, the BE /ʌ/ is spectrally close to the short Dutch vowel /ɑ/, and even slightly closer to the long Dutch /a/.[19]

There is anecdotal evidence that as Dutch speakers become more experienced in their L2, they continue to identify English /ʌ/ with a vowel(s) of Dutch. van Heuven (1986) indicated that Dutch L2 Learners identify BE /ʌ/ with the Dutch /œ/; and Collins and Mees (1984) indicated that even though the mid-high front rounded Dutch vowel /œ/ and BE /ʌ/ are "very different" inexperienced Dutch learners of English substitute the Dutch /œ/ for English /ʌ/ and experienced Dutch L2 learners tend to substitute the short Dutch vowel /ɑ/ for /ʌ/.[20] Data reported by Schouten (1975) also suggests that interlingual identification continues. Dutch students identified /ʌ/ correctly less often than /æ/ (41% of instances, as compared to 80% for synthetic /æ/s). There was only a small difference in the rates for /ʌ/ obtained for advanced and beginning students (48% versus 32%).

Classification of the vowel in the word *hot*, represented here as /ɒ/, is complicated by the fact that it is realized as a central, unrounded vowel (/ɑ/) in AE but as a slightly rounded *back* vowel (/ɒ/) in checked syllables in BE (Wells 1982). Figure 3 shows that AE /ɑ/ is similar spectrally to the long Dutch vowel /a/, but tests performed by Disner (1983) indicated that these vowels had significantly different F_1 and F_3 (but not F_2) frequencies. Since AE /ɑ/ is more distant from the short than the long Dutch /ɑ/, it is likely that acoustic differences between Dutch /ɑ/ and AE /ɑ/ would also be significant.

It appears then, that from the standpoint of Dutch, AE /ɑ/ should be regarded as a similar vowel. Figure 4 shows the acoustic relationship of /ɒ/ — the BE equivalent to AE /ɑ/ — to Dutch vowels. BE /ɒ/ is close to Dutch /ɑ/ in the F_1-F_2 space, but is considerably longer (see Holtse, 1972) than Dutch /ɑ/, which Nooteboom (1973) suggests is represented centrally by Dutch speakers as being half the length of /a/. It is probably because of this temporal mismatch that even highly proficient Dutch L2 Learners continue to substitute Dutch /ɔ/ for BE /ɒ/ (Collins and Meese, 1984).[21]

9. Methods

9.1 *Subjects*

9.1.1 *Talkers*

The study examined English vowels spoken by 50 native Dutch talkers (25 males, 25 females) whose production and perception of English stops was examined in an earlier study (Flege and Eefting, 1987a). The Dutch talkers were individuals between the ages of 20 and 25 years who began learning English at about the age of 12 years in school. Forty of the students were majoring in English at the University of Utrecht, all of whom spoke English quite well. The remaining 10 students were majoring in engineering at a technical school in Delft. They had not studied English beyond the six years required in high school, and were consequently less proficient in English than the English majors.

Of the eight native speakers of BE selected to define the "norm" for English, four (all femals) were recorded in Birmingham, Alabama and four (all males) were recorded in Amsterdam. None of these talkers could speak Dutch; all could be described as speaking General RP.[22]

9.1.2 *Listeners*

The vowels were identified by three native speaker each of BE and AE. The responses of both BE and AE listeners were collected because dialect discrepancies between talkers and listeners may inflate the number of vowel identification errors (Macchi, 1980). AE can be heard in the Netherlands on television and in popular music, but BE is taught in the school (sometimes by native BE talkers). Consequently, Dutch speakers of English often seem to have a "British" accent to Americans.

The AE listeners (A1-A3) were native speakers of General AE. A3 was the author; A1 and A2 were part-time research assistants who participated in the experiment as part of their ordinary duties.[23] The three BE listeners (B1-B3) were not speech researchers and were, accordingly, paid a nominal sum for participating.[24] None of the listeners spoke Dutch or indicated familiarity with Dutch-accented English. None of the AE or BE listeners spoken with a marked regional accent.

9.2 Speech materials

The talkers produced test words formed by inserting six vowels (/ i,I,ɑ,u,ʌ,æ/ into a single consonantal frame (/h_t/), which yielded six real words: *heat, hit, hot, hoot, hut,* and *hat.* The words were read from a randomized list at the end of a the carrier phrase *Sip through a__.* The utterances were recorded using high-quality equipment (Sony Model TCD5M with Nakamichi CM-300 microphone). Three tokens of each word from the middle of the list were low-pass filtered at 5 kHz, digitized at a 12 kHz rate with 12-bit amplitude resolution, and stored on disk.

A waveform editor was used to discard all but the periodic portion (or "vowel", for short) from each stored waveform to avoid lexical bias effects in the subsequent identification experiment.[25] Removing the noise associated with the initial /h/ and the stop gap and release burst for the final /t/ was considered preferable to having the talkers try produce *isolated* vowels because English lax vowels are not permitted to occur in open syllables. Moreover, prolonged, isolated vowels often have offglides not seen in CVCs. One disadvantage of the editing was that it was likely to decrease the overall rate of correct identifications, due in part to the loss of temporal information (see e.g., Bond, 1976).

9.3 Procedures for the intellibility test

9.3.1 Response categories

The listeners were told to identify the English vowels using 14 keywords listed on a response box in the following order: *heat, hoat*, foot, hit, hat, hoot, hate, hot, hurt, hite, hout*, het*, hut, hoit*.* The four orthographic response categories marked by an asterisk are not real words in English, but all of the keywords conformed to English spelling conventions. Note that potentially confusable items such as *heat* and *hit* were not juxtaposed. The keywords represented all AE vowels except for /ɔ/ and /ə/. Schwa was excluded because it, like the Dutch schwa, does not occur in stressed syllables; and /ɔ/ was excluded because it did not contrast with /ɑ/ in the dialect of the AE listeners.

9.3.2 *Pre-Test*

Owing to the large number of response categories, it was necessary to familiarize the listeners with the testing procedures before data collection began. The listeners always produced the keywords with the expected vowel when asked to read them (e.g., *hoit* was read as [ho^{I}t]). They were given rhyming words for keywords that might be confused (e.g., *boy* for *hoit*). Next, the listeners were asked to point to keywords on the response box in response to the experimenter's live voice presentation of isolated vowels found in the 14 keywords.

Once the listeners were able to respond correctly and confidently to the isolated live-voice vowels, they participated in a formal pre-test. Isolated test vowels were prepared using the procedures described above. The pre-test consisted of the randomized presentation of three tokens of all 14 vowels (each edited from /hVt/ words). The vowels presented to AE listeners were edited from words read by a native speaker of AE; those presented to the BE listeners were from words spoken by a native speaker of BE. To be allowed to participate, a listener could make only two errors on the 42-item pre-test on the first and second days of testing (the errors could not be errors on the same vowel). One BE listener was unable to pass the pre-test and was replaced; another British listener passed the pre-test but was unable to complete the experiment, and so was also replaced.

9.3.3 *Instructions*

The listeners were told that they would hear vowels edited from /hVt/ words that had been spoken by an unspecified proportion of native speakers of Dutch and BE. Unlike the AE listeners, the BE listeners were unaware that the talkers had actually spoken only six /hVt/ words, not all 14 words listed on the response box. However, both the AE and the BE listeners were told to use all 14 response categories, as appropriate, and to guess if uncertain.

To signal their response, the listeners positioned the lever on the response box next to one of the 14 keywords. Each vowel was presented 1.0 sec after a response had been received for the preceding vowel.

9.3.4 *Stimulus presentation*

The 1044 vowel stimuli were normalized for overall RMS intensity and presented over headphones (TDH-49) at a comfortable level (76 dB SPL-A peak syllable intensity). The 6 vowels x 3 tokens = 18 stimuli for each talker were randomly presented three times each in a single block. The order of the talkers was counterbalanced across listeners. About eight talkers were presented per day over an approximately two-week period. At least one native English talker was presented along with the Dutch talkers on each day of testing. This yielded a total of 3,132 responses from each listener (58 talkers x 6 vowels x 3 replicate tokens x 3 randomized presentations).

9.3.5 Evaluating degree of foreign accent

The experimental design called for grouping the Dutch talkers according to their pronunciation of English.

The foreign accent scores obtained for the Dutch talkers in a previous study (Flege and Eefting 1987a) were used for this purpose. In the earlier study, the 50 Dutch talker and five native speakers of BE produced sentences containing sounds known to be problematical for Dutch speakers of English: *I can read this for you*; *The good shoe fits Sue*; *The red book was good*. The sentences were digitized and randomly presented three times each to eight native speakers of BE residing in Birmingham, Alabama. In evaluating the 165 sentences, the listeners positioned a lever on a response box between endpoints marked "Strong Foreign Accent" and "No Foreign Accent". The lever was connected to a linear potentiometer which, in turn, was connected to an 8-bit A-D converter that returned values ranging from 1 to 256 (that is, the higher the score the higher the degree of authenticity and the less the foreign accent).

The foreign accent scores obtained in this way averaged 239 (SD = 9) for the native BE talkers, 178 (SD = 36) for the 40 Dutch talkers majoring in English, and just 86 (SD = 29) for the 10 Dutch engineers. The Dutch talkers who received the 16 lowest scores were designated the "Strong Foreign Accent" group. The 16 Dutch talkers with the highest scores were designated the "Mild Foreign Accent" group even though two of them received scores in the native English range. The "Moderate Foreign Accent" group consisted of 16 talkers from the middle of the range.[26]

It is likely that the Dutch talkers with mild foreign accents had more English-language experience than those with strong accents. This assumption was supported by an analysis of stop consonant production. In Dutch, /t/ is implemented as a voiceless unaspirated stop with short-lag VOT values. Flege and Eefting (1987a) found that the 50 Dutch talkers' foreign

accent scores correlated positively with the VOT measured in their productions of English /t/. The better their overall pronunciation of English, the
more closely the Dutch students approximated the phonetic norm of English for /t/.[27] Moreover, a language background questionnaire revealed that
the engineering students, who were all rated as having strong accents, had
less access to native speakers of English and spoke English far less frequently than the students majoring in English.

9.3.6 *Analyses*

The listeners' responses were stored on disk and later tabulated automatically. The dependent variable for each listener was the percentage of times,
out of maximum of 9 responses (3 tokens x 3 presentations), that each of
the six vowels spoken by the 58 talkers was identified as intended. Mean
percent correct scores were then calculated for the three BE and three AE
listeners. These scores, which were based on 27 forced-choice identification
judgments for each vowel, were analyzed in mixed-design Group x Vowel
ANOVAs. Separate analyses were carried out for the AE and BE listeners
because only the AE listeners had speech training, and only they were
aware of the vowels the talkers had identify of the six intended to produce.[28]

10. Results of the intelligibility test

10.1 *American listeners*

The results are summarized separately for each of the three American listeners in Table 2. The mean percentage scores presented here are based on
the frequency with which each of the six vowels was identified as intended.
The phonetic symbols indicate error responses, that is, vowels heard
instead of the intended vowels in more than five percent of instances.

Figure 5 (top) shows the mean percent correct scores for vowels spoken by the native BE speakers and the Dutch talkers with strong, moderate, and mild accents. The data shown here were averaged over the three
AE listeners, who varied somewhat in the overall rate of correct identifications.[29] Averaged across all six vowels, the correct identification rate was
greater for native than nonnative talkers (94% versus 86%). Four vowels (/

Table 2. *The mean rate at which three American listeners (A1-A3) identified vowels in six English words spoken by native speakers of British English (n = 8) and Dutch (n = 50). The numbers indicate the percentage of times each vowel was identified correctly. The phonetic symbols in parentheses indicate the vowels heard instead of the intended vowel in more than 5% of instances; their ordering indicates relative frequency of occurrence.*

	heat /i/		hit /I/		British English talkers hoot /u/		hot /ɒ/		hat /æ/	hut /ʌ/		M
A1	99(	)	99(	)	100(	)	96(	)	86(ʌ,ɛ)	99(	)	97
A2	99(	)	100(	)	96(	)	99(	)	82(ʌ)	64(ɑ	)	90
A3	99(	)	100(	)	·99(	)	99(	)	88(aᵁ)	81(ɑ,æ)		94
M	99(	)	100(	)	98(	)	98(	)	85(ʌ)	81(ɑ	)	94

	heat /i/		hit /I/		Dutch talkers hoot /u/		hot /aa/		hat /æ/	hut/ʌ		M
A1	99(	)	100(	)	84(U	)	82(ʌ	)	63(ɛ,ʌ)	87(ɑ	)	86
A2	100(	)	100(	)	97(	)	88(ʌ	)	69(ʌ,)	75(ɑ	)	88
A3	98(	)	100(	)	81(U	)	80(ʌ	)	69(ɛ,ʌ)	79(ɑ,æ)		85
M	99(	)	100(	)	87(U	)	83(ʌ	)	67(ʌ,ɛ)	80(ɑ	)	86

i/, /I/, /u/, /aa/) produced by the native BE talkers were identified at near-perfect rates, but two of their vowels (/æ/, /ʌ/) were identified in less than 90% of instances.

The native BE talkers' /æ/s tended to be misidentified as /ʌ/ by the AE listeners; and their /ʌ/s tended to be misheard as /ɑ/. The relatively poor intelligibility of /æ/ and /ʌ/ as spoken by the BE talkers agrees with results obtained previously for AE talkers' production of these vowels (see Table 1). However, the AE listeners identified the vowel in *hot*, which is implemented as /ɒ/ in BE, somewhat better than the vowel that Americans produce in this word (viz. /ɑ/) has been identified previous vowel identification experiments.

As for the native BE talkers, The Dutch talkers' /i/s and /I/s were also identified at near-perfect rates, and their /æ/s and /ʌ/s were identified relatively poorly. The greatest difference between the native and Dutch talkers was for /u/ and /ɑ/. The Dutch talkers' vowels were less intelligible than the native talkers' because their /u/ was heard as /U/ and their /ɑ/ (/ɒ/) was heard as /ʌ/. Other common substitutions heard in the Dutch-accented English were /ʌ/-for-/æ/ and /ɛ/-for-/æ/, and /ɑ/-for-/ʌ/. The only important difference in substitution errors heard for the native and Dutch talkers was

American Listeners

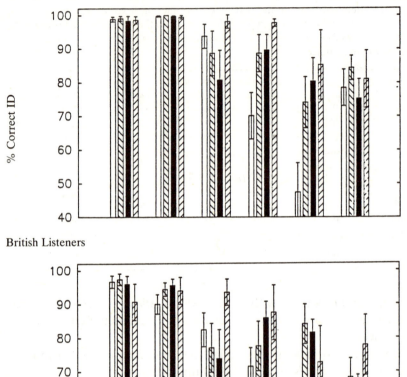

British Listeners

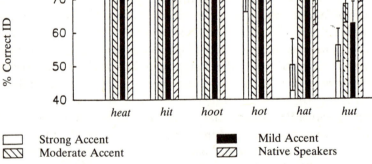

Figure 5. *(top) The mean rate at which American English listeners correctly identified six English vowels (/i/, /I/, /u/, /ɒ/, /æ/, /ʌ/) spoken by Dutch talkers who spoke English with relatively strong, moderate, or mild foreign accents (16 per group) and by native speakers of British English (n = 8); (bottom) the results obtained for three British English listeners. The error bars enclose +/− one standard error.*

that the Dutch talkers' /æ/ attempts were sometimes heard as /ɛ/. The /ɛ/ variants were likely to have been the result of cross-language phonetic interference, for /ɛ/ seems to be the Dutch vowel that is closest to English /æ/.

Figure 5 (top) shows that there were systematic differences between the three Dutch groups for certain vowels but not others. Between-group differences did not exist for either /i/ or /I/ because these vowels were identified consistently at near-perfect rates. The rate for /ʌ/ was about 80% correct for all three Dutch groups. For /aa/ and /æ/, the percent correct scores increased as a function of how well the Dutch talkers spoke English. For /ɒ/, the Dutch talkers with strong, moderate, and mild foreign accents had percent correct scores of 70%, 87%, and 90%, respectively. For /æ/, the percent correct scores were 47%, 74%, and 80%. Conversely, the scores for /u/ seemed to *decrease* as a function of how well the Dutch subjects pronounced English. The percent correct scores for the Dutch talkers with relatively strong, moderate, and mild foreign accents were 94%, 87%, and 81%, respectively.

To determine which, if any, of the three Dutch groups differed from the native BE talkers, the percent correct scores obtained for the AE listeners were submitted to a mixed-design ANOVA. The significant Group x Vowel interaction obtained $[F(15,260) = 2.64, p < 0.001]$ was followed by tests of simple main effects, which suggested that learning had taken place for two of the six English vowels. The Group effect was significant for /ɒ/ $[F(3,52) = 4.09, p = 0.011]$ and /æ/ $[F(3,52) = 4.48, p = 0.007]$ but was non-significant for the other four vowels examined $(p > 0.10)$. Post-hoc tests (Newman-Keuls, $\alpha = 0.05$) revealed that for both /æ/ and /ɒ/, the Dutch talkers with moderate and mild foreign accents had higher correct identification rates than those with strong accents but these two groups did *not* differ from the native BE talkers.

The present experiment was undertaken to test the speech learning model outlined in earlier sections. In this context it is important to note that the results for the new vowel /æ/ were predicted by the SLM, but not the results for the similar vowel /ɒ/.[30]

10.2 *British English listeners*

The misidentifications of the three BE listeners are summarized in Table 3. The mean rates at which these listeners identified vowels spoken by native

Table 3. *The mean rate at which three native British English listeners (B1-B3) identified vowels in English words spoken by native speakers of British English (n = 8) and Dutch (n = 50). The numbers indicate the percentage of times each vowel was identified correctly. The phonetic symbols in parentheses indicate the vowels heard instead of the intended vowel in more than 5% of instances; their ordering indicates relative frequency of occurrence.*

	heat /i/	hit /I/	hoot /u/	hot /aa/	hat /æ/	hut/ʌ/	M
	British English talkers						
B1	85( )	82(e^I,ʒ)	82(U,o)	82(ʌ)	86(a^U)	76(a^U,æ)	82
B2	95( )	100( )	99( )	96( )	57(ʌ,ɛ)	85(ɒ)	89
B3	93( )	100( )	100( )	85(ʌ)	75(ɛ,a^U)	72(ɒ,æ)	88
M	91( )	94( )	94( )	88(ʌ)	73(ʌ,|,a^U)	78(ɒ,æ,a^U)	86
	Dutch talkers						
	heat /i/	hit /I/	hoot /u/	hot /aa/	hat /æ/	hut/ʌ/	M
B1	94( )	83(e^I)	66(U,o)	73(a^U,ʌ)	80(a^U,ʌ)	55(a^U,æ)	75
B2	99( )	96( )	82(U,o)	78(ʌ)	60(ɛ,ʌ)	71(ɒ,U,æ)	81
B3	97( )	100( )	85(U)	86(ʌ)	76(ɛ,ʌ)	62(æ,ɒ)	84
M	97( )	93( )	78(U,o)	79(ʌ)	72(ʌ,ɛ,)	63(æ,a^U,ɒ)	80

BE talkers and talkers in the three Dutch groups are shown in Figure 3 (bottom).

The BE listeners were expected to be better able than the AE listeners to identify vowels spoken by their fellow countrymen, but the rates of correct identification of vowels was actually lower for for the BE than AE listeners (86% vs. 94% correct). The most likely explanation for this paradoxical finding is a methodological difference. Recall that the AE but not the BE listeners were aware that the talkers had actually intended to produce just six vowels, not all 14 vowels shown on the response box.

In support of this explanation, Table 3 reveals that the BE listeners used a wider range of response variants in identifying vowels than the AE listeners. One response variant used by the BE but not the AE listeners in identifying /ɒ/ (/ɑ/ in AE[31]) was /ʌ/. In addition to hearing /ʌ/-for-/æ/ substututions, the BE listeners also heard /ɛ/-for-/æ/ substitions. And in addition to hearing /ɒ/ (/ɑ/)-for-/ʌ/, the BE listeners also heard /æ/-for-/ʌ/. In general, however, the misidentifications of the BE and AE listeners were similar. The BE listeners misheard /æ/ as /ʌ/. They heard /ʌ/ as either /ɒ/ or /æ/, /u/ as /U/, and /ɒ/ as /ʌ/.

The BE listeners also identified fewer vowels spoken by the Dutch talkers than the AE listeners (80% vs. 86%). As shown in Figure 5 (bottom), they identified the Dutch talkers' attempts at /i/ and /I/ most of the time (97% and 93% correct, respectively). The BE listeners identified the Dutch talkers' /u/s and /ɒ/s less often (78%, 79%) than the Dutch talkers' high front vowels, and identified their /æ/ and /ʌ/ attempts even more poorly (72%, 63% correct).

There were between-group differences in intelligibility for all six vowels. Somewhat surprisingly, the /i/s produced by the Dutch talkers in all three groups were uniformly higher than the native BE talkers' /i/s. There was a small increase in the rate of correct /I/ identifications as a function of accent. The rates for the Dutch subjects with strong, moderate, and mild accent were 90%, 94%, and 96%, respectively. A similar pattern was evident for /ɒ/ (72%, 78%, and 86%), /æ/ (50%, 84%, 82%) and /ʌ/ (56%, 68%, 65%). For /u/, on the other hand, performance seemed to deteriorate slightly along with improvements in accent (82%, 77%, 74%).

As expected, the ANOVA yielded a significant Group x Vowel interaction [$F(15,260) = 2.34$, $p = 0.004$]. The simple main effect of Group was significant for /æ/ [$F(3,52) = 6.42$, $p < 0.001$] but non-significant for all other vowels, including /ɒ/. Post-hoc tests revealed that the Dutch talkers with moderate and mild foreign accents had higher scores for /æ/ than those with strong accents ($p < 0.05$). The moderately and mildly-accented Dutch talkers did not differ significantly from the native BE talkers.

These results supported the prediction of the SLM for /æ/. It is important to note that, for the BE listeners, the Dutch subjects did not show a significant improvement in /ɒ/ intelligibility (the result obtained earlier for AE listenrs).

To understand better why the AE listeners but not the BE listeners registered a significant improvement for /ɒ/, which was classified as a similar vowel, the variants that the BE and AE listeners gave in identifying the vowel in *hot* as spoken by mildly and strongly-accented Dutch talkers were tabulated. The AE listeners used fewer error variants, and applied those variants to fewer Dutch talkers in the Mild than Strong Foreign Accent group.[32] Unlike the AE listeners, the BE listeners did not give fewer error variants for talkers in the Mild than Strong Foreign Accent groups, but they did show a decrease in the number of talkers to whom they applied the error variants they used.

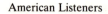

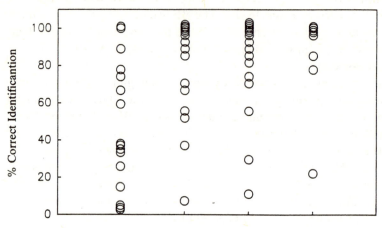

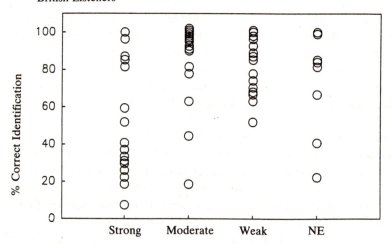

Figure 6. *The mean rate of correct identifications of /æ/ as spoken by Dutch talkers who spoke English with strong, moderate, or mild foreign accents (16 per group) and eight native speakers of British English ("NE"). The top panel shows results obtained from native American English listeners; the bottom panel shows results obtained for British English listeners. Each data point is based on 27 judgments (3 tokens x 3 presentations x 3 listeners).*

10.3 Individual talkers' production of the new vowel /æ/.

The SLM generated the prediction that Late L2 learners will produce a new L2 vowel authentically once they recognize it to be new. Since little is known at present concerning how long such recognition may take, Figure 6 was prepared to show the correct identification rates for the /æ/s spoken by 48 individual Dutch talkers.

Figure 6 (top) shows the rates obtained from the AE listeners; and Figure 6 (bottom) shows the rates obtained for the BE listeners. Note that some talkers in all three Dutch subgroups produced the new vowel /æ/ well, and some produced it poorly. The AE listeners seldom identified one native BE talker's /æ/s correctly, frequently hearing his intended /æ/ tokens as /a^U/ or /ʌ/. This talker was a 25-year-old male from Preston, England who was living in Amsterdam. According to James (1989), this individual had been exposed to a "northwest regional influence (i.e., Lancashire)" which might be expected to have caused a backing and/or lowering of his /æ/. The range of correct identifications for the remaining BE talkers was 78%-100% correct.

All three subgroups of Dutch talkers showed a wide range for /æ/. Just three of the 16 strongly accented Dutch talkers had rates exceeding 75% correct, whereas 11 moderately accented and 12 mildly accented Dutch talkers had rates above this level.

The range of percent correct scores for the native BE talkers was wider in the data obtained from the BE than the AE listeners. The one native BE talker whose /æ/ was poorly identified by the AE listeners was also poorly identified by the BE listeners (22% correct for both listener groups). However, several talkers' /æ/s were identified less often by the BE than the AE listeners. One talker's identification rate for /æ/ dropped from 100% to 40% correct because the BE listeners heard his /æ/ attempts as /ɛ/; another talker's /æ/ rate dropped from 96% to 67% because the BE listeners heard /ʌ/.

11. Acoustic measurements

The intelligibility study supported the SLM's prediction that a new vowel (English /æ/) would be produced authentically by at least the most proficient Dutch speakers of English. However, it provided little support for the model's prediction concerning English vowels classified as "similar" (viz. (/ i/, /u/, /ʌ/, /ɒ/). It was predicted that the Dutch talkers would produce the similar English vowels in a Dutch-like manner; Since the similar Dutch vowels diverged from the phonetic norm of English for corresponding English vowels, they were expected to be less intelligible when produced by even by highly proficient Dutch speakers of English than by native BE talkers. However, this prediction was not supported.

The possibility exists that persistent differences between native and non-native speakers did exist for the similar vowels, as predicted, but that the intelligibility test did not have a sufficiently fine resolution to reveal the differences. After all, the intelligibility scores were based on the percentage of correct *identifications*, and identification implies the reduction (or elimination) of fine-grained stimulus characteristics. An acoustic analysis was therefore carried out to further test the prediction of the SLM concerning similar vowels.

11.1 *Procedures*

Fourteen linear prediction coefficients were computed to estimate the center frequency of the first two formants (F_1, F_2) in vowels spoken by the 10 Dutch males with the best accents and the 10 Dutch males with the poorest accents. For the LPC analysis, a 25.6-ms Hamming window was placed at the acoustic midpoint of the vowels in *heat, hit, hat, hot, hut,* and *hoot*.

To provide a sufficiently large number of BE talkers to permit statistical comparisons of native and Dutch talkers, the data reported by Holtse (1972) for six male native speakers of standard RP was added to data obtained for the four BE males who participated in the present study. Holtse measured formants in the vowels found in *heat-heed, hit-hid, hat-had, cut-cud, heart-hard,* and *coot-cooed* as spoken by six male native speakers of RP. Most of the subjects were students or faculty members at the University of Copenhagen. Holte's (1972) study differed from the present one in several respects. Vowels were measured spectographically rather than by LPC analysis; means were based on a larger number of tokens (viz. 10-16); and some of the lexical items examined in the two studies differed. However, the data for the four BE males from this study did not appear to differ systemmatically from Holtse's six BE male subjects.

11.2 Results and discussion of the acoustic analysis

The mean values (in Hz) for the four groups of male talkers are presented in Table 4. The mean values are plotted in a Mel scale in Figure 7, which shows that the Dutch subjects with a relatively good English pronunciation more closely approximated the native BE talkers' vowel system than the Dutch subjects with relatively poor accents. Most of the difference between the native and Dutch speakers, and between the two Dutch groups, was confined to the new vowel /æ/ and the similar vowels /ʌ/ and /ɒ/ (/ɑ/). There seemed to be little difference between groups for the two similar vowels /i/ and /u/.

To determine which, if any, of these differences was significant, the 30 mean F_1 values (3 groups x 10 subjects) for each of the six vowels were submitted to separate ANOVAs, as were the mean F_2 values. The alpha level was set at 0.008 to obtain a per-experiment error rate of 0.05 for the F_1 and F_2 tests. The difference between groups was non-significant for the new vowel /æ/. As expected from previous cross-language research (Disner, 1983), the between-group differences for the identical vowel /I/ were non-significant. It is noteworthy, however, that the magnitude of the non-significant acoustic differences between groups for this vowel were about the same as those for the similar vowels /i/ and /u/.

Table 4. *The mean first and second formants frequencies (in Hz) for six English vowels spoken by 10 male native speakers of British English (4 from the present study and 6 from Holtse, 1972), 10 native Dutch males with good accents in English, and 10 native Dutch males with relatively poor (i.e., strong) accents in English.*

	/i/	/I/	/æ/	/ʌ/	/ɒ/	/u/
Native speakers of English						
F_1	270(56)	405(43)	715(93)	681(85)	649(103)	294(40)
F_2	2410(74)	2033(141)	1644(178)	1294(101)	1021(113)	1232(236)
Dutch with, good accents in English						
	/i/	/I/	/æ/	/ʌ/	/ɒ/	/u/
F_1	283(29)	390(21)	638(85)	572(89)	526(50)	336(27)
F_2	2255(186)	1895(129)	1482(96)	1217(57)	961(85)	1102(94)
Dutch with poor accents in English						
	/i/	/I/	/æ/	/ʌ/	/ɒ/	/u/
F_1	281(33)	389(33)	604(186)	531(125)	516(83)	324(20)
F_2	2215(227)	1884(132)	1615(131)	1296(91)	1018(120)	1078(162)

F₂ Frequency in Mels

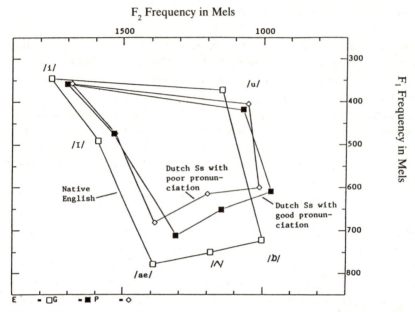

Figure 7. *The mean F₁ and F₂ frequencies (in Mels) in six English vowels spoken by native speakers of English and by Dutch subjects differing in degree of foreign accent (see Table 4 legend).*

As predicted by the SLM, a between-group difference was obtained for the F_1 values in the similar vowels /ʌ/ and /ɒ/ [$F(2,27)$ = 5.86, 8.24]. Newman-Keuls post-hoc tests revealed that the native BE talkers' F_1 frequencies were significantly higher than those of both Dutch groups. The differences for the other two similar vowels (/i/, /u/) were non-significant, however, as were all of the between-group differences for F_2.

The acoustic results partially confirmed the SLM's prediction that similar vowels will represent a persistent pronunciation problem for late L2 learners. One reason why between-group differences were not seen for two of the four similar vowels may have been that the acoustic differences between the two similar English vowels and their counterparts in Dutch were too small to detect reliably.

12. General discussion

The present study tested a speech learning model (SLM) by examining the intelligibility of identical, similar, and new English vowels spoken by native speakers of British English (BE) and Dutch talkers who spoke English with relatively strong, moderate, and mild foreign accents. As expected from previous vowel intelligibility studies (see Table 1), the high English vowels /i/, /ɪ/, and /u/ were identified more often than the non-high vowels /ɑ/, /æ/, and /ʌ/. The between-vowel differences were not significant for the native BE talkers, either when their vowels were assessed auditorily by fellow native speakers of British English or by native speakers of American English.

It came as no surprise that English /ɪ/ was as intelligible when spoken by talkers in all three Dutch subgroups as when spoken by the native BE talkers. This vowel was classified as "identical" to the /ɪ/ of Dutch because previous research had shown little or no difference between the /ɪ/ of Dutch and that of English. A different pattern of results was obtained for English vowels classified as new and similar, however.

12.1 The production of new vowels

Important between-vowel differences existed for Dutch talkers with mild, moderate and strong foreign accents. The SLM predicted that in early stages of learning, Late L2 learners may initially fail to produce new L2 sounds authentically, but will eventually do so as a result of establishing phonetic categories for them. In support of this, the Dutch talkers with moderate and mild foreign accents produced /æ/ significantly more intelligibility than Dutch talkers with strong foreign accents. The intelligibility of English /æ/ as spoken by the moderately and mildly-accented Dutch talkers did not differ significantly from that for the native /æ/s spoken by BE talkers. The Dutch talkers with strong accents produced /æ/ significantly less intelligibly than /ɪ/, /i/, or /u/ whereas the intelligibility of the /æ/s produced by the Dutch talkers with moderate and mild foreign accents did not differ from that of the high vowels.

The result for /æ/ agrees with the finding by Bohn and Flege (1991) that Germans are able to learn English /æ/. Taken together with that finding, the results presented here show that phonetic learning remains possible beyond early childhood, and support an important prediction of the SLM, namely that L2 vowels occupying a portion of the phonetic space not exploited by the L1 vowel system can be "learned", that is, produced authentically, by Late L2 Learners.

There are three reasons for caution, however. The first is that Dutch has English loanwords with /æ/ such as *fan* and *dancing*, and that the vowels in these words may be realized with a slightly lower quality than the Dutch /ɛ/ (James, 1989). One might argue, then, that /æ/ wasn't really a new vowel.

A second reason for caution is that the Dutch talkers who succeeded in producing /æ/ authentically had first begun learning English in school at the age of 12 years. One might argue that they had not yet passed a "critical period" and that they should not be classified as late L2 learners. However, data reported by Flege and Fletcher (1991) suggests that the offset of the critical (or sensitive) period for human speech learning occurs long before the age of 12 years.

The third reason for caution is that the Dutch subjects who succeeded in producing English /æ/s authentically were all students majoring in English at the University of Utrecht. Perhaps they succeeded because of some special training or talent. If so, then the results may not generalize to other L2 learners who are equally experienced in English. Many Dutch L2 learners examined here produced English /æ/s that were identified in 100% of instances by both American (AE) and British English (BE) listeners but, contrary to the SLM's prediction, some talkers in all three Dutch groups — including the Mild Accent group made up exclusively of students majoring in English — produced /æ/ poorly. This leads one to ask "Why did some Dutch subjects but not others succeed in learning /æ/?"

12.2 *The production of similar vowels*

An hypothesis of the SLM is that category formation for similar L2 sounds is blocked by equivalence classification. This generates the prediction that Late L2 Learners will phonetically approximate the phonetic norm for similar L2 vowels but will never produce such vowels authentically.

In agreement with this, there was not a significant difference in intelligibility between the Dutch talkers with strong, moderate, and mild foreign accents for three of the similar L2 vowels examined (/i/, /u/, and /ʌ/). However, contrary to hypothesis, the Dutch groups did not differ from native speakers of English for these vowels; and improvement with L2 experience was noted for the similar vowel /ɒ/. Intelligibility for /ɒ/ was higher for the moderately and mildly accented Dutch talkers than for the strongly accented Dutch talkers.

One might argue that the improvement for /ɒ/ did not provide counterevidence to the SLM's prediction about similar vowels because /ɒ/ is used to produce words like *hot* in British English whereas /ɑ/ is the most common vowel used in such words in American English. An improvement in the Dutch talkers' /ɒ/ production was noted in the data obtained for British English (BE) but not American English (AE) listeners. However, the lack of a difference between the Dutch and native speakers for the similar vowel /ɒ/ represents a more serious challenge to the model.

The SLM hypothesizes that similar L2 vowels pose a persistent problem for Late L2 Learners because they continue to be identified with vowels in the L1 as the result of equivalence classification. This led to the prediction that similar English vowels spoken by the Dutch subjects, even those with very good overall accents, would differ from those produced by native speakers of English. More specifically, it was predicted that the Dutch talkers would show "compromise" acoustic values representing an assimilation of the phonetic properties of the corresponding L1 and L2 vowels that were equated at a phonetic category level.

The present study failed to show a significant difference in intelligibility between native and Dutch talkers for any of the similar vowels examined, but an acoustic analysis supported partially the prediction concerning similar vowels. It revealed significant formant frequency differences in the production of the similar vowels /ɒ/ and /ʌ/ between native speakers and Dutch L2 learners, both those with good and relatively poor accents. These two similar English vowels were probably more distant from their closest Dutch counterparts than the other two similar English vowels (viz. /i/, /u/) that did not yield a native versus nonnative difference.

Even if there were a difference between the native and nonnative speakers' /i/s and /u/s, as predicted, acoustic measurement resolution may have been too coarse-grained to show it. That is, the similar English vowels /i/ and /u/ may be so close to the corresponding Dutch vowels that even the unmodified substitution of a Dutch vowel for a similar English vowel might not reduce intelligibility or be detectable in acoustic analysis. The possibility exists that a more fine-grained auditory analysis, such as the paired comparison of Dutch and English /i/s (and /u/s) in an accent-detection test (see Flege, 1984), would support the prediction of a continued difference between native and nonnative speakers for the similar L2 vowels. Whatever the outcome of such a test, it is clear that the larger the L1 vs. L2 difference in similar vowels, the easier they are to measure acoustically (and probably to detect auditorily).

One trend seen for both the BE and AE listeners is worthy of further comment. According to Collins and Mees (1984), the production of English /u/ may deteriorate as Dutch speakers gain experience in English. They stated that experienced Dutch speakers of English begin to substitute /yu/ for English /u/. The present study showed that percent correct scores for /u/ decreased non-significantly as foreign accents improved. Perhaps the Dutch talkers with the best English pronunciations had begun reproducing the very fronted, [y]-like realizations of /u/ used by native speakers of BE (Bauer, 1985). If so, the vowel of *boot* may have been misidentified by native BE and AE listeners when presented in isolation. A question for future study is whether an apparent deterioriation is the production of English /u/ would be noted if vowel tokens were presented in context (see Section 5).

This chapter provided a more explicit operational definition of the distinction between similar and new vowels than has been offered in earlier work still, an important question that remains to be answered is "How much must an L2 vowel differ from vowels in the L1 to be regarded as new?" It remains to be determined if there is an absolute phonetic difference threshold that, once crossed, triggers the formation of a new phonetic category. Future research may show that the new vs. similar vowel distinction, can be defined only on the basis of an individual learner's vowel system, not generalizations drawn for a whole population (i.e. a language). Patterns of inter-lingual identification may also be influenced by as-yet undefined individual modes of phonetic processing.

Acknowledgments

This research was supported by NIH grant DC00257. The author expresses gratitude to the colleagues who recorded subjects in The Netherlands (W. Eefting, A. James) and provided information about Dutch (B. Elsendoorn, V. van Heuven), the research assistants who helped with various phases of the project (B. Hartley, L. Skelton, and H. Slocom), and especially the British English listeners who made so many visits to the Bicommunication Research Laboratory for testing. Thanks are also extended to O.-S. Bohn for comments on a previous draft of this chapter.

Notes

1.   One might question whether the English subjects had to learn something in order to pro-
      duce French stops authentically for it is likely that, as adults, they produced English /d/
      with short-lag VOT and, as children, they implemented English /t/ with short-lag VOT
      values (Zlatin and Koenigsknecht, 1976).

2.   The earliest version of the SLM (Flege, 1981) was called the "phonological translation"
      hypothesis because it was then believed that interlingual identification occurred at a
      phonemic level. The model's name has been changed owing to the current belief that
      interlingual identification occurs at a *phonetic* level of analysis (see below). Another
      change made since the first statement of the model is that age of learning is now regarded
      as a crucial factor in determining how authentically certain L2 sounds will be produced.

3.   It appears that not all phonetic contrasts will be lost in the absence of environmental
      stimulation. Best et al (1988) found that infants being reared in an English-speaking envi-
      ronment remained able to discriminate Zulu click contrasts even though clicks are not
      found in English. These authors hypothesized that both the acoustic nature of a novel
      phonetic contrast and its relation to phonetic categories and contrasts in the language spo-
      ken around an infant, play a role in determining which phonetic contrasts will be lost.

4.   An alternative to the use of prototypes in a developmentally-oriented model of speech
      perception was recently described by Jusczyk (1989). Prototype models assume the exis-
      tence of an abstract, underlying representation to which incoming phones are matched.
      During speech learning, the prototype is refined by adding additional detail and/or by re-
      specifying the weighting of various properties. According to a multiple-trace model, on
      the other hand, phones are identified by comparison to multiple individual instances.
      Experience leads to the addition of individual traces, which are based on exemplars used
      collectively in recognition. Such an approach might provide a perceptual basis for the dif-
      ferent phonetic realization rules Late L2 learners use to distinguish similar L1 and L2
      sounds in the absence of different phonetic categories (see below).

5.   It appears that the "tuning" hypothesized by Aslin and Pisoni (1980) referred to experi-
      ence-based modifications of phonemic categories. Best et al. (1988) also hypothesize that
      the detection of divergences from the phonetic norms of a language occurs at a phonemic
      level.

6.   This procedure for estimating a perceptual norm for L2 vowels must be regarded as a first
      approximation, and must be used with caution. It is conceivable, for example, that talkers
      could produce a vowel in a way that differs from their internal perceptual representation
      by using a realization rule. This caution is especially applicable to production data
      gathered in a formal experiment, where maximally clear, careful speech is likely to be eli-
      cited.

7.   The difference in symbols is by no means trivial, for it leads to different expectations con-
      cerning L2 learning. For example, symbolizing the lax vowel as /I/ suggests that it will be
      regarded as a new vowel by Spanish learners of English whereas symbolizing it as a short
      /i/ suggests that it will be regarded as a *similar* vowel.

8.   Direct magnitude estimation might be used to estimate the phonetic similarity of vowels
      in L1 and L2. The potential problem with this method is that listeners might evaluate dis-

tances using an auditory metric (Pols et al, 1969), a phonetic metric, or some combination of both (see Kewley-Port and Atal, 1989).

9. New sounds might require a longer time to identify than similar sounds in a speeded classification test. Similar sounds might be easier to remember than new vowels in a list learning experiment.

10. These predictions concerning the production of similar L2 stop consonants are founded on two important assumptions: additional realization rules with which to produce similar L2 stops can be established even though additional categories cannot; and substantial VOT differences between L1 and L2 stops cannot be achieved through the use of realization rules.

11. It should be noted, however, that the equally experienced French learners of English showed only a non-significant difference in the expected direction from English monolinguals in producing English /u/. The seemingly divergent results for the French and English subjects was surprising since the subjects in both groups had lived in an L2-speaking environment for about 12 years on the average.

12. Portuguese does not have a phoneme whose most characteristic allophone is [æ]. Portuguese has an /e/ and /ɛ/. Acoustic data (Godinez, 1978) suggest that Portuguese /ɛ/ is produced with a wide range of variants. It overlaps the Portuguese /e/ category in an F1-F2 space. Portuguese /ɛ/ seems to occupy a portion of the acoustic space occupied by English /æ/, but an even larger portion of the space occupied by English /ɛ/.

13. The finding just reported is based on my own analysis of data reported by Major (1987), which were obtained at the Biocommunication Research Laboratory.

14. Interestingly, the /æ/s and /ʌ/s (and also /I/s) produced by a wide range of text-to-speech devices are also misidentified at relatively higher rates (Logan et al, 1989).

15. Such variation also seems to exist in L2 speech production. Ma and Herasimchuk (1971, cited by Amastae, 1978) found that English /æ/ was produced correctly by Puerto Ricans in only about half of instances. The expected Spanish "interference" variant (/a/) was used in about 30% of instances, and an /ɛ/ "approximation" variant was used in about 20% of instances. The interference variant was more frequent in the most formal speaking context than in less formal contexts.

16. A high correct identification rate can be obtained under certain circumstances, however, even when the listener is offered as many as 15 response alternatives. Verbrugge et al (1976) cite a study by Abramson and Cooper (1959) which yielded a 96.0% identification rate with 15 response alternative. The vowel tokens in that study were carefully selected, the listeners were personally familiar with the talkers, there were relatively few talkers (8), and the total number of vowels produced by each talker was relatively large (15).

17. The ellipses are drawn through four points located two standard deviations from the intersection of axes defining the two principal components of variation.

18. Elsendoorn (1986) offered the same view. Data reported by Schouten (1975) supports the belief that L2 learners may not recognize immediately the identity of L1 and L2 vowels.

In that study, 77 native Dutch students majoring in English at the University of Utrecht identified synthetic vowels with a fixed 175-ms duration using 15 phonêtic symbols and keywords. The synthetic English /I/s were identified correctly in only 71% of instances, probably because of difficulty using phonetic symbols, or because the fixed duration was more appropriate for Dutch /e/ than /I/ (van Heuven, 1986). The /I/s were misidentified as /e^I/ in 13% of instances, and as /ɛ/ in 12% of instances.

19.   It should be noted, however, that a great deal of variation exists in the production of BE /ʌ/ (Collins and Meese, 1984). Barry (1974) indicated that there are two distinct "norms" for /ʌ/, one for RP English and another, more centralized regional English variant. This observation was later confirmed by a study comparing acoustic values obtained in a number of studies examining English /ˆ/ (Bauer, 1985).

20.   Holtse (1972, p. 9) noted the presence of additional low amplitude formants in BE /ʌ/ which, although not classified as F_1 or F_2, might cause this vowel to be perceived as "closer in quality" than might be suggested by its position in an F_1-F_2 space. According to Elsendoorn (1986), BE /ʌ/ is perceptually close to the Dutch schwa but would probably not be identified with it because the Dutch schwa occurs only in unstressed syllables.

21.   Collins and Meese (1984) report that Dutch /ɔ/ differs perceptually as well as acoustically from BE /ɒ/. According to Collins and Meese (1984), native speakers of BE identify Dutch /ɑ/ with BE /aa/.

22.   Of these subjects, one was born in Glasgow, Scotland; one in Preston, England; and one in London (for whom biographical data is not available). These talkers were described (James, 1985b) as speaking a form of English free of any of "class-defining" or "regional accent" features. The female talkers all held advanced degrees. Their birthplaces were Oxford, Darley, Liverpool, and Kenya (Africa).

23.   Listener A1 was a female, aged 31, who was born and raised in San Francisco; A2 was a female, aged 26, from the Washington, D.C.; A3 was a male, aged 37, from Cincinnati, Ohio. Listeners A1 and A2 were newly arrived in Birmingham, whereas A3 had lived there for six years, and had lived for two years in Western Europe.

24.   Listener B1 was a 39-year-old male scientist at the University of Alabama at Birmingham who had arrived in Birmingham just prior to the experiment. B1 was born in London and had lived in the London area (Hertfordshire, St. Albans) up to the age of 18 years. He had lived in a variety of places in Great Britain (Liverpool-3 years, Cambridge-3 years, Leicester-3 years) and had completed a two-year post-doctoral fellowship in Raleigh, NC. B1 characterized his speech as a "London" accent. Listener B2 was a 30-year-old male UAB scientist who had lived in Bristol until the age of 18 years. After three years of university work at Cambridge, he spent the following six years earning a Ph.D. in Biochemistry at the State University of New York at Stoneybrook. Listener A3 was an 18-year-old male Londoner who was spending a summer in Birmingham prior to beginning his university studies. He reported having lived in Wiltshire and Berkshire.

25.   Previous research (e.g., Ganong, 1980) suggests that listeners would tend to identifiy a vowel token that was ambiguous between /ɛ/ and /æ/ as hat rather than het because, of these two choices, only hat is a lexical item of English. Smaller response biases might result from differences in familiarity among real-word responses.

222   JAMES EMIL FLEGE

26. Data for two Dutch talkers were excluded to ensure an equal number of talkers in all three subgroups.

27. Another possibility is that both global pronunciation and specific aspects of segmental articulation depend on some general speech learning ability rather than amount of L2 experience. However, this seems unlikely since all 10 of the engineering students were assigned to the Strong Foreign Accent group, and all 10 of these talkers produced English /t/ with Dutch-like short-lag VOT values.

28. The same results were obtained when the values were transformed using an arcsine transformation recommended by Kirk (1968), and therefore will not be reported here.

29. The average rate for vowels spoken by native BE talkers ranged from 90% to 97% correct (listeners A2 and A1, respectively); and the rate for the Dutch talkers ranged from 85% to 88% (listeners A3 and A2, respectively).

30. The vowel effect was nonsignificant for the native BE talkers [$F(5,35) = 2.41$, p $= 0.056$]. As expected, they seem to have been equally successful in producing all six vowels. The effect of Vowel was significant, however, for the Dutch talkers with strong, moderate, and mild accents [$F(5,35) = 15.7, 4.16, 4.07$; p < 0.01]. Post-hoc tests showed that for the Mild Accent group, /ʌ/ was less intelligible than /i/ and /I/. For the Moderate Accent group, /ɒ/ but not /ʌ/ was less intelligible than /i/ and /I/. For the Strong Accent group, both /ʌ/ and /ɒ/ were less intelligible than /i/ and /I/. In addition, /ʌ/ and /ɒ/ were less intelligible than /u/; and /æ/ was less intelligible than all other vowels.

31. The BE listeners' use of the keyword *hot* is marked as /ɒ/ whereas the AE listeners' use of the same keyword is marked as /ɑ/.

32. For the AE listeners, the number of talkers showing the following variants for the Mild Accent group were: /ʌ/-3 talkers, /o/-2 talkers, /U/-1 talker; in the Strong Accent group it was: /ʌ/-8, /o/-3, /U/-1, /æ/-1). For the BE listeners the number of talkers in the Mild Accent group was /ʌ/-4, /aᵁ/-3, /o/-1, /æ/-1, /U/-1, and in the Strong Accent group it was /ʌ/-8, /aᵁ/-6, /o/-4, /æ/-1, /U/-1). There was not a significant difference in the rate at which the six vowels spoken by the native BE talkers were identified [$F(5,35) = 2.43$, p > 0.10], but a Vowel main effect was obtained for the Dutch talkers with mild, moderate and strong accents [$F(5,35) = 7.68, 4.24, 17.7$, p < 0.01]. For the mildly-accented talkers, /ʌ/ was identified less often than /i/ and /I/, their /ʌ/s were identified less often than /ɒ/ or /æ/, and their /u/s were identified less often than the /i/ or /I/. For the moderately-accented talkers, /ʌ/ was identified less often than /i/ and /I/. For the Dutch talkers with strong accents, both /ʌ/ and /æ/ were identified less well than /i/, /I/, /u/ and /ɒ/; and /ɒ/ was identified less often than /i/ or /I/.

References

Amastae, J. 1978. "The acquisition of English vowels." *Papers in Linguistics* 11, 423-457.

Anderson-Hsieh, J. and Koehler, K. 1989. "The effect of foreign accent and speaking rate on native speaker comprehension." *Language Learning* 38, 561-614.

Anglin, J. 1977. *Word, Object, and Conceptual Development.* New York: Norton.

Aslin, R. and Pisoni, D. 1980. "Some developmental processes in speech perception." *Child Phonology, Vol. 2, Perception.* ed. by G. Yeni-Komshian, J. Kavanagh, and C. Ferguson, 67-98. New York: Academic.

Assman, P. Nearey, T. and Hogan, J. 1982. "Vowel identification: Orthographic, perceptual, and acoustic aspects." *Journal of the Acoustic Society of America* 71, 975-989.

Barry, W. 1974. "Language background and the perception of foreign accent." *Journal of Phonetics* 2, 65-89.

Bauer, L. 1985. "Tracing phonetic change in the received pronunciation of British English." *Journal of Phonetics* 13, 61-82.

Benson, B. 1988. "Universal preference for the open syllable as an independent process in interlanguage phonology." *Language Learning* 38, 221-242.

Best, C., McRoberts, G. and Sithole, N. 1988. "Examination of perceptual reorganization for nonnative speech contrasts: Zulu clock discrimination by English-speaking adults and infants." *JEP:HPP* 14, 345-360.

Bennett, D. 1968. "Spectral form and duration as cues in the recognition of English and German vowels." *Language & Speech* 11, 64-85.

Black, J. 1976. "Speech Intelligibility: Assessments and determinants." *Lectures in Speech Sciences.* ed. by A. Huckleberry. Department of Speech and Hearing, Ball State Univ.

———. 1990. "Interlingual identification and the role of foreign language experience in L2 vowel perception." *Applied Psycholing*, 11, 303-328.

Bohn, O.-S. and Flege, J. 1991. "The production of new and similar vowels by German speakers of English." *Journal of Phonetics*, under review.

Bond, Z. 1976. "The identification of vowels excerpted from neutral and nasal contexts." *Journal of the Acoustic Society of America* 59, 1229-1232.

Borden, G., Gerber, A. and Milsark, G. 1983. "Production and perception of the /r/-/l/ contrast in Korean adults learning English." *Language Learning* 33, 499-526.

Bornstein, M. 1975. "Qualities of color vision in infancy." *Journal of Exp. Child Psychology* 19, 401-419.

Bornstein, M. 1987. "Sensitive periods in development: Definition, existence, utility, and meaning." *Sensitive Periods in Development.* ed. by M. Bornstein, 3-18. Hillsdale, N.J.: Lawrence Erlbaum Assoc.

Burnham, D. 1986. "Developmental loss of speech perception: Exposure to and experience with a first language." *Applied Psycholinguistics* 7, 207-240.

Brady, S., Shankweiler, D., and Mann, V. 1983. "Speech perception and memory coding in relation to reading ability." *Journal of Exp. Child Psychology* 35, 345-367.

Bradley, L., and Bryant, P. 1983. "Categorizing sounds and learning to read — a causal connection." *Nature* 301, 419-421.

Briere, E. 1966. "An investigation of phonological interference." *Language* 42, 769-796.

Bruner, J. 1964. "The course or cognitive growth." *American Psychologist* 19, 1-15.

Bruner, J., Oliver, R., and Greenfield, P. 1966. *Studies in Cognitive Growth.* New York: Wiley.

Carlson, R., Granstöm, B. and Fant, G. 1970. "Some studies concerning perception of isolated vowels." *Quarterly Progress and Status Report*. 2-3, Royal Institute of Technology (KTH), Stockholm.

Carney, A., Widin, G. and Viemeister, N. 1977. "Non-categorical perception of stop consonants differing in VOT." *Journal of Acoustic Society of America* 62, 961-970.

Chomsky, N. and Halle, M. 1968. *The Sound Patterns of English*. New York: Prentice-Hall.

Christensen, J. 1984. "The perception of voice onset time: A cross language study of American English and Danish." *ARIPUC* 18, 163-185 (Annual Report of the Inst. of Phonetics, Univ. of Copenghagen).

Collins, B. and Mees, I. 1984. *The Sounds of English and Dutch*. Leiden: Leiden University Press.

Danchev, A. 1987. "The stressed vowels in the Bulgarian English Interlanguage." *Tagungsberichte des Anglistentags* 8, ed. by R. Böhn, 287-305. Giessen: Hoffman.

Delattre, P. 1964. "Comparing the consonantal features of English, German, Spanish, and French." *International Review of Applied Linguistics* 2, 155-203.

Delattre, P. 1969. "An acoustic and articulatory study of vowel reduction in four languages." *International Review of Applied Linguistics* 7, 295-323.

diBenedetto, M.-G. 1989. "Vowel representations: Some observations on temporal and spectral properties of the first formant." *Journal of the Acoustic Society of America* 86, 55-66.

Disner, S. 1983. *Vowel Quality: The Relation between Universal and Language Specific Factors*. UCLA Working Papers in Phonetics, 58.

Ekstrand, L. 1982. "English without a book revisited: The effect of age on second language acquisition in a formal setting." *Child-Adult Differences in Second Language Acquisition*, ed. by S. Krashen, R. Scarcella and M. Long, 123-135. Rowley, MA: Newbury House.

Eguchi, S and Hirsh, I. 1969. "Development of speech sounds in children." *Acta Oto-Laryngologica*, Suppl. 257, 1-51.

Elsendoorn, B. 1986. Personal communication.

Ferguson, C. 1986. "Discovering sound units and constructing sound systems: It's child's play." *Invariance and Variability in Speech Processes*, ed. by J. Perkell and D. Klatt, 36-57. Hillsdale, N.J.: Erlbaum.

Flege, J. 1980. "Phonetic approximation in second language acquisition." *Language Learning* 30, 117-134.

———. 1981. "The phonological basis of foreign accent." *TESOL Quarterly* 15, 443-455.

Flege, J. 1984. "The detection of French accent by American listeners." *Journal of the Acoustic Society of America* 76, 692-707.

———. 1987a. "The production of 'new' versus 'similar' vowels in a foreign language: Evidence for the effects of equivalence classification." *Journal of Phonetics* 15, 47-65.

———. 1987b. "A critical period for learning to pronounce foreign languages?" *Applied Linguistics* 8, 162-177.

———. 1988a. "Factors affecting degree of perceived foreign accent in English sentences." *Journal of the Acoustic Society of America* 84, 70-79.

————. 1988b. "The production and perception of foreign language speech sounds." *Human Communication and Its Disorders, A Review — 1988*, ed. by H. Winitz, 224-401. Norwood, N.J.: Ablex.

————. 1988c. "The development of skill in producing word-final /p/ and /b/: Kinematic parameters." *Journal of the Acoustic Society of America* 84, 1639-1652.

————. 1989a. "Chinese subjects' perception of the word-final English /t/-/d/ contrast: Performance before and after training." *Journal of the Acoustic Society of America*, 86, 1684-1697.

————. 1989b. Differences in inventory size affects the location but not the precision of tongue positioning in vowel production, *Language Speech*, 32, 123-147.

————. 1991a. "Age of learning affects the autenticity of voice onset time (VOT) in stop consonants produced in a second language." *Journal of the AcousticalSociety of America* 89, 395-411.

————. 1991b. "The production of English vowels by native speakers of Spanish." MS in preparation, Department of Biocommunication, Univ. of Alabama at Birmingham.

Flege, J. and Fletcher, K. 1991. Talker and listener effects on the perception of degree of perceived foreigh accent. *Journal of the Acoustical Society of America*, to appear.

Flege, J. and Davidian, R. 1985. "Transfer and developmental processes in adult foreign language speech production." *Journal of Applied Psycholinguistics Research* 5, 323-347.

Flege, J. and Eefting, W. 1986. "Linguistic and developmental effects on stop perception and production by native speakers of English and Spanish." *Phonetica* 43, 155-171.

————. 1987a. "Cross-language switching in stop consonant production and perception by Dutch speakers of English." *Speech Communication* 6, 185-202.

————. 1987b. "The production and perception of English stops by Spanish speakers of English." *Journal of Phonetics* 15, 67-83.

————. 1988. "Imitation of a VOT continuum by native speakers of English and Spanish: Evidence for phonetic category formation." *Journal of the Acoustic Society of America* 83, 729-740.

Flege, J. and Hammond, R. 1982. "Mimicry of non-distinctive phonetic differences between language varieties." *Studies in Second Language Acquisition* 5, 1-18.

Flege, J. and Hillenbrand, J. 1984. "Limits on pronunciation accuracy in adult foreign language speech production." *Journal of the Acoustic Society of America* 76, 708-721.

Flege, J. and Wang, C. (1990). "Native-language phonotactic constraints affect how well Chinese subjects perceive the word-final English /t/-/d/ contrast." *Journal of Phonetics*, 17, 299-315.

Flege, J., McCutcheon, M. and Smith, S. 1987. "The development of skill in producing word-final English stops", *Journal of the Acoustic Society of America* 82, 433-447.

Fletcher, H., and Steinberg, J. 1929. "Articulation testing methods." *Bell Syst. Tech. Journal* 8, 806-854.

Florentine, M. 1985. "Speech perception in noise by fluent, non-native listeners." *Journal of the Acoustical Society of America* 77, S106(A).

Ganong, W.F, III 1980. "Phonetic categorization in auditory word perception." *JEP:HPP* 6, 110-125.

Gass, S. and Varonis, E. 1984. "The effect of familiarity on the comprehensibility of nonnative speech." *Language Learning* 34, 65-89.

Gibson, E. 1969. *Principals of Perceptual Learning and Development.* New York: Appleton-Century-Crofts.

Godinez, M. 1978. "A comparative study of some Romance vowels." UCLA Working Papers in Phonetics 41, 3-19.

Gottfried, T. and Beddor, P. 1988. "Perception of temporal and spectral information in French vowels." *Language & Speech* 31, 57-75.

Green, B., Logan, J. and Pisoni, D. 1986. "Perception of synthetic speech produced by rule: Intelligibility of eight text-to-speech systems." *Behavioral Research Methods, Instruments, & Computers* 18, 100-107.

Greenberg, S. and Roscoe, S. 1988. "Echoic memory interference and comprehension in a foreign language." *Language Learning* 38, 209-219.

Grieser, D. 1984. *The Internal Structure of Vowel Categories in Infancy: The Effects of Stimulus 'Goodness'.* Unpubl. Ph.D. thesis, Univ. of Washington.

Grieser, D. and Kuhl, P. 1989. "The categorization of speech by infants: Support for speech-sound prototypes." *Developmental Psychology*, 25, 577-588.

Hillenbrand, J. 1983. "Perceptual organization of speech sounds by infants." *Journal of Speech & Hearing Research* 26, 268-282.

Hillenbrand, J. 1984. "Speech perception by infants: Categorization based on nasal consonant place of articulation." *Journal of the Acoustic Society of America* 75, 1613-1622.

Holden, K. and Nearey, T. 1986. "A preliminary report on three Russian dialects: Vowel perception and production." *Russian Language Journal* 40, 3-21.

Holtse, P. 1972. "Spectrographic analysis of English vowels." ARIPUC 7, 1-48 (Annual Report of the Inst. of Phonetics, Univ. of Copenhagen).

Hudgins, C. and Numbers, F. 1942. "An investigation of the intelligibility of the speech of the deaf." *Genetic Psychology Monographs* 25, 289-392.

Inhelder, B. and Piaget, J. 1969. *The Early Growth of Logic in the Child.* New York: Norton.

Jaeger, J. 1986. "Concept formation as a tool for linguistic research." *Experimental Phonology*, ed. by J. Ohala and J. Jaeger, 211-238. London: Academic Press.

James, A. 1984. "Syntagmatic segment errors in non-native speech." *Linguistics* 22, 481-505.

James, A. 1985a. "Phonetic transfer and phonological explanation: Some theoretical and methodological issues." *Cross-language influence in Second Language Acquisition.* ed. by E. Kellerman and M. Sharwood. Oxford: Pergamon Press

———. 1985b. Personal communication.

———. 1989. Personal communication.

Johnson, J. and Newport, E. 1989. "Critical period effects in second language learning: The influence of maturational state on the acquisition of English as a second language." *Cognitive Psychology* 21, 69-99.

Jusczyk, P. 1985. "On characterizing the development of speech perception." *Neonate Cognition: Beyond the Blooming, Buzzing Confusion*, ed. by J. Mehler and R. Fox, 199-229, Hillsdale, NJ: Lawrence Erlbaum Assoc.

———. 1986. "Toward a model of the development of speech perception." *Invariance and Variability in Speech Processes*, ed. by J.Perkell and D. Klatt, 1-35, Hillsdale, NJ: Lawrence Erlbaum Assoc.

———. 1989. "Developing phonological categories from the speech signal." Paper presented at the International Conference on Phonological Development, Stanford University, September 22, 1989.

Jusczyk, P., Friederici, A., and Wessels, J. 1989. "Infants' recognition of foreign versus native language words." MS in preparation.

Kalikow, D., Stevens, K. and Elliot, L. 1977. "Development of a test of speech intelligibility in noise using sentence materials with controlled word predictability." *Journal of the Acoustic Society of America* 61, 1337-1351.

Keating, P. 1984. "Phonetic and phonological representation of stop consonant voicing." *Language* 60, 286-319.

Kent, R. 1974. "Auditory-motor formant tracking: A study of speech imitation." *Journal of Speech & Hearing Research* 17, 203-222.

Kent, R. and Forner, L. 1979. "Developmental study of vowel formant frequencies in an imitation task." *Journal of the Acoustic Society of America* 65, 208-217.

Kewley-Port, D. and Preston, M. 1974. "Early apical stop reproduction: A voice onset time analysis." *Journal of Phonetics* 2, 195-210.

Kewley-Port, D. and Atal, B. 1989. "Perceptual differences between vowels located in a limited phonetic space." *Journal of the Acoustic Society of America* 85, 1726-1740.

Kirk, R. 1968. *Experimental Design: Procedures for the Behavioral Sciences*. Belmont, CA: Brooks/Cole.

Kirtley, C., Bryant, P., MacLean, M., and Bradley, L. 1989 "Rhyme, Rime, and the Onset of Reading." *Journal of Experimental Child Psychology*, 48, 224-245.

Klatt, D. 1979. "Speech perception: A model of acoustic-phonetic analysis and lexical access." *Journal of Phonetics* 7, 279-312.

Koopmans-van Beinum, F. 1980. *Vowel Contrast Reduction*. Amsterdam: Academische Pers B.V..

Koster, C. 1987. *Word Recognition in Foreign and Native Language*. Dordrecht: Foris.

Kuhl, P. 1979. "Speech perception in early infancy: Perceptual constancy for spectrally dissimilar vowel categories." *Journal of the Acoustic Society of America* 66, 1668-1679.

Kuhl, P. and Padden, D. 1983. "Enhanced discriminability at the phonetic boundaries for the place feature in macaques." *Journal of the Acoustic Society of America* 73, 1003-1010.

Labov, W. 1981. "Resolving the neogrammarian controversy." *Language* 57, 267-309.

———. 1986. "Sources of inherent variation in the speech process." *Invariance and variability in speech processes*. ed. by J. Perkell and D. Klatt, 402-425. Hillsdale, N.J.: Erlbaum.

Ladefoged, P. 1975. *A Course in Phonetics*. New York: Harcourt, Brace, and Jovanovich.

———. 1980. "What are linguistic sounds made of?" *Language* 54, 485-502.

———. 1983. "The limits of biological explanation in phonetics." *Abstracts of the Tenth International Congress of Phonetic Sciences*, ed. by A. Cohen and M. v.d. Broecke. Dordrecht, The Netherlands: Foris.

Leather, J. 1983. "Second-language pronunciation learning and teaching." *Language Teaching* 16, 198-219.

Liberman, I., Shankweiler, D., Fisher, F., and Carter, B. 1974. "Explicit syllable and phoneme segmentation in the young child. *Journal of Experimental Child Psychology* 18, 201-212.

Lieberman, P. 1970. "Towards a unified phonetic theory." *Linguistic Inquiry* 1, 307-321.

Linell, P. 1982. "The concept of phonological form and the activities of speech production and perception." *Journal of Phonetics* 10, 37-72.

Logan, J., Green, B., and Pisoni, D. 1989. "Segmental intelligibility of synthetic speech produced by rule." *Journal of the Acoustic Society of America* 86, 566-581.

Logan, J., Lively, S. and Pisoni, D. 1989. "Training Japanese listeners to identify /r/ and /l/: A first report." *Research on Speech Perception*, Progress Report 14.1-25 (Dept. of Psychology, Indiana U.).

Ma, R. and Herasimchuk. 1971. "The linguistic dimensions of a bilingual neighborhood." *Bilingualism in the Barrio*. ed. by J. Fishman, R. Cooper, and R. Ma, 349-479. Bloomington: Indiana Univ. Press.

Macchi, M. 1980. "Identification of vowels spoken in isolation versus vowels spoken in consonantal context." *Journal of the Acoustic Society of America* 68, 1636-1642.

Mack, M. 1989. "Consonant and vowel perception and production: Early English-French bilinguals and English monolinguals." *Perception & Psychophysics* 46, 187-200.

Mack, M. and Lieberman, P. 1985. "Acoustic analysis of words produced by a child from 46 to 149 weeks." *Journal of Child Language* 12, 527-550.

Macken, M. and Barton, D. 1980a. "A longitudinal study of the the acquisition of voicing contrast in American-English word-initial stops." *Journal of Child Language* 7, 41-74.

———. 1980b. "The acquisition of the voicing contrast in Spanish: A phonetic and phonological study of word-initial consonants." *Journal of Child Language* 7, 433-458.

Maddieson, I. 1984. *Patterns of Sounds*. Cambridge: Cambridge University Press.

Major, R. 1987. "Phonological similarity, markedness, and rate of L2 acquisition." *Studies in Second Language Acquisition*, 9, 63-82.

Mann, V. (1984). "Reading skill and language skill." *Developmental Review* 4, 1-15.

———. 1986. "Phonological awareness: The role of reading experience." *Cognition* 24, 65-92.

Massaro, D. and Cohen, M. 1983. "Evaluation and integration of visual and auditory information in speech perception." *JEP: HPP* 9, 753-771.

———. 1984. "Categorical or continuous speech perception: A new test." *Speech Communication* 2, 15-35.

Massaro, D. and Oden, G. 1980. "Evaluation and integration of acoustic features in speech perception." *Journal of the Acoustic Society of America* 67, 996-1013.

Matthei, E. 1989. "Crossing boundaries: More evidence for phonological constraints on early multi-word utterances." *Journal of Child Language* 16, 41-54.

McGarr, N. 1978. *The differences between experienced and inexperienced listeners in understanding the speech of the deaf.* Unpubl. Ph.D. thesis, City Univ. of New York.

McLaughlin, B. 1978. *Second Language Acquisition in Childhood.* Hillsdale, N.J.: Lawrence Erlbaum Assoc..

———. 1984. *Second-Language Acquisition in Childhood: Vol. 1. Preschool Children*, 2nd ed. Hillsdale, N.J.: Lawrence Erlbaum Assoc.

Menn, L. 1982. "Development of articulatory, phonetic, and phonological capabilities." *Language Production*, Volume 2, ed. by B. Butterworth, 3-50. New York: Academic Press.

Miller, J. 1989. "Auditory-perceptual interpretation of the vowel." *Journal of the Acoustic Society of America* 85, 2114-2134.

Miller, G., Heise, G. and Lichten, W. 1951. "The intelligibility of speech as function of the context of the test materials." *JEP* 41, 329-335.

Miranda, S. and Strange, W. 1989. "The role of spectral, temporal, and dynamic cues in the perception of English vowels by native and non-native speakers." *Journal of the Acoustic Society of America*, Suppl 1, 85.S53(A).

Morais, J., Cary, L., Alegria, J. and Bertelson, P. 1979. "Does awareness of speech as a sequence of phones arise spontaneously?" *Cognition* 7, 323-331.

Moulton, W. 1962. "The vowels of Dutch: Phonetic and distributional classes." *Lingua* 11, 294-312.

Mullennix, J., Pisoni, D. and Martin, C. 1989. "Some effects of talker variability on spoken word recognition." *Journal of the Acoustic Society of America*, 85, 365-368.

Nabèleck, A. and Donahue, A. 1984. "Perception of consonants in reverberations by native and non-native listeners." *Journal of the Acoustic Society of America* 75, 632-634.

Nelson, K. 1974. "Concept, word, and sentence: Interrelationship in acquisition and development." *Psycholgoy Review* 81, 267-285.

Nooteboom, S. 1972. *Production and Perception of Vowel Duration, A study of Durational Properties of Vowels in Dutch.* Ph.D. thesis, Univ. of Utrecht.

———. 1973. "The perceptual reality of prosodic durations." *Journal of Phonetics* 1, 25-45.

Nooteboom, S. and Slis, A. 1972. "The phonetic feature of length in Dutch." *Language Speech* 15, 301-316.

Obler, L. and Albert, M. 1978. "A monitor system for bilingual language processing." *Aspects of Bilingualism*, ed. by M. Paradis. Columbia, S.C.: Hornbeam Press.

Oden, G. and Massaro, D. 1978. "Integration of featural information in speech perception." *Psychology Review* 85, 172-191.

Oller, D. and Eilers, R. 1983. "Speech identification in Spanish- and English-learning two-year-olds." *Journal of Speech & Hearing Research* 26, 50-53.

Oller, J. and Ziahosseiny, S. 1970. "The contrastive analysis hypothesis and spelling errors." *Language Learning* 20, 183-189.

Olson, L., and Samuels, J. 1973. "The relationship between age and accuracy of foreign language pronunciation." *Journal of Education Research* 66, 263-267.

Pisoni, D., Aslin, R., Perey, A. and Hennessey, B. 1982. "Some effects of laboratory training on identification of voicing contrasts in stop consonants." *JEP:HPP* 8, 297-314.

Pisoni, D., Nusbaum, H. and Green, B. 1985. "Perception of synthetic speech generated by rule." *Proceedings of the IEEE* 73, 1665-1676.

Peterson, G. and Barney, H. 1952. "Control methods used in a study of the vowels." *Journal of the Acoustic Society of America* 24, 175-184.

Politzer, R. and Weiss, L. 1969. "Developmental aspects of auditory discrimination, echo response, and recall." *Modern Language Journal* 53, 75-85.

Pollock, K. and Keiser, N. 1990. "AN examination of vowel errors in phonologically disordered children." *Clinical Linguistics & Phonetics* 4, 161-178.

Pols, L., van der Kamp, L. and Plomp, R. 1969. "Perceptual and physical space of vowel sounds." *Journal of the Acoustic Society of America* 46, 458-467.

Pols, L., Tromp, H. and Plomp, R. 1973. "Frequency analysis of Dutch vowels from 50 male speakers." *Journal of the Acoustic Society of America* 53, 1093-1101.

Reed, C., Delhorn, L. and Durlach, D. 1987. "Tactile reception of fingerspelling and sign language", *Journal of the Acoustic Society of America*, Suppl. 1, 82, S24(A).

Remez, R., Rubin, P., Pisoni, D., and Carrell, T. 1981. "Speech perception without traditional cues." *Science* 212, 947-950.

Repp, B. 1981. "Two strategies in fricative discrimination." *Perception & Psychophysics*, 30 217-227.

———. 1976. "Identification of dichotic fusions." *Journal of the Acoustic Society of America* 60, 456-469.

Repp, B., Healy, A., and Crowder, R. 1979. "Categories and contexts in the perception of isolated steady-state vowels." *Journal of Experimental Psychology: Human Perception Peformance* 5, 129-145.

Robson, B. 1982. "Teaching English pronunciation to speakers of Korean." *Focus* 11, 1-9 (National Clearinghouse for Bilingual Educ., Washington, DC).

Rosch, E. 1975. "Universals and cultural specifics in human categorization." *Cross-Cultural Perspectives on Learning*, ed. by R. Brislin, S. Bochner and W. Lonner. New York: Halsted Press.

Rubin, J. 1983. *Static and Dynamic Information in Vowels Produced by the Hearing Impaired*. Unpubl. Ph.D. thesis, City Univ. of New York (Available from the Indiana Univ. Ling. Club).

Samuel, A. 1977. "The effect of discrimination training on speech perception: Non-categorical perception." *Perception & Psychophysics* 22, 321-330.

———. 1982. "Phonetic prototypes." *Perception & Psychophysics* 31, 307-314.

Schouten, M.. 1975. *Native-language Interference in the Perception of Second-Language Vowels*. Utrecht: Drukkerij Elinkwijk.

Scovel, T. 1981. "The recognition of foreign accents." *Proceedings of the 5th Congress of the Int. Assoc. of Applied Linguistics*, ed. by J.-G. Savard and L. Laforge. Quebec: Univ. of Laval Press.

Sinnott, J. 1989. "Detection and discrimination of synthetic English vowels by Old World monkeys (Cercopithecus, Maccaca) and humans." *Journal of the Acoustic Society of America* 86, 557-565.

Smith, B. 1977. "Temporal aspects of English speech production: A developmental perspective." *Journal of Phonetics* 6, 37-69.

Snow, C. 1988. "Relevance of the notion of a critical period to language acquisition." *Sensitive Periods in Development, Interdisciplinary Perspectives*, ed. by M. Bornstein, 183-210. Hillsdale, N.J.: Lawrence Erlbaum Assoc.

Snow, C. and Hoefnagel-Höhle, M. 1977. "Age differences in the pronunciation of foreign sounds." *Language Speech* 20, 357-365.

——. 1982. "Age differences in the pronunciation of foreign sounds." *Child-Adult Differences in Second Language Acquisition*, ed. by R. Scarcella and M. Long, 84-92. Rowley, MA: Newbury House.

Spolsky, B., Sigurd, B., Sako, M., Walker, E. and Atterbrun, C. 1968. "Preliminary studies in the development of techniques for testing overall second language proficiency." *Language Learning* 18, 79-101.

Stevens, K. and House, A. 1963. "Perturbation of vowel articulations by consonant context: An acoustical study." *Journal of Speech & Hearing Research* 6, 111-128.

Stockwell, R. and Bowen, J. 1965. *Sounds of English and Spanish*. Chicago: University of Chicago Press.

Strange, W. 1989. "Dynamic specification of coarticulated vowels spoken in sentence context." *Journal of the Acoustic Society of America* 85, 2135-2153.

Strange, W., Verbrugge, R., Shankweiler, D., and Edman, T. 1976. "Consonant environment specifies vowel identity." *Journal of the Acoustic Society of America* 60, 213-224.

Tahta, S., Wood, M. and Loewenthal, K. 1981. "Foreign accents: Factors relating to transfer of accent from the first language to a second language." *Language & Speech* 24, 265-272.

Trubetzkoy, N. 1939/1969. *Grudzuge der Phonolgie*. Travaux du Cercle Linguistique de Prague 7. English translation by C. Baltaxe. Berkeley, CA, Univ. of California Press.

van Balen, C. 1980. *Intelligibility of Speech Fragments*. Utrecht: Drukkerij Elinkwijk.

van Heuven, V. 1986. *Personal communication*.

Varonis, E. and Gass, S. 1982. "The comprehensibility of nonnative speech." *Studies in Second Language Acquisition* 4, 114-136.

Verbrugge, R., Strange, W., Shankweiler, D. and Edman, T. 1976. "What information enables a listener to map a talker's vowel space?" *Journal of the Acoustic Society of America* 60, 198-212.

Weinreich, U. 1953. *Languages in Contact: Findings and Problems*. The Hague: Mouton.

Wells, J. 1982. *Accents of English, Vol. 1, An Introduction*. Cambridge: Cambridge Univ. Press.

Werker, J. 1986. "Phonetic discrimination and perceptual reorganization in human infants." Paper presented at the Int. Conf. of Infant Studies, Los Angeles, CA.

Werker, J. and Logan, J. 1985. "Cross-language evidence for three factors in speech perception." *Perception & Psychophysics* 37, 35-44.

Werker, J. and Tees, R. 1982. "Perceptual reorganization in the first year of life." Paper presented at Canadian Psych. Assoc., Montreal, June, 1982.

———. 1983. "Developmental changes across childhood in the perception of non-native speech sounds." *Canadian Journal of Psychology* 37, 278-286.

———. 1984a. "Cross-language speech perception: Evidence for perceptual reorganization during the first year of life." *Infant Behaviour Development* 7, 49-63.

———. 1984b. "Phonemic and phonetic factors in adult cross-language speech perception." *Journal of the Acoustic Society of America* 75, 1866-1878.

Williams, H. and Nottebohm, F. 1985. "Auditory responses in avian motor neurons: A motor theory for song perception in birds." *Science* 229, 279-282.

Wode, H. 1977. "The L2 acquisition of /r/." *Phonetica* 34.200-217.

———. 1978. "The beginning of non-school room L2 phonological acquisition." *International Review of Applied Linguistics* 16, 109-125.

Zlatin, M. and Koenigsknecht, R. 1976. "Development of the voicing contrast: A comparison of voice onset time in stop perception and production." *Journal of Speech & Hearing Research* 19, 93-111.

Chapter 6

Speech intelligibility in the hearing impaired: Research and clinical implications

Mary Joe Osberger
Indiana University School of Medicine

The intelligibility of hearing-impaired children's speech has been studied extensively over the years. It has been a topic of great interest and concern to professionals and parents because intelligibility data provide an estimate of the viability of oral communication for hearing-impaired children. Research in this area has quantified the intelligibility of the speech of hearing-impaired children with varying degrees of hearing loss, examined different methods to measure intelligibility, and identified variables that affect intelligibility scores.

The largest body of research data reports the intelligibility of hearing-impaired talkers in terms of a performance measure. That is, a percent intelligibility score is obtained, or a numerical rating is assigned to a sample of speech. The advantage of this technique is that it lends itself to analyzing group data and it can provide important descriptive information. The limitation of this approach is that no information is obtained about the underlying causes for reduced intelligibility. Information of this nature is crucial for developing intervention programs to improve a hearing-impaired talker's intelligibility.

During recent years, there has been a move toward the use of procedures that provide more diagnostic information than can be obtained from

* Reprinted from *Topics in Language Disorders*, Vol. 6, No. 4, p. 40, with permission of Aspen Publishers, Inc., © 1986.

performance measures. From a research standpoint, interest has shifted toward using measures that provide more than a single index of performance. Emphasis now is placed on examination of the speaker's ability to convey specified phonetic contrasts and identification of the acoustic properties underlying the phonetic contrasts. This information is necessary to understand how specific phonetic and acoustic distortions affect intelligibility, and to develop improved computer-based aids for speech assessment and training. From a clinical perspective, the need for diagnostic intelligibility tests became apparent with the introduction of Public Law 94-142 which required the development of Individualized Education Plans (IEP) for all handicapped children. Consequently, there was a need for procedures that identified areas of strength and weakness for individual children to assist in formulating goals and objectives for the IEP.

Another factor that has influenced the way in which intelligibility is measured, at least clinically, is the emphasis in the child language literature on pragmatics and *communication effectiveness*. In this context, intelligibility is defined as the ability to use speech to communicate effectively in everyday situations rather than being specified as the number of words correctly understood by a panel of listeners.

The first part of this chapter will review information on traditional methods to assess intelligibility, recent modifications in assessment methods, and the factors that affect intelligibility scores. The second part of the chapter describes training and assessment procedures that are intended to assist the clinician in gaining a better understanding of a child's speech intelligibility in everyday situations, and in identifying appropriate intervention strategies to improve speech intelligibility.

Methods of measuring intelligibility

Two methods have been used to assess the intelligibility of hearing-impaired talkers: item identification and scaling. These methods are not unique to assessing the speech of hearing-impaired talkers but have been used to study the speech of other clinical populations as well (see, e.g., Kent, Weismer, Kent, and Rosenbeck, 1989). A brief description of each method and its application in measuring the speech of hearing-impaired talkers is presented first. However, as noted by Kent et al. (1989), an intelligibility score cannot be interpreted without taking into consideration the specific conditions under which the data were collected. Therefore, a more extensive review of the data collected on the speech of hearing-impaired talkers with each type of method is presented in the following section in conjunction with a discussion of the factors that affect intelligibility scores.

Item identification

Traditionally, item identification has used an open-set response format in which a panel of listeners write down what they think the child has said. A recent modification is the use of a closed-set, multiple-choice format similar to that used in speech perception experiments.

Open-set intelligibility tests

A speech sample, consisting of words or sentences, is read by the speaker, audio-recorded, and subsequently randomized, and played back to a panel of listeners. The listeners are instructed to write down what they believe the talker has said, and their responses are scored in terms of the percentage of words correctly understood. Most often sentence material is scored in terms of key words correctly understood in each sentence (e.g., Smith, 1975), although in some cases all of the words in the sentence are scored (e.g., Magnan, 1961), or intelligibility is expressed in terms of the percentage of sentences completely understood by the listener (Hudgins & Numbers, 1942). Another approach is to use a weighting system in which words in sentences are given different values depending on their contribution to the linguistic message conveyed. The scheme developed by Monsen (1978) assigned content words a relatively higher value than function words. Brannon (1964) scored the number of words correctly understood in an elicited speech sample rather than in a read one. This technique, however, does not permit the examiner to score the words understood by the listener in terms of the words intended by the talker.

The advantage of using open-set item identification, or a write-down procedure, is that it has high face validity (Samar and Metz, 1988). The disadvantage is that data collection and analyses are time consuming, making this technique difficult to use in clinical situations. Further, the outcome is a single index of performance, the intelligibility score, with no information about the underlying causes for reduced intelligibility.

Closed-set intelligibility tests

With this approach, the listener is given a set of possible alternatives from which to choose the word spoken by the talker. The forced-choice procedures developed for use with hearing-impaired speakers are designed to assess the talker's ability to convey specific phonetic contrasts to the listener. The strength of these procedures is that performance is quantified in terms of the speaker's ability to transmit a message even though the productions may not conform to those produced by normal-hearing talkers. Another strength of this approach is that data can be examined to identify those features of speech that are not accurately conveyed by the talker. This information can then be used to formulate a speech intervention program.

The first person to apply this approach was Monsen (1981), who developed a closed-set response test for teachers and clinician's to use. The test, referred to as the Speech Intelligibility Evaluation (SPINE), consists of 10 subtests with four CVC words in each subtest. The four words contrast one or more phonetic or acoustic features. The choice of contrasts is based on Monsen's extensive research on the speech of hearing-impaired talkers (Monsen, 1978). The features examined are vowel height and place, consonant voicing, and production of liquids and semivowels. Each subtest consists of 10 decks of cards with each deck containing an equal number of cards with one of the four different words printed on them. The examiner selects ten cards from each deck, and the child is asked to read the word on each card. The examiner must then decide which of the four possible words in each subtest that the child has said. This procedure is repeated for all ten subtests. Performance is scored in terms of the percentage of words on each subtest that are perceived correctly by the examiner. Monsen (1981) reported a correlation of .86 between the subjects' scores on the SPINE test and the scores obtained on an open-set sentence intelligibility test, indicating that the SPINE test is highly predictive of speech intelligibility.

The procedure developed by Boothroyd (1985a; 1988), the Speech Pattern Contrast (SPAC) test, consists of monosyllabic words which contain pairs of phonetic contrasts. Listeners are given four response alternatives for each test utterance, providing the possibility for independent errors along two phonetic dimensions. The following contrasts are evaluated: vowel height (high vs. low), vowel place (front vs. back), initial consonant voicing, initial consonant continuance (stop vs. continuant), initial consonant place, final consonant voicing, final consonant continuance, and final consonant place. Performance is scored in terms of the percentage of time that a contrast is perceived correctly by the listener (chance level of performance = 50%).

Boothroyd (1985a) evaluated the speech production abilities of 16 profoundly hearing-impaired adolescents between the ages of 13 to 19 years with the SPAC. The subjects in Boothroyd's study demonstrated better ear pure-tone thresholds (3-frequency average) ranging from 82 dB HL to 110 dB HL, with a median of 102 dB HL. Two groups of subjects listened to the hearing-impaired subjects' production of the SPAC utterances. One group consisted of persons experienced in listening to the speech of the hearing impaired and the other group consisted of inexperienced listeners. In our laboratory, the SPAC has been administered to a group of 7 hearing-impaired children, ranging in age from 8 to 12 years, with the three-frequency pure tone average in the better ear ranging from 92 dB HL to 107 dB HL, with a median of 98 dB HL. The SPAC productions were evaluated by three listeners who had some experience in listening to the speech of profoundly hearing-impaired talkers. Note that the hearing levels of the subjects in our sample were slightly better than those in Boothroyd's study and the subjects were younger. Also, half of the subjects in our study had acquired hearing losses, and two of the subjects with acquired deafness did not lose their hearing until almost 5 years of age. Boothroyd did not state the age of onset of hearing loss in his sample, although given the population tested, it is assumed that the majority of subjects had congenital losses, or losses of early onset.

Figure 1 shows the SPAC scores for each contrast for the two groups of subjects, averaged across subjects and listeners. It is important to keep in mind that the number of utterances produced by the speakers in the two studies (12 tokens per subtest by each speaker in the Boothroyd study and 32 tokens per subtest by each speaker in our study) differed. The raw scores from both groups of data have been corrected for guessing, as described by Boothroyd (1988:314). The correction formula is:

$$S_c = (S_u - S_g)/(100 - S_g)*100$$

where Sc is the corrected score in percent, S_u is the uncorrected score in percent, S_g is the mean score expected from guessing (i.e., 50%). The data in Figure 1 reveal the following trends. First, the subjects in both studies produced the vowel contrasts better than the consonant contrasts. Secondly, the subjects in our study were able to convey all contrasts more

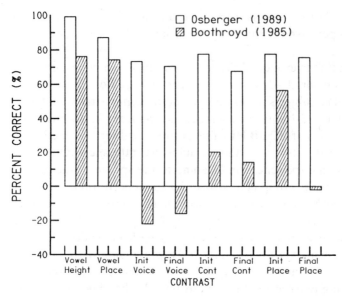

Figure 1.*Scores obtained by two groups of profoundly hearing-impaired sub-jects on the Speech Pattern Contrast (SPAC) test. Scores have been averaged across 16 subjects in Bootroyd's (1985) sample and across 7 subjects in the Osberger (1989) study.*

effectively than the subjects in the Boothroyd study. This presumably reflects the better hearing levels and later onset of deafness of some of the subjects in our study. All consonant contrasts were conveyed relatively well by the speakers in our study and there was negligible difference between the scores as a function of type of consonant contrast produced. In contrast, the subjects in Boothroyd's study had difficulty producing nearly all the consonant contrasts. The exception to this pattern is their ability to convey initial consonant place with about 60% accuracy. These data highlight the differences in the speech production abilities among subjects with profound hearing losses, and the effect that variables such as degree of hearing loss and age of onset of hearing loss have on speech.

The SPAC also contains a subtest that assesses the talker's ability to convey contrastive stress, and a subtest that examines the ability of a talker to convey an utterance as a statement or a Yes-No question (Boothroyd, 1988). The contrastive stress subtest requires the talker to emphasize one of three words in a short phrase, and then the listener must decide which word has been stressed (chance performance = 33.33%). The Question vs. Statement subtest requires the talker to produce a short phrase with a falling or rising intonation (chance performance = 50%). Boothroyd (1985a) reported no data for his subjects on these subtests. The mean score, corrected for guessing, for the 7 subjects in our study on the subtest evaluating contrastive stress was 94%, and 80% on the Question vs. Statement subtest.

Boothroyd (1985a) compared the scores obtained on the SPAC to open-set sentence intelligibility scores for the 16 subjects in his study and he found that the composite contrast score accounted for about 70% of the variance of the sentence measure. He concluded that although the contrast score was not a perfect predictor of intelligibility, there was a strong relationship between the skills assessed on the contrast test to those assessed when producing sentences.

Data collected from procedures such as the SPAC, however, do not tell the examiner why a particular feature has not been transmitted effectively by the talker. For example, a speaker may omit a final consonant or substitute one containing a feature other than the targeted one. There is no way to determine which type of error has been made without performing a phonetic transcription of the utterances.

Sentence material also can be used with a closed-set format. Carney (1986) had profoundly hearing-impaired children produce selected sentences from the Test of Syntactic Abilities (Quigley, Steinkamp, Power, and Jones, 1978), and then allowed listeners to choose the target sentences from a closed-set of sentences. The use of a closed-set format is particularly useful for talkers whose intelligibility is so reduced that their scores on open-set measures would be zero. Data collected in our laboratory, comparing the intelligibility scores obtained with an open- and closed-set format are presented later in the chapter.

Scaling

The scaling technique used most frequently to rate the intelligibility of hearing-impaired talkers' speech employs an interval scale. This approach has been employed extensively by Subtelny (1977) and colleagues at the National Technical Institute for the Deaf to rate the intelligibility of the speech of young, profoundly hearing-impaired adults who attend the school. In the classic Subtelny (1977) study, a panel of five listeners rated the speech (a paragraph of prepared text) of 156 profoundly hearing-impaired talkers on a 9-half point, discrete rating scale. Test-retest analyses revealed the intra-judge reliability coefficient to be .97. Open-set sentence intelligibility was assessed and compared to the rating data to examine the validity of the rating scale used. A validity coefficient of .87 was observed, which led Subtelny to conclude that the use of a rating scale system to evaluate speech intelligibility was valid for clinical and research purposes.

The conclusion reached by Subtelny (1977) regarding rating-scale validity was challenged later by Samar and Metz (1988), who replicated and extended the Subtelny study. Samar and Metz obtained reliability and validity coefficients similar to those reported by Subtelny, but they also found that the distribution of estimation error over the full range of rating-scale values revealed violations of measurement prediction within the midrange of speech intelligibility. Specifically, the overall accuracy of prediction of speech intelligibility, as measured by the write-down sentence procedure, was roughly 3.0 times greater from directly measured write-down scores than from rating-scale measurements. These data suggest that distinctions among individuals whose speech intelligibility falls in the midrange (i.e., between 20 and 80%) may not be apparent if intelligibility is assessed with an interval rating scale. This is an important consideration to keep in mind when selecting an evaluation protocol for clinical or research purposes, given that the majority of intelligibility scores for hearing-impaired talkers will fall within the mid-range of intelligibility.

An alternative to the use of interval rating scales is to use direct magnitude estimation. Unlike interval scaling, which requires the listener to assign a number along a linear scale, direct magnitude estimation allows the listener to assign each stimulus a value representing the ratio of that stimulus to a standard. Schiavetti, Metz, and Sitler (1981) examined the appropriateness of direct magnitude estimation and interval scaling procedures for assessing the speech intelligibility of hearing-impaired talkers. Their findings showed better construct validity for direct magnitude estimation than for interval scaling. The use of scaling procedures to assess intelligibility is discussed in geater detail by Schiavetti (this volume).

Factors affecting intelligibility measures

Speech intelligibility scores are affected by at least three major variables: the speech material used, the characteristics of the listeners who perform the intelligibility evaluations, and the characteristics of the talkers whose speech is under study. The effect of these variables on the measurement of speech intelligibility in hearing-impaired talkers is discussed below.

Speech material

Contextual cues

The variable which has been manipulated most often in intelligibility studies is the degree of context and linguistic redundancy in the speech stimuli produced by the talker. It has been demonstrated that listeners' ability to understand speech which has been degraded by noise or filtering is better when words are heard in sentences than when words are heard in isolation (see, e.g., Miller, Heise, and Lichten, 1951). This same interaction between degree of linguistic context and intelligibility has been demonstrated with listeners who hear the speech of hearing-impaired talkers. A consistent finding in the literature is that sentence-intelligibility scores are higher than single-word intelligibility scores (Thomas, 1963; Brannon, 1964; McGarr, 1983; Sitler, Schiavetti, and Metz, 1983). When speech is degraded, as it is by the presence of a profound hearing loss, the listener is able to use multiple acoustic, linguistic, and phonological cues in sentence material to assist in decoding what the speaker has said. These same cues, however, are not present when the listener hears only isolated words. The results of several investigations which have examined the effect of context have shown that isolated word-intelligibility scores range from 17 to 31% correct whereas sentence-intelligibility scores range from 30 to 50% correct, depending on the particular words and sentences used (Thomas, 1963; Brannon, 1964; McGarr, 1983; Sitler et al., 1983).

McGarr (1983) extended the work of previous investigators and examined the interaction between degree of linguistic context and intelligibility. Sentences were constructed to lend either high predictability (high-context sentences) or low predictability (low-context sentences) to a key word in each sentence. McGarr found that scores were significantly higher for the test words with high-context than for those with low context. Scores for key words in high-context sentences were approximately 16% higher than for those in low-context sentences.

Sitler and colleagues (Sitler et al., 1983) observed an interaction between degree of context and the overall intelligibility of the talker's speech. They found that sentence intelligibility was superior to isolated-word intelligibility only for the most intelligible talkers whereas sentence and word-intelligibility scores were equivalent for the least intelligible talkers. That is, the speech of the most unintelligible deaf talkers was so degraded that the listeners were unable to use even contextual cues to decode what had been said.

Phonologic and syntactic complexity

A review of the literature reveals large differences in sentence intelligibility scores reported by investigators. A frequent finding is that the average sentence-intelligibility of profoundly hearing-impaired children's speech is about 20% (Brannon, 1964; John and Howarth, 1965; Markides, 1970; Smith, 1975). That is, only about one out of every five words they say can be understood by a listener who is unfamiliar with the speech of hearing-impaired talkers. Monsen (1978), however, reported an average sentence intelligibility score of 76% for profoundly hearing-impaired children. Monsen attributed the difference in intelligibility scores between his and other studies to differences in the speech material which the children produced. The sentences in Monsen's study were shorter, had more familiar vocabulary, and were syntactically less complex than those used by other investigators.

In a follow-up investigation, Monsen (1983) found an interaction between sentence complexity and the overall intelligibility of the talker on the intelligibility score. The effect of consonant clusters, polysyllabic words, and syntactic complexity was greatest for the least intelligible talkers, with differences in sentence-intelligibility as large as 17%. These data suggest that Sitler et al. (1983) might not have observed an interaction between context and overall intelligibility of the speaker if they had used simple sentences.

Monsen (1983) also found that intelligibility scores improved approximately 7%, on the average, if listeners heard two presentations, rather than only one, of the test sentence. Further, the average percent correct for sentences heard with verbal context (i.e., a sentence providing information about the test sentence) was approximately 14% higher than for sentences heard without context.

Characteristics of the listener

Listener experience

One of the most important factors which influence intelligibility judgments is the past experience that the listener has had in hearing profoundly hearing-impaired people talk. Numerous studies have shown consistently that persons experienced in listening to the speech of the hearing impaired obtain higher intelligibility scores than do listeners who are inexperienced in listening to the speech of this population (Thomas, 1963; Monsen, 1978; McGarr, 1983; Monsen, 1983). This effect has been observed irrespective of the speech material produced, although the effect is greater for sentences than for words (Thomas, 1963; McGarr, 1983) and for the less intelligible than more intelligible talkers (Monsen, 1983). A finding of particular significance is that an experienced listener does not require personal knowledge of the speaker to understand his or her speech better. Rather, the ability to understand the speech of the hearing impaired is generalized across hearing-impaired talkers.

The explanation for the superior ability of experienced listeners to understand the speech of the hearing impaired is not obvious. Hudgins and Numbers (1942) posed two hypotheses to account for this effect. The first hypothesis was that experienced listeners gradually learn to interpret the articulatory patterns characteristic of the speech of profoundly hearing-impaired talkers. This is not an unreasonable assumption because numerous studies have shown common error patterns in the speech of profoundly hearing-impaired talkers (Levitt and Stromberg, 1983). If this assumption were true, however, experienced listeners would be better able than inexperienced listeners to understand poorly articulated words produced by hearing-impaired talkers. This finding was not observed in a study designed to test this hypothesis (McGarr, 1983).

A second hypothesis posed by Hudgins and Numbers (1942) was that experienced listeners were better able to make use of contextual information than inexperienced listeners. Hudgins and Numbers argued that naive listeners were so distracted by the unusual quality of the speech produced by profoundly hearing-impaired talkers that they failed to attend to relevant contextual information. McGarr (1983) observed, however, that intelligibility scores for both experienced and inexperienced listeners were higher for sentences with high than low context. That is, there was no significant interaction between listening skill and degree of contextual information. Thus, it does not appear that the higher intelligibility scores obtained by experienced listeners can be explained simply by access to enhanced contextual cues. If this was so, then McGarr should have observed an interaction between degree of context and listener experience. Context, however, must contribute in some manner to the phenomenon of better understanding of profoundly hearing-impaired talkers' speech by experienced listeners because the relative advantage of experience is negligible when the hearing-impaired talker produces isolated words rather than sentences (McGarr, 1983; Boothroyd, 1985a).

Identifying the underlying basis for experienced listeners' superior ability to understand the speech of hearing-impaired talkers is important because this information has implications for developing improved intervention programs. Such information could be used to identify those errors which should be corrected first in a child's speech, or identify communicative strategies which are effective to use with people who are unfamiliar with the speech of the hearing impaired. An encouraging finding is that the advantage that experienced listeners demonstrate in decoding the speech of hearing-impaired talkers is acquired rather quickly, evidenced by a decrease in the difference between the scores of experienced and inexperienced listeners as the latter hear more examples of hearing-impaired speakers (Monsen, 1983).

Access to auditory and visual cues

Another factor that affects the ability of listeners to understand the speech of the hearing impaired is whether they are allowed to see as well as hear the speaker. Speechreading is typically viewed as a skill that is used only by hearing-impaired people to enhance *their* speech perception abilities. The higher intelligibility scores obtained when listeners are able to see, as well as hear the hearing-impaired speaker, demonstrate that this is a strategy used by people to help *them* understand the speech of the hearing-impaired talker. The average improvement in the intelligibility of hearing-impaired talkers' speech between the listen-only and look-plus-listen condition has been reported to be roughly 15% (Thomas, 1963; Monsen, 1983).

Characteristics of the speaker

Degree of hearing loss

In general, it has been found that as hearing level increases, speech intelligibility decreases (see, e.g., Smith, 1975). The speech of children with moderate-to-severe hearing losses (i.e., hard of hearing children), has been found to be more intelligible than the speech of children with profound losses (Markides, 1970; Monsen, 1978). The systematic relationship between degree of hearing loss and intelligibility breaks down, however, once the hearing level reaches 85 dB HL (Smith, 1975; Monsen, 1978). This situation is reflected in the common observation that some deaf children develop intelligible speech whereas others do not.

The most obvious explanation for the above observation is that some children with profound hearing losses demonstrate more residual hearing than other children. Smith (1975) observed that children who had residual hearing through 3000 Hz had significantly higher intelligibility scores than those who did not. The children with the most reduced speech intelligibility in Smith's study had no measurable hearing above 1000 Hz and were probably responding to auditory stimuli on the basis of vibrotactile sensation. These data, as well as clinical observation, suggest that a child is most likely to develop intelligible speech if residual hearing is present in the higher frequencies (i.e., above 2000 Hz). Of course, differences in the speech intelligibility of children with profound hearing losses also might reflect factors such as consistency of hearing aid use and the quality and consistency of training. The importance of residual hearing in learning to talk is highlighted by the data of Boothroyd (1985b) which indicated that 5 dB of hearing is worth 1.5 years of instruction in terms of the influence on speech intelligibility.

The role of hearing in speech production also needs to be examined in terms of the speech perception abilities of the hearing-impaired talker. Smith (1975) found that profoundly hearing-impaired children's performance on a phoneme recognition task was more highly correlated with intelligibility than with hearing level. Stark and Levitt (1974) examined production and perception of selected suprasegmental contrasts in children with profound hearing losses, and found that those children who scored high on the perception test did not necessarily score well on the production test. Children who did well on the production test, however, always scored at an average-to-above average level on the perception test. Thus, good

perceivers did not always turn out to be good producers, but good producers wer almost always good perceivers.

Linguistic competence

Speech intelligibility can be influenced by the linguistic competence of the
hearing-impaired talker. An utterance which is produced with articulatory
and prosodic distortions is more likely to be intelligible if word order and
other grammatical features conform to those of the spoken language than if
lingusitic errors are present. A distorted utterance may be relatively unintelligible if, however, the listener is unable to use his or her knowledge of
the rules of the language to decode what has been said. Subtelny (1977)
compared the rated speech intelligibility of hearing-impaired talkers based
on production of prepared text and speech elicited using a picture description. A significant difference was observed between the two types of speech
samples, with the speech intelligibility of the read sample higher than that
of the spontaneous sample. Carney (1986) compared hearing-impaired children's production of the sentences on the Test of Syntactic Abilities (Quigley, et al., 1978) to their comprehension of the syntactic structures sampled
on the test. She found that speech intelligibility varied as a function of the
syntactic ability of the subject. In everyday communication situations, it is
likely that the linguistic deficits of most hearing-impaired talkers interact
with aritculatory and prosodic production skills to affect the intelligibility of
their speech.

Child's age

The speech of adolescents with profound hearing losses has been reported
to be more intelligible than that of younger, school-age children (Smith,
1975; McGarr, 1983). After the age of 12 years, however, Boothroyd
(1985b) reported only limited improvement in speech intelligibility for children with severe and profound hearing losses. A study of particular significance involved a four-year longitudinal evaluation of the speech skills of 80
children with profound hearing losses, which began when the children were
10 years of age (McGarr, 1987). The results of this study showed essentially
no change in the subjects' speech intelligibility over the four-year period.

Age of onset hearing loss

Intuitively, one might expect that the speech of children who experienced some period of normal hearing before the onset of a hearing loss would be more intelligible than the speech of children who have not heard before. An important factor, however, is whether or not the child is left with some residual hearing after the onset of the hearing loss. The interaction between degree of hearing loss and age of onset of deafness is illustrated in Figures 2 and 3, which show the SPAC scores for three subjects with acquired deafness. These data were collected in the same manner described earlier in the chapter. The onset of SBP's loss was at 2.5 years of age secondary to meningitis. She retained some hearing in one ear after the meningitis, demonstrating thresholds between 90 to 100 dB HL from 500 Hz to 4000 Hz. SBP was approximately 12 years of age when these data were collected.

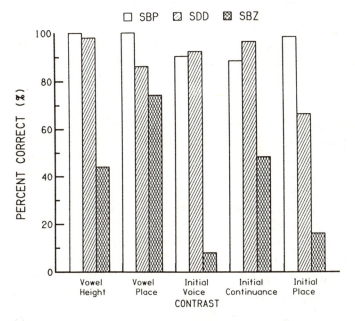

Figure 2. *Scores on 5 contrasts on the Speech Pattern Contrast test (SPAC) for three subjects with acquired deafness. SBP lost her hearing at 2.5 years of age whereas SDD and SBZ lost their hearing at 5 years of age. Subjects SBP and SDD have some residual hearing whereas SBZ does not.*

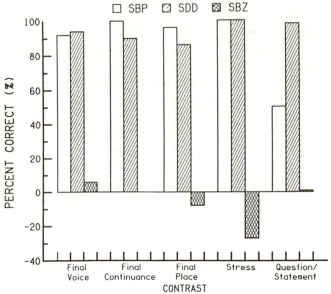

Figure 3. *Scores for the remaining 5 subtests of the Speech Pattern Contrast for three subjects with acquired deafness (see above legend).*

In contrast, Subjects SDD and SBZ lost their hearing when they were about 5 years of age. SBZ lost his hearing secondary to meningitis whereas the onset of SDD's loss occurred secondary to renal complications. Subject SDD was 9 years old when these data were collected whereas SBZ was about 6 years of age. In her better ear, SDD demonstrated thresholds between 90 — 115 dB from 500 to 2000 Hz with no measurable hearing above 2000 Hz. SBZ, on the other hand, showed no response to sound at any frequency under earphones or with powerful hearing aids.

There are several striking findings in the data shown in Figures 2 and 3. First, both SBP and SDD are able to convey the contrasts on the SPAC to the listeners with a high degree of accuracy even though SBP had normal hearing for only the first two-and-one-half years of life whereas SDD heard normally for five years. It might be that SBP's better hearing sensitivity compensates for the shorter period of time that she had normal hearing. That is, SBP was able to use her residual hearing to learn the contrasts after the onset of her hearing loss, or retain them if they had been acquired before the onset of her deafness. The only contrast that appeared more difficult for SBP than SDD to produce was the Question vs. Statement, which requires the production of a rising or falling intonation pattern. The SPAC scores of SBZ are in sharp contrast to those of either of the other two subjects. His reduced speech production abilities presumably reflect total absence of auditory feedback for speech monitoring purposes. The only contrast which SBZ was able to convey effectively was that involving vowel place. Data collected in our laboratory show that absence of residual hearing has an even more profound effect on speech production abilities when the loss occurs before three years of age. These data show a high degree of similarity between the speech of children who heard normally for two or even three years before becoming totally deaf and the speech of children with total, congenital deafness.

Effect of speech errors on intelligibility

The effect that particular types of speech errors have on the intelligibility of the speech of profoundly hearing-impaired talkers has been studied rather extensively. Identification of those errors which have the greatest impact on intelligibility is important because this information could be used to design improved speech training programs. That is, the errors that would be targeted first to correct in a child's speech might be those known to have the greatest influence on intelligibility. Although a number of errors have been found to be highly correlated with intelligibility, our knowledge is far from complete in this area. Research in this area is complicated by the method used to examine the relationship between types of errors and intelligibility. Correlational analysis is the technique used most often. This is the most practical approach but it is problematic to infer a causal relationship between intelligibility and errors identified through correlational analyses. The findings are further complicated by the fact that many speech features are not independent of one another. A more direct way to examine the effect that different errors have on intelligibility is to use digital speech processing techniques to correct specific errors and then measure the changes that occur in intelligibility. This approach is extremely time consuming, and a more complete description of many of the acoustic characteristics of the speech of profoundly hearing-impaired talkers is needed before parameters for synthesis and correction can be identified.

Correlational studies

In these studies, error types as determined from phonetic transcription have been correlated with open-set sentence intelligibility. Generally, as the frequency of segmental or phonemic errors increases in the speech of hearing-impaired talkers, intelligibility decreases (see, Osberger and McGarr, 1982). The number of segmental errors alone, however, does not totally account for reduced intelligibility. Smith (1975) observed that some subjects with approximately the same frequency of segmental errors had speech intelligibility scores that differed by as much as 30%. She hypothesized that the intelligibility differences were related to the presence of suprasegmental errors that interacted in a complex manner with segmental errors to reduce intelligibility. The segmental errors that have been found to have a negative effect on intelligibility are omission of phonemes in the word-initial position, consonant substitutions involving a change in the manner of articulation, substitutions of non-English phonemes, such as a glottal stop, and unidentifiable or gross distortions of the intended phoneme (Levitt and Stromberg, 1983). At the suprasegmental level, correlational analyses have shown that errors caused by poor phonatory control resulting in excessive and inappropriate changes in pitch have a strong negative effect on intelligibility.

Another approach has been to examine the relationship between acoustic deviations and intelligibility. Monsen (1978) found that of four acoustically measured variables of consonant production, three acoustic variables of vowel production, and two measures of prosody, three measures accounted for 73 percent of the variance among intelligibility scores. These variables were the difference in voice-onset time between /t/ and /d/, the difference in second format location between /i/ and /ɔ/, and the acoustic characteristics of nasal and liquid consonants. Metz, Samar, Schiavetti, Sitler, and Whitehead (1985) extended the work of Monsen and attempted to circumvent the problem of intercorrelated predictor variables by first performing a factor analysis on the acoustic variables followed by a multiple regression analysis on the factor scores. Two factors were found to be strongly related to speech intelligibility. One factor primarily reflected segmental production processes, whereas the other factor reflected prosodic production, namely control of overall sentence duration.

Causal studies

This approach was first used by Osberger and Levitt (1979) who manipulated the temporal characteristics of digitized utterances originally produced by profoundly hearing-impaired talkers. The study was extended by Maassen and Povel (1984a,b) who modified and corrected intonation as well as temporal distortions. The results of these investigations showed that correction of timing and intonation errors resulted in small, but statistically significant improvements in intelligibility. The largest change in intelligibility, however, was observed in a subsequent study by Maassen and Povel (1985) when vowel errors were corrected in the speech of hearing-impaired children. These data, as well as those collected from correlational studies, suggest that phonemic or segmental errors have a greater effect on intelligibility than do suprasegmental or prosodic errors. This should not be interpreted to mean that speech training programs need not incorporate training on prosodic speech features. In fact, many of the underlying articulatory skills needed to effect segmental distinctions rely on the same gestures involved in prosodic feature production. Although methods of analysis exist that, on the surface, separate phonemic and prosodic features, production of relatively few features of speech are totally independent of one another.

Summary

The information presented above highlights the complexity of assessing and describing the speech intelligibility of hearing-impaired talkers. Speech intelligibility is influenced by many factors, some of which are under the control of the examiner, such as the degree of context and linguistic complexity of the speech material, whereas other variables are not, such as the degree of hearing loss or age of the speaker. The interaction between key variables and speech intelligibility is apparent particularly for speakers with the most reduced speech production abilities. Under some conditions, the poorest speakers may be totally unintelligible whereas under other conditions, such as with enhanced contextual cues or when experienced listeners serve as judges, the speaker may be able to communicate effectively using only speech. There are situations, then, in which even talkers with the most limited production skills can be understood. Likewise, there are situations in which the most intelligible talkers will not be understood, such as when background noise is present. Too often, however, a bimodal system is used to describe the intelligibility of hearing-impaired talkers: intelligible or unintelligible. The many factors that influence intelligibility scores need to be considered before judgments are made about a child's ability to communicate with speech. The information presented in the next section illustrates how this can be accomplished.

Development of speech training and assessment procedures

The typical speech training programs for hearing-impaired children emphasize drill work on selected features of speech embedded in nonsense syllables or words (see, e.g., Ling, 1976). There is certainly a need for this type of training to assist the hearing-impaired child in learning how to produce the segmental and suprasegmental features of speech. Clinical experience has shown, however, that the greater the degree of hearing loss, the less likely that skills, established with nonsense syllables, will transfer to other linguistic contexts (Osberger, 1983). The following training suggestions are designed to provide the child with practice using a range of speech materials in a variety of communication contexts. The training suggestions have been developed within a diagnostic teaching framework, providing both the child and the clinician with feedback about the skills which need to be developed as well as performance information. First, several assessment procedures are described.

Comparison of open- and closed-set intelligibility tests

A current project in our laboratory involves the evaluation of the speech intelligibility of profoundly hearing-impaired children who use a cochlear implant or vibrotactile aid as their primary sensory aid. These children use an implant or tactile aid because they have no residual hearing and receive essentially no benefit from conventional hearing aids. Evaluating the speech of these children has been a challenge because they demonstrate a wide range of production abilities (Osberger, 1989). Some children, who did not acquire their hearing losses until 5 or 6 years of age, demonstrated substantially better speech production skills than those children who were born deaf. Further, the speech of the children with implants and tactile aids is compared to the speech of children with profound hearing losses who do benefit from hearing aids. The hearing aid subjects have been selected to include children who have residual hearing between 90-105 dB HL through at least 2000 Hz. Typically the hearing aid subjects demonstrate speech production skills superior to those of the subjects in the experimental groups who use an implant or tactile aid. Thus, the procedures we selected to evaluate intelligibility had to be sensitive to a wide range of intelligibility performance.

Ten sentences, developed by Monsen (1983), formed the corpus of sentences produced by the subjects. The sentences, which are shown in Table 1, were selected to cover a range of articulatory and linguistic complexity, as described by Monsen. The sentences were elicited from the subjects on an imitative basis. The subjects were shown a card with the target sentence printed on it at the same time that they heard and saw the examiner's production of the target sentences. The sentences were digitized, randomized, and played to a panel of three judges. Each set of 10 sentences produced by one child was heard by one panel of three judges. Each sentence was played two times for the judges. The judges had no prior experience in evaluating the speech of hearing-impaired talkers, and, the majority of them were undergraduate students. The sentences were played to the judges using both an open- and closed-set format. First, the judges were instructed to write down what they thought the child had said. The sentences were then re-played and the judges were shown the list of 10 possible sentences and instructed to select the sentence they thought had been produced.

Data have been analyzed from 27 subjects who used either conventional hearing aids, an implant, or tactile aid at the time of testing. The sub-

Table 1. *Ten sentences used to assess intelligibility*

Can he stop them?
You got a nice haircut.
My dog is mean.
My grandmother is beautiful.
The house is white
Did she bring it?
Did you find some?
We made a good birdhouse.
Can he make any?
That elephant was dangerous.

jects ranged from 8 to 16 years of age. The listeners' responses which were collected during the open-set testing were scored two ways. One method used the weighting system, described by Monsen (1983), which assigned a higher value to content words than to function words. The second method, referred to as the unweighted method, assigned equal value to all words in the sentence. Specifically, a percent score was calculated by dividing the number of words correctly understood by the total number of words in each sentence. The responses obtained with the closed-set procedure were scored in terms of the number of sentences correctly identified. Data have been averaged across subjects for each method of scoring (weighted, unweighted, and closed set) to illustrate differences as a function of scoring method. These data are shown in Table 2. A one-way analysis of variance revealed a significant difference among scoring procedures ($p < .001$). As the data in Table 2 show, the mean open-set scores were essentially the same for the weighted and unweighted scoring systems. In contrast, the mean score obtained with the closed-set procedure was over two times as high as the open-set scores. These data suggest that there was no particular advantage in using the weighted over the unweighted scoring system, at least for the speech samples analyzed in our study.

The difference in performance between open- and closed-set testing is more striking when the data for individual subjects are examined. Figure 4 shows the intelligibility scores for three subjects, SAZ, SBU, and SCD, who obtained scores of 10% or less when an open-set, write-down approach was used. Based on these data, it might be concluded that the speech of these subjects could never be understood by listeners. However, the closed-set scores indicate that the speech of at least two of the subjects (SBU and SCD) could be understood if additional cues were provided to the listeners. In contrast, the closed-set score of SAZ shows that his speech remained highly unintelligible even when additional cues were present.

Table 2. *Mean intelligibility scores in percent correct for 27 subjects*

	Mean	SD
Weighted	34	35
Unweighted	33	35
Closed Set	78	26

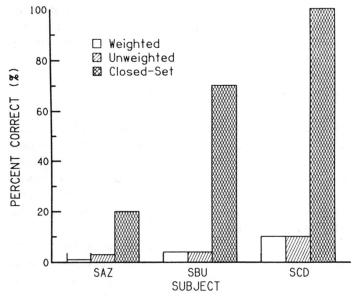

Figure 4. *Intelligibility scores for three subjects with limited speech production abilities.*

These data suggest that using a closed-set sentence task may provide more meaningful information about intelligibility than can be obtained with an open-set format when the subject has limited speech production abilities. To avoid a ceiling effect, like that demonstrated by SCD's closed-set score, the difficulty of the task can be increased by providing a greater number of alternatives from which to choose. The alternatives can include words similar to those in the target sentences to prevent the listeners from using a key-word identification strategy. Further, the closed-set strategy need not require panels of listeners to serve as judges. Rather, a clinician can make up key sentences, write each one on a card, shuffle the cards, and have the child select cards, one at a time, and read each sentence. The clinician can then guess which sentence the child has produced. This technique is similar to the one described by Monsen (1981) to assess intelligibility, but the stimuli can be changed for each child. For children who cannot read, picture cards can be used. The child could be required to name what is on the card, or make up a sentence about it. The advantage of this approach is that the stimuli can be selected so that the child experiences some success with the task. At the same time, the child is given practice in assuming responsibility for making his or her speech understood. This lays the foundation for developing those skills necessary for the child to function as a *partner* in communicative interchanges.

Development of the meaningful use of speech scale

A scale has been developed to evaluate hearing-impaired children's use of speech in everyday situations. The need to assess use of speech in everyday situations has become apparent in our work with children who use Total Communication as their primary mode of communication. In our experience, the majority of these children are seldom, if ever, required to communicate without signs even though they could be successful using their oral skills under the appropriate conditions.

The Meaningful Use of Speech Scale (MUSS) scale has been developed using the framework developed by Robbins (1989) to quantify hearing-impaired children's ability to use speech in a meaningful way in everyday situations. The purpose of the MUSS is to determine if a: (1) child uses speech without the support of gestures, signs or other nonvocal cues to communicate, (2) child's use of speech varies as a function of listener familiarity with the child's speech, and (3) child uses appropriate repair and clarification strategies when his or her speech is not understood. There are 10 probes, which appear in Table 3. Information is obtained from parents or teachers using an interview technique rather than asking the questions directly. The responses to each probe are scored on a scale from 0 to 4, based on the frequency of reported behavior (i.e., 0=never, 1=rarely, 2=occasionally, 3=frequently, 4=always). For example, in response to the first probe, a value of 0 would be assigned if the child never used his or her voice spontaneously while communicating. A value of 4 would be assigned if the child always used his or her voice during communication, irrespective of the intelligibility of the vocalizations. For the second probe, a value of 0 would be assigned if the child used speech *inappropriately* to attract the attention of others, and a value of 4 would be assigned if the child consistently *and* appropriately used speech to attract the attention of others. The goal of the MUSS is to determine how often and how effectively a child uses speech for communication, and to identify areas where improvement needs to be made. The MUSS is currently being administered to children who use hearing aids, implants, and tactile aids to assess their use of speech in everyday situations.

Table 3. *Ten probes on the meaningful use of speech scale (MUSS)*

1. Vocalizes during communicative interactions
2. Uses speech to attract others' attention
3. Vocalizations vary with content and intent of message
4. Is willing to use speech *only* (or primarily) to communicate with familiar people on known topics
5. Is willing to use speech *only* (or primarily) to communicate with unfamiliar people on known topics
6. Is willing to use speech *only* (or primarily) to communicate with familiar people on novel topics or with reduced contextual information
7. Is willing to use speech *only* (or primarily) to communicate with unfamiliar people on novel topics or with reduced contextual information
8. Message understood by people familiar with child's speech
9. Message understood by people unfamiliar with child's speech
10. Uses appropriate repair and clarification strategies

Diagnostic intervention strategies

The goal of the training approach described below is to provide a child practice in communicating using auditory and speech skills, and to identify those conditions which have the greatest effect on the intelligibility of the child's speech. The approach to training is based on that described by Erber (1982) to develop auditory training goals. Erber suggested systematic manipulation of the speech stimuli presented to the child and the child's response task. Our application of this approach to speech training, involves systematic manipulation of the amount of *listener* experience in hearing the speech of the child and amount of *contextual* support, as illustrated in Figure 5. The experience of the listener can be systematically manipulated, beginning with the least difficult situation of having someone highly experienced with the particular child's speech, such as a parent or the child's teacher, serve as the listener. The most difficult situation would involve listeners who have no prior experience in listening to the speech of the hearing impaired, such as a clerk in a store. Contextual support can be manipulated in terms of the availability of linguistic or non-linguistic cues. Manipulation of linguistic cues might involve production of familiar sentences with simple vocabulary and high linguistic predictability. Manipulation of non-linguistic cues would involve use of speech during familiar routines when

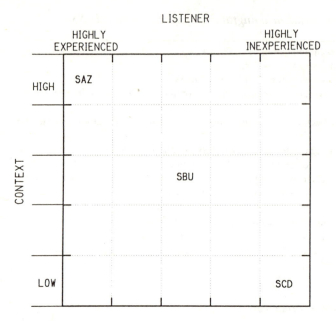

Figure 5. *Framework to select appropriate speech training goals. Suggested points for initiating training are illustrated for three subjects, SAZ, SBU, and SCD.*

situational cues are present to help the listener understand what the child has said (e.g., have the child ask for milk and cookies during snack time). Figure 5 illustrates where practice might begin for the three subjects whose speech intelligibility scores were shown in Figure 4.

At the same time that degree of listener experience and context are manipulated, other environmental conditions can be manipulated. The setting in which the training takes place can vary from highly structured (e.g., one-on-one training session) in which the child is in a "ready" set to use his or her best speech to an unstructured situation (e.g., in the classroom). The acoustic environment in which the communication takes place can range from quiet (e.g., small room) to noisy (e.g., classroom with other children talking). Further, the cues available to the *listener* could include auditory plus visual or only auditory.

An important part of this training is to help the child learn appropriate strategies to use when his or her speech is not understood. When this happens, hearing-impaired children often are at a loss as to what to do next. Children who do not learn effective repair and clarification strategies often develop one of two inappropriate strategies: they either gain control of the conversation, preventing others from participating, or they make no attempt to repair the conversational break-down, bringing the communicative interchange to a complete halt. Parents and clinicians often fail to help the child learn effective strategies because they often assume the child's role in the communication situation, failing to let the child go through the normal process of learning to repeat what was not understood, or discovering other effective strategies.

Tables 4 and 5 illustrate a checklist that can be used to record the strategies used by hearing-impaired children in discourse situations. These checklists are based on the approach described by Moeller, Osberger, and Eccarius (1986) to promote question comprehension in hearing-impaired children. The checklist in Table 4 can be used when examining the child's *speech perception* skills in a discourse situation whereas the checklist in Table 5 is designed to be used when the effectiveness of the child as the *talker* in a conversation is examined. A hierarchy of communication strategies is listed, beginning with the least desirable (i.e., no response when noncomprehension occurs) to the provision of specific information for clarification. Table 5 also illustrates the conditions under which the communication takes place, as well as the use of various discourse strategies. The difficulty of the task can be manipulated by using a familiar or a novel topic.

A final technique that can be used to promote conversational speech skills is the use of connected discourse tracking. This technique, developed by De Filippo and Scott (1978) was originally intended to train and evaluate the *reception* of ongoing speech. A team of two people is required. One person serves as the talker, or sender, and the other serves as the receiver. The talker reads successive segments from a prepared text, and the receiver must repeat verbatim what has been said. Performance is measured in number of words of text repeated correctly per unit of time. This performance measure (words per minute) can then be used as an index of efficiency of communication. Osberger, Johnson, and Miller (1987) used the tracking technique to train the *production* of speech skills. With this application, the profoundly hearing-impaired child served as the sender and the clinician served as the receiver. Performance was evaluated in terms of the number of words produced by the child that were correctly understood and repeated by the clinician. Tracking was conducted with each of 5 children in

Table 4. *Checklist to record communication strategies used when hearing-impaired child is the listener in a discourse situation* (Adapted from Moeller, et al. (1986: 37-50) based strategies to use with hearing-impaired students with comprehension deficits.)

Communication strategy Familiar topic	Unfamiliar topic	or topic shift
Fails to seek clarification No response	_____	_____
Inappropriate response	_____	_____
Indicates noncomprehension Nonverbally	_____	_____
Verbally asks for repetition	_____	_____
says/signs "what?"	_____	_____
shifts topic inappropriately	_____	_____
Requests clarification (e.g. "I didn't hear what you said", "please repeat what you said"	_____	_____
Requests specific clarification (e.g., "What does ___mean?" "What did you say about ___?"	_____	_____

Conditions

Acoustic: _____ Quiet _____ Noisy

Setting: _____ Structured _____ Semi-structured _____ Unstructured

Visual cues: _____ With Visual Cues _____ Without Visual Cues

Table 5. *Checklist to record communication strategies used when the hearing-impaired child is the talker in a discourse situation.* (Adapted from Moeller, et al. (1986: 37-50): Cognitively based strategies for use with hearing-impaired students with comprehension deficits.)

Communication strategy	Familiar topic	Novel topic
Fails to respond when listener shows noncomprehension	_____	_____
Responds when listener shows noncomprehension Nonverbally	_____	_____
Verbally (repeats utterance) Shifts topic inappropriately	_____	_____
Queries listener for specifics (e.g. "What didn't you understand?")	_____	_____
Provides specific clarification (e.g., repeat specific word, describe, modify message with synonyms or analogies)	_____	_____
Use of discourse strategies *Negotiates new topic*	_____	_____
Appropriate presupposition	_____	_____
Appropriate topic shifts	_____	_____
Correct use of elaborated and restricted codes	_____	_____

Conditions

Acoustic: _____ Quiet _____ Noisy

Setting: _____ Structured _____ Semi-structured _____ Unstructured

Listerner: _____ Very familiar _____ Mod familiar _____ Unnfamiliar

8-minute blocks on 16 different days. On the average, the difference in tracking rate between the first session and the last session was only about 5 words per minute but the relative gain suggested that about one-third more of what the children said could be understood during the last than the first session. One of the most important outcomes of the study was that the children enjoyed performing the tracking and were highly motivated to perform the task. Some of the children were surprised that their speech was intelligible to the clinician. Also, some of them reportedly developed increased awareness of the error patterns in their speech, demonstrated by self-correction of articulation errors. The students also learned to use a number of different repair and clarification strategies when they were not understood, including repetition paraphrasing, chunking, defining, or spelling missed words.

In summary a variety of approaches can be used to promote the use of speech by profoundly hearing-impaired children. Techniques such as the ones described above have the advantage in that they also provide the child practice in learning to use various strategies to enhance communication effectiveness. One of the most important features of these suggested activities is that they can be employed with children who demonstrate a range of speech production abilities. Use of these procedures provides the clinician with a realistic estimate of each child's speech intelligibility under various conditions. At the same time, the child learns under what conditions his or her speech is likely to be understood.

Note

The author acknowledges the helpful comments of Stacey Berry, Sue Todd, and Amy McConkey Robbins. Preparation of this manuscript was supported, in part, by grant DC000423 from NIH-NIDCD.

References

Boothroyd, A. 1985a. "Evaluation of speech production of the hearing impaired: Some benefits of forced-choice testing." *Journal of Speech Hearing Research* 28, 185-196.
Boothroyd, A. 1985b. "Residual hearing and the problem of carry-over in the speech of the deaf." *AHSA Reports* 15, 8-14.
Boothroyd, A. 1988. "Perception of speech pattern contrasts from auditory presentation of voice fundamental frequency." *Ear and Hearing* 9, 313-321.

Brannon, J. B. 1964. "Visual feedback of glossal motions and its influence on the speech of deaf children." Unpublished Ph.D. diss, Northwestern Univ.

Carney, A. 1986. "Understanding speech intelligibility in the hearing impaired." *Topics Land Disord.* 6, 47-59.

De Filippo, L. & Scott, B. 1978. "A method for training and evaluating the reception of ongoing speech." *Journal of the Acoustic Society of America* 63, 1186-1192.

Erber, N. 1982. *Auditory Training.* Washington, DC: A.G. Bell Association for the Deaf.

Hudgins, C. V. & Numbers, F. C. 1942. "An investigation of the intelligibility of the speech of the deaf. *Gen Psych Mono* 25, 289-392.

John, J.E.J. & Howarth, J. 1965. "The effect of time distortions on the intelligibility of deaf children's speech." *Language and Speech* 8, 127-134.

Kent, R. D., Weismer, G., Kent, J., F., & Rosenbek, J. C. 1989. "Toward phonetic intelligibility testing in dysarthria." *Journal of Speech & Hearing Disorders* 54, 482-499.

Levitt, H. & Stromberg, H. 1983. "Segmental characteristics of the speech of hearing-impaired children: Factors affecting intelligibility." *Speech of the Hearing Impaired: Research, Training, and Personnel Preparation*, ed. by I. Hochberg, H. Levitt & M. J. Osberger, 53-74. Baltimore: University Park Press.

Ling, D. 1976. *Speech and the Hearing-Impaired Child: Theory and Practice.* Washington, DC: A.G. Bell Association for the Deaf.

Maassen, B., & Povel, D. J. 1984a. "The effect of correcting temporal structure on the intelligibility of deaf speech." *Speech Communications* 3, 123-135.

———. 1984b. "The effect of correcting fundamental frequency on the intelligibility of deaf speech and its interaction with temporal aspects." *Journal of the Acoustic Society of America* 76, 1673-1681.

———. 1985. "The effect of segmental and suprasegmental corrrections on the intelligibility of deaf speech." *Journal of the Acoustic Society of America* 78, 877-886.

Magnan, K. 1961. "Speech improvement through articulation testing." *American Annals Deaf* 106, 391-396.

Markides, A. 1970. "The speech of deaf and partially hearing children with special reference to factors affecting intelligibility. *British Journal of Audiology* 11, 51-58.

McGarr, N. 1983. "The intelligibility of deaf speech to experienced and inexperienced listeners." *Journal of Speech & Hearing Research* 26, 451-458.

———. 1987. "Communication skills of hearing-impaired children in schools for the deaf. *Language and Communication Skills of Deaf Children*, ed. by H. Levitt, N. S. McGarr, & D. Geffner, *ASHA Monographs, 26*. Washington, DC: American Speech-Language-Hearing Association.

Metz, D., Samar, V., Schiavetti, N., Sitler, R. & Whitehead, R. 1985. "Acoustic dimensions of hearing-impaired speakers' intelligibility." *Journal of Speech & Hearing Research* 28, 345-355.

Miller, G. A., Heise, G. A., & Lichten, W. 1951. "The intelligibility of speech as a function of the context of the test materials." *Journal of Exp Psychology* 41, 329-335.

Moeller, M. P., Osberger, M. J., & Eccarius, M. 1986. "Cognitively based strategies for use with hearing-impaired students with comprehension deficits." *Topics in Language Disorders* 6, 37-50.

Monsen, R. B. 1978. "Toward measuring how well hearing-impaired children speak." *Journal of Speech & Hearing Research* 21, 197-219.
———. 1981. "A usable test for the speech intelligibility of deaf talkers." *Amer. Annals Deaf* 126, 845-852.
———. 1983. "The oral speech intelligibility of hearing-impaired talkers." *Journal of Speech & Hearing Disorders* 48, 286-296.
Osberger, M. J. 1983. "Development and evaluation of some speech training procedures for hearing-impaired children." *Speech of the Hearing Impaired: Research, Training, and Personnel Preparation*, ed. by I. Hochberg, H. Levitt, & M. J. Osberger, 338-348. Baltimore: University Park Press.
———. 1989. "Speech production in profoundly hearing-impaired children with reference to cochlear implants." *Cochlear Implants in Young Deaf Children*, ed. by E. Owens & D. Kessler, 257-282. Boston: College-Hill Press, A Division of Little, Brown, and Co.
Osberger, M. J., Johnson, D., & Miller, J. D. 1987. "Use of connected discourse tracking to train functional speech skills." *Ear and Hearing* 8, 31-36.
Osberger, M. J. & Levitt, H. 1979. "The effect of iming errors on the intelligibility of deaf children's speech." *Journal of the Acoustic Society of America* 66, 1316-1324.
Osberger, M. J. & McGarr, N. 1982. "Speech production characteristics of the hearing impaired." *Speech and Language: Advances in Basic Research and Practice*, Volume 8, ed. by Norman Lass, 221-283. New York: Academic Press.
Quigley, S. P., Steinkamp, M., Power, D. J., & Jones, B. W. 1978. *Test of Syntactic Abilities*. Beaverton, OR: Dormac, Inc.
Robbins, A. M. 1989. "Meaningful auditory integration scale (MAIS)." Unpublished report, Indiana University School of Medicine, Indianapolis, IN.
Samar, V. & Metz, D. 1988. "Construct validity of speech intelligibility rating-scale procedures for the hearing-impaired population." *Journal of Speech & Hearing Research* 31, 307-316.
Sitler, R., Schiavetti, N., & Metz, D. **1983?????**. "Contextual effects in the measurement of hearing impaired speakers' intelligibility. *Journal of Speech & Hearing Research* ????? **26, 30-35.**?????
Schiavetti, N., Metz, D., & Sitler, R. **1981????**. "Construct validity of direct magnitude estimation and interval scaling of speech intelligibility." *Journal of Speech & Hearing Research* ?????? **26, 30-35.**????
Smith, C. R. 1975. "Residual hearing and speech production in deaf children." *Journal of Speech & Hearing Research* 18, 795-811.
Stark, R., & Levitt, H. 1974. "Prosodic feature reception and production in deaf children." *Journal of the Acoustic Society of America* 55, S23.
Subtelny, J. 1977. "Assessment of speech with implications for training." *Childhood Deafness*, ed. by Fred H. Bess, 183-196. New York: Grune & Stratton.
Thomas, W. 1963. "Intelligibility of the speech of deaf children." *Proceedings of the International Congress on the Education of the Deaf. Document No. 106*, 245-261. Washington, DC: Library of Congress.

Chapter 7

Intelligibility measurement as a tool in the clinical management of dysarthric speakers*

Kathryn M. Yorkston, Patricia A. Dowden &   David R. Beukelman
University of Washington   *University of Nebraska*

Intelligibility can be broadly defined as the understandability of speech. Implicit in the definition is a task in which a speaker produces a message and a listener who does not know the content of message attempts to comprehend and/or reproduce it. Although the model for intelligibility tasks is a simple one, these tasks have considerable potential for the development of both assessment and intervention approaches for dysarthric speakers. Intelligibility is a particularly straightforward indicator of the adequacy of dysarthric speech because the distortion in the signal arises from a movement problem rather than from word retrieval or other language-related problems. Measures of intelligibility have long played a role in the description and evaluation of dysarthric speakers. Estimates (Darley, Aronson, and Brown, 1975; and Enderby, 1983) and actual measures of intelligibility of connected speech (Yorkston and Beukelman, 1978, 1981) have served as overall indicators of speech adequacy. The clinical use of intelligibility tasks has also found support in the research literature. As a measure of severity, intelligibility has been related to information transfer (Beukelman and Yorkston, 1979), articulatory function (Platt, Andrews, and Howie, 1980;

* This chapter was supported in part by Grant #H133B80081 from the National Institute of Disability and Rehabilitation Research, Department of Education, Washington, D.C. The authors wish to thank Vicki Hammen, for her assistance.

and Platt, Andrews, Young and Quinn, 1980) and fine motor control (Barlow and Abbs, 1986).

This chapter will focus on intelligibility tasks as they are currently applied in the clinical setting to make intervention decisions rather than on tasks that may be used to answer research questions. First, tasks used to measure the level and pattern of disability will be described. A rationale driven by clinical requirements and constraints will be provided for the selection of sentence, word, and phoneme intelligibility tasks. Next, intelligibility tasks will be discussed which are used to identify factors important for the improvement of functional performance of dysarthric speakers. These include the identification of optimum speaking rate, documentation of the impact of management of the velopharyngeal incompetence using palatal lifts, identification of candidates for behavioral training aimed at increasing articulatory precision, and intervention to improve listeners' ability to interpret severely dysarthric speech. Finally, the complex interactions among the various factors impacting intelligibility will be discussed.

Measurement of the level and pattern of disability

One of the primary functions of clinical intelligibility tasks is to provide an overall indication of the severity of the dysarthria. Few measures other than intelligibility of connected speech allow the clinician to evaluate the sum of the interacting processes that are involved in dysarthric speech production. Any number of tasks or combinations of speaker and listener activities can be used to measure intelligibility. The tasks selection is to a large extent dependent upon the nature of the questions being asked. Readers will note that the term, "intelligibility" rarely appears in this chapter without an adjective as a modifier. That is, we will be describing "sentence," "word," or "phoneme" intelligibility tasks. This use of terminology reflects our belief that modifiers are needed to clarify the tasks that the speakers and or listeners are being asked to perform. Because each task has been developed for specific purposes, none are sufficient alone to address all pertinent clinical questions.

Sentence intelligibility

Sentence intelligibility has traditionally been used to answer the question, "How severe is the problem?" Sentence intelligibility when combined with a measure of speaking rate, provides information about "the distance from the norm." Such information is critical in the clinical setting when one is evaluating a mildly dysarthric individual and attempting to distinguish the performance of that individual from non-impaired speakers. It is also critical when monitoring the clinical course of the dysarthria, whether it be progressive, stable, or improving. When evaluating a more severely dysarthric speaker, sentence intelligibility measures provide information that helps the clinician determine whether or not the speaker is sufficiently understandable to be a functional communicator in a variety of natural settings.

Many different intelligibility tasks could be used to assess the severity of the disorder. Table 1 contains a listing of the features of three different intelligibility tasks commonly used for clinical measurement of dysarthric speech. Note that the stimuli for sentence intelligibility measurement (Yorkston, Beukelman, and Traynor, 1984) are sentences of varying word lengths that are randomly selected from a large pool of alternatives. Dysarthric speakers are audio-recorded as they read or imitate these sentences. The samples are timed and listeners, who have not been involved in the recording process, attempt to orthographically transcribe the messages they hear. Results are reported in percentage of words correctly transcribed, speaking rate (words per minute, WPM) and rate of intelligible speech (IWPM).

A number of constraints dictate the selection of this task for the measurement of intelligibility in the clinical setting. For example, one may legitimately ask, if the goal is to provide a functional indicator, why use a reading rather than spontaneous speaking activity? A reading task was selected because consistency across samples is important in monitoring a potentially changing clinical course. One limitation of the reading tasks is the fact that, for a small number of dysarthric speakers, sentence reading or imitation is markedly different from spontaneous speech. Although some clinical judgment must be exercised in making firm statements about the relationship between spontaneous productions and reading or imitation tasks, use of spontaneous speech for measurement would also be problematic. Spontaneous speech varies so widely in content and utterance complexity that these variables would no doubt contribute to large variability if not controlled in some way.

Table 1. *Features of intelligibility tasks utilized in clinical settings*

	Sentence intelligibility	Word intelligibility with & without semantic context	Phoneme intelligibility
Stimulus	Randomly selected sentences (5-15 words)	Single words selected from semantic-related words lists	Single words (CVC) selected from phonetically-similar word lists
Speaking task	Reading or imitation	Reading or imitation	Reading or imitation
Transmission system	Audio-tape	Audio-tape	Audio-tape
Listener task	Orthographic transcription	Orthographic transcription	Broad phonetic transcription (with level of listener certainty)
Measures obtained	–Percentage of words correct –Speaking rate –Intelligible words per minute	Percent of words correct (with & without context)	Phonemes correct initial vs. final vowel vs. cons. consonant type
Functions of the measures	Functional level – mod. & mild speakers –Optimum speaking rate	Functional level for severely involved speaker	Pattern of articulatory errors

Another task selection decision involves the listener's or judge's task. In the case of sentence intelligibility, this task involved orthographic transcription of the sample. In the clinical setting, no doubt the quickest way of obtaining an indication of a speaker's intelligibility would be to listen to a sample of speech and either estimate its intelligibility on assign it a rating on some simple scale. Although orthographic transcription is more time-consuming than simple estimates of intelligibility, such estimates are problematic because they are influenced by factors such as the familiarity of the listener with the passage (Beukelman and Yorkston, 1980). Judges familiar with the passage tend to overestimate the intelligibility of moderately dysarthric individuals. In an effort to circumvent some of the problems inherent in estimates of intelligibility, we sought to "objectify" the measure of sentence intelligibility by requiring that judges who are naive to the content of the message orthographically transcribe what they hear.

Word intelligibility with and without semantic context

Sentence intelligibility based on orthographic transcription of sentences read by a dysarthric speaker is a clinically useful task, but clearly does not provide a complete picture of functional performance for dysarthric speakers at every level of severity. Because it is a physiologically demanding task requiring production of long utterances, a sentence intelligibility task often produces scores that are near zero for severely dysarthric individuals. Although these individuals are clearly in need of augmentative communication approach in some situations, their natural speech may also be an important component of communication. Because of task difficulty, sentence intelligibility may underestimate the functional usefulness of severely dysarthric speech. We frequently evaluate individuals in our augmentative communication clinic who are referred to us by consultants from the education or vocational settings. It is not uncommon for families to question the referral indicating that natural speech is "just fine." When questioned in more detail, it is clear that they understand speech at home in situations where the messages are highly predictable. However, when attempting to communicate in less predictable academic or vocational settings, natural speech of these individuals falls far short of being functional. Clinically, it is important to document the functional level of natural speech despite its highly distorted nature. By documenting intelligibility with and without context, we are able to suggest that both referring agencies and families may be correct in their perception of the usefulness of natural speech. Families see speech as functional in limited situations and professionals in academic or vocational settings see that augmentation as a necessary component of independence in other situations.

In an effort to mimic some of the features of predictable, conversational settings, a contextual intelligibility task was developed (Dowden, Yorkston and Stoel-Gammon, 1987; Yorkston, Dowden and Honsinger, 1988) (See Table 1). Severely dysarthric speakers are audio-recorded as they read or imitated a list of words. These words were randomly selected from groups of semantically related words (e.g. the colors, items of clothing, things to drink, etc.). Judges first listened to the tapes and attempted to transcribe these words orthographically. After doing this, the samples were scored a second time. During the second judging, the listeners are provided with semantic context. At times, the contexts are rather narrow, for example, "a day of the week." Other contexts are much broader, "an animal" or "something you might by in a drug store." During the second judging the listeners are given context but are asked not to guess simply on the basis of context alone. Rather, they are asked guess only if the word in context gives them some basis for the guess.

As with all of the intelligibility tasks described in this chapter, the characteristics of the population and clinical process impose constraints on task selection. Single words were chosen because sentence material may be physically exhausting for severely dysarthric individuals. Semantic context was chosen in an effort to mimic, at least to some extent, what may happen in a natural communication situation where the listener often has information regarding the situation. A random sample generation process was again employed so that equivalent samples could be administered judging over time.

The potential impact of semantic context on the word intelligibility of severely dysarthric individuals is both statistically significant and clinically important. Figure 1 illustrates the results of this task in a group of 13 severely dysarthric adults. For the majority of these individuals, dysarthria was the result of cerebral palsy (N = 11), and in the remaining two individuals dysarthria was the result of traumatic brain injury. Scores reflect measures averaged across three judges. Note that these speakers are severely dysarthric with single word intelligibility ranging from zero to 21 percent without semantic context. In all cases, when context was provided during the judging, scores substantially improved. Without semantic con-

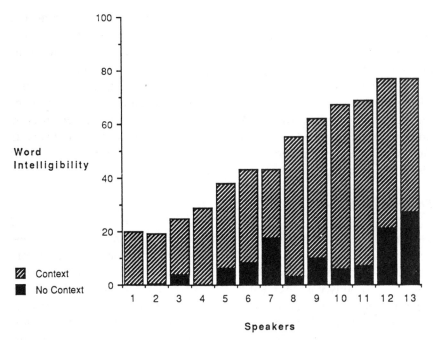

Figure 1. *Word intelligibility for 13 severely dysarthric speakers with and without semantic context* (Yokston, Dowden & Honsinger, 1988)

text, word intelligibility averaged 8.6 percent (S. D. = 8.5); with context, scores averaged 48.5 percent (S. D. 20.7).

Examination of Figure 1 also suggests that there is considerable variability from one speaker to another in terms the impact of semantic context on intelligibility. Yorkston, Dowden, and Honsinger (1988) reviewed some of the factors that may allow some severely dysarthric individuals to benefit from context cues and not others. While conducting the perceptual judging needed to complete this project, we were struck by the differences among these severely dysarthric individuals. All severely dysarthric speakers do not sound the same. Some are able to approximate at least some speech sounds and others appear to be unable to do so. Some have good respiratory/phonatory control and are able to produce voicing and signal syllables consistently; others are unable to do so. Some are highly consistent in their disordered productions and others appear to produce words differently on each attempt or produce words with extraneous yet inconsistent audible elements that have a tendency is mislead the listener. Any of these factors singly or in combination may impact word intelligibility. For example, knowing the the number of syllables in a word is certainly not sufficient to insure intelligibility when no context is provided. However, together some gross phoneme approximations, it may be sufficient to insure intelligibility when semantic context is provided. Further investigation of speech characteristics of severely dysarthric individuals would appear to be necessary in order to design more adequate intervention programs for these individuals and to better understand how these individuals are able to use their highly distorted speech functionally.

Phoneme intelligibility

Thus far, the emphasis of this chapter has been on sentence and word intelligibility (with and without semantic context). From these measures, information about the functional level of performance can be obtained. Sentence intelligibility measurement tasks in particular, give little information regarding the nature of articulatory error patterns in dysarthric individuals. According to Kent, Weismer, Kent and Rosenbek (in press), intelligibility measures that provide only a single overall score give little information about why intelligibility is poor. Such information is necessary if one is to understand the nature of the deficit. In an effort to more adequately describe the pattern of articulatory disability, the intelligibility task can be modified so that the targeted information is a phoneme rather than a word or group of words. Choice of an intelligibility task rather than a more traditional articulatory testing, in which judges phonetically transcribe known productions, was made based on the nature of articulatory error pattern seen in dysarthric individuals. The traditional articulatory testing approach is problematic for a number of reasons when applied to dysarthric speech. First, distortions are the most frequent type of error in dysarthria (Johns and Darley, 1970). Frank substitutions are relatively rare. Research reported elsewhere suggests that clinicians tend to overestimate the adequacy of production especially in the moderately severe dysarthric population (Yorkston, Beukelman, and Traynor, 1988). Good diacritical marking systems for dysarthric speech are not frequently reported in the literature.

As with other clinical intelligibility tasks, our samples containing targeted units are randomly generated from pools of phonetically similar words. In the case of phoneme intelligibility, the targeted units are singleton consonants, vowels and diphthongs. Speakers are audio-recorded as they read or imitate a list of 57 CVC words. Forty-one consonants (22 pre-vocalic and 19 postvocalic) and 16 vowels and diphthongs are sampled. When judging the sample, listeners who are naive to the identity of the target phoneme are presented with a word frame such as "ma __" and are asked to identify the missing phoneme. Judges also give an indication of the level of confidence they have in their response. All word frames are con-structed so that judges are selecting from multiple, real-word options. In the case of the word frame "ma __," possible options include mad, mat, mack, match, mash, etc. Scatterplots of target versus perceived phonemes are generated and scores may be reported in a variety of ways — for exam-ple, accuracy of vowel versus consonants, initial versus final consonants, pressure consonants versus nasals/glides. To a large extent, the data reported are dependent upon the clinical issues being addressed. For exam-ple, intervention with a severely involved flaccid dysarthric speaker may focus on lip strengthening exercises in order to achieve bilabial closure. The phoneme intelligibility task would allow for the monitoring of changes in the perceived adequacy of bilabial sound production. In another example, intervention with a severely dysarthric individual with poor respiratory sup-port who is recovering from traumatic brain injury may focus on inclusion of final consonants. The phoneme intelligibility task would allow for the monitoring of change over time in final consonants as compared with changes in non-treated sounds.

Identifying factors impacting intelligibility

Clinicians are faced with the task of understanding the extent and nature of the impairment experienced by their clients. However, this may be viewed as the first step in the clinical process of attempting to identify and imple-ment intervention strategies to improve intelligibility. The clinician must also ask the question, "What strategies, techniques, or clinical approaches will make a difference?" Intelligibility tasks can be structured in order to provide an answer to this question.

Rate control

Slowing a dysarthric speaker's rate is among the most frequently employed strategies in the clinician's arsenal. In addition to the documentation of the severity of the disability, sentence intelligibility can serve to assist in clinical management decisions in the area of rate control. For example, data related to intelligibility and speaking rate indicate whether the speaker's rate is appropriate given the level of motor impairment. Speaking rate is a particularly important issue in at least two dysarthric populations. The first population includes individuals with Parkinson's disease whose speech is characterized by reduced movements and rapid rushes of speech. A sub-group of Parkinsonian speakers are unique in that their speech is more rapid that non-impaired individuals. The impact of rate control has been well documented in this group (Hanson and Metter, 1980, 1983; Yorkston, Beukelman, and Bell, 1988). The other clinical population for whom rate control is important are individuals with ataxic dysarthria. In this group, slowing their speaking rate may allow them to better hit the articulatory targets and thus increase speech intelligibility (Yorkston and Beukelman, 1981).

Appropriateness of speaking rate can be assessed in a number of ways. The first is to compare single word and sentence intelligibility. If all else is equal, sentence intelligibility should be higher than single word intelligibility because sentences provide contextual information that may assist the listener in "filling in the gaps" when attempting to understand the distorted production. No such context is available when words are produced in isolation. Thus, when sentence intelligibility is considerably lower than single word intelligibility, clinicians should be alerted to the potential benefits of reducing speaking rate.

Recently, a more direct means of assessing the impact of rate reduction of speech intelligibility has become available (Beukelman, Yorkston, and Tice, 1988). Using Pacer/Tally software, speech can be paced at rates below the habitual rate and impact on intelligibility and naturalness can be assessed. Figure 2 illustrates the relationship between speaking rate and sentence intelligibility for two dysarthric speakers. The first speaker is an individual with predominantly ataxic dysarthria as the result of a traumatic brain injury. Note that his habitual rate of 72 wpm is less than 40 percent of a normal rate for this task. Intelligibility at this rate is only 39 percent. When speaking rate paced at 60 percent of habitual, intelligibility improves

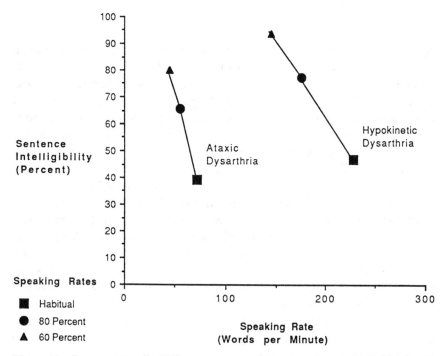

Figure 2. *Sentence intelligibility versus speaking rate for an individual with ataxic dysarthric and one with hypokinetic dysarthria. Sentence intelligibility was measured at habitual speaking rates and at 80 and 60 percent of habitual rates.*

to 80 percent. The second speaker illustrated in the figure is quite different from the first in that his pattern is typical of an individual with Parkinson's disease. His habitual rate is faster than normal at 228 wpm. At this rapid rate, sentence intelligibility is only 46 percent. When this speaker is slowed to 145 wpm (60 percent of habitual), sentence intelligibility improves to 94 percent. Thus, slowing the speaking rate has a marked impact on the intelligibility of these two individuals. Data related to the impact of rate control on intelligibility and naturalness of a larger group of dysarthric speakers can be found elsewhere (Hammen, Beukelman, and Iraynor; 1990).

Palatal lift fitting

Velopharyngeal dysfunction is a common characteristic of dysarthria. It may range from mild problems in the timing of closure during speech to complete inability to achieve closure regardless of speaking rate and phonetic context. At times, velopharyngeal dysfunction is disproportionately impaired compared to other aspects of motor speech production; at other times it is consistent with other problems. When velopharyngeal deficits are severe they can exaggerate and complicate other aspects of speech production. For example, air leakage as the result of severe velopharyngeal incompetence may exaggerate the impact of poor respiratory support on overall speech production. Inability to build up oral air pressure because of velopharyngeal incompetence may exaggerate poor oral control. Management of velopharyngeal incompetence with palatal lift fitting has a long clinical history (Yorkston, Beukelman, and Bell, 1988). Results of this intervention are frequently documented with either subjective measures of satisfaction with the lift or with highly specific, physiological measures such as changes in velopharyngeal resistance.

We have found that measurement of phoneme intelligibility is useful in answering specific questions related to the speech production process in the area of velopharyngeal function. Data from this task may be used to distinguish severely dysarthric individuals with a pattern of consistent velopharyngeal incompetence from dysarthric individuals who are hypernasal but who are able to achieve adequate velopharyngeal closure at times. (Yorkston, Beukelman, Honsinger, and Mitsuda, 1989). Clinically, we have used the task to identify potential candidates for palatal lift fitting, and to document the impact of lift fitting at both the time of the initial fitting and on follow-up (Yorkston, Honsinger, Beukelman, and Taylor, 1989). Figure 3 illustrates such data for a 28-year-old woman who was 8 years post-onset traumatic brain injury when she was fitted with a palatal lift. Prior to palatal lift fitting, this client exhibited a classical pattern of velopharyngeal incompetence. Her respiratory support was good, but pronounced nasal emission was noted on all attempts to produce pressure consonants. Perceptual measures of articulatory adequacy were consistent with these aerodynamic findings. At 96 months post onset (MPO), habitual productions of pressure consonants were identified correctly less than 10 percent of the time, while productions of nasal and glides were identified with over 80 percent accuracy. After lift fitting and a period of accommodation to the

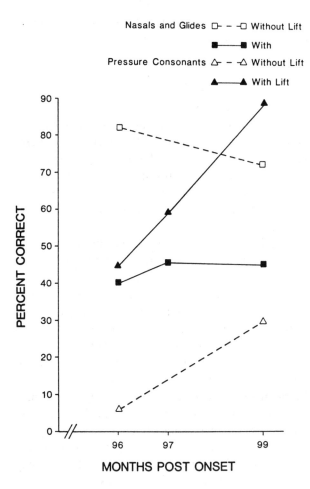

Figure 3. *Measures of phoneme intellibility (with and without the palatal lift) for a 28-year-old woman who was 8 years post onset traumatic brain injury. These measures were obtained at 96 months post onset (MPO) and during follow-up evaluation at 97 MPO and 99 MPO* (from: Yorkston, Honsinger, Beukelman, & Taylor, 1989).

lift and speech intervention, the accuracy with which judges were able to identify pressure consonants improved to 90 percent.

Behavioral modification

Intelligibility tasks may also be used to assess the speaker's ability to modify unintelligible productions. Knowing whether or not an individual is capable of volitional change is vital in clinical treatment of dysarthria where there are few treatment candidacy guidelines. Unless a dysarthric speaker is able to modify faulty productions voluntarily, many routinely applied behavioral interventions are unlikely to succeed. In the clinical setting, the instructions to modify productions is often carried out using intelligibility drills, tasks similar to those used in assessment.

Intelligibility tasks in which the dysarthric speaker produces a message and the listener attempts to understand the message are a frequent intervention approach. This approach has an important place in clinical intervention for a number of reasons (Yorkston, Beukelman, and Bell, 1988). First, the difficulty levels of intelligibility tasks may be adjusted to meet the speaker's needs. For example, a severely dysarthric individual in the process of making the transition to natural speech after a brain stem stroke may be severely involved and only be able to signal the difference between grossly differing syllables; VC, V, and CV. Intelligibility tasks may be targeted with the development of the speaker's ability to signal the presence or absence of initial or final consonants. With the less severely involved speaker, the contrast may be increasingly finer. Use of intelligibility tasks in treatment is also attractive because they do not require specific instructions to the speaker about how to produce the sound. Rather, they depend on the speaker's ability to compensate for the motor impairment and to find ways to produce a perceptually acceptable sound. In the clinical setting, the clinician rarely has detailed information about movement control and movement patterns of the various articulators. Even if such information were available, it may or may not change what is done in clinical practice. For example, the speaker simply may not be able to modify a severely impaired lip movement, and instead, may need to compensate for such impairment by making a complex series of adjustments in the movements of other structures. Tasks such as intelligibility drills allow the speaker to attempt compensation in the presence of perhaps the most important kind of feedback — knowledge of whether or not the listener has understood the attempt.

Evidence is only now beginning to accumulate (Till and Toye, 1988) to suggest that dysarthric speakers are able to modify acoustic features such as voice onset time after specific feedback. Even neurologically stable dysarthric speakers are able to modify productions of sound that were not understood on the first attempt. We reported the results of a project in which two linguistically-intact speakers with adult onset dysarthria were asked to read a series of single words generated as part of the phoneme intelligibility task (Yorkston, Hammen, and Minifie, 1988). After the dysarthric speakers produced the word, a listener who was naive to the target phoneme, attempted to identify the target phoneme by repeating the word that the listener had understood the speaker to be saying. If the listener correctly identified the phoneme, no further analysis was conducted. If the listener had misunderstood the phoneme, then the dysarthric speaker was asked to "Say the word one more time so that your listener can understand it." Thus, we were analyzing only episodes of actual misunderstanding. Later, the first and second attempts at words which were initially misunderstood were digitized for preparation of perceptual judging tapes. Tapes were constructed from the digitized samples so that first and second attempts were randomly placed within the judging tape. Six speech/language pathologists experienced in dysarthria treatment served as judges. Judges were both naive to the target phoneme and naive to whether the utterance was the first or second attempt. Our question was: "Do perceptual measures based on phoneme intelligibility task indicate improvement from first to second attempt?" The following is the percentage of phonemes correctly identified across judges for the first and second attempts of our dysarthric speakers:

	Sp 1	Sp 2
First Attempt	9.7%	13.2%
Second Attempt	47.3%	38.7%

A review of these data suggests that both speakers are making sufficient modification in the productions of initially misunderstood phoneme to improve listeners' ability to understand the productions. This ability to modify performance suggests that intervention to stabilize the "best performance" of dysarthric speakers may result in improvements in performance.

Partner training

In the clinical setting, changes in intelligibility can, of course, be brought about by improving dysarthric speakers' production of the utterance.

Changes in intelligibility may also result from an improvement in the listener's ability to interpret the distorted signal. Clinical experience has suggested that partners familiar with severely dysarthric speakers tend to vary extensively in their ability to understand highly distorted speech. Some are remarkably good at interpreting utterances that are completely unintelligible to most others; others have skills that are no different from any other partner unfamiliar with the dysarthric speaker. When attempting to identify and implement factors that may impact intelligibility, an understanding of why some listeners are more effective than others would appear to be critical. The goal, of course, would be to find the identifying factors that contribute to the making of a "good listener" and to develop training procedures in an effort to create more good listeners.

The area of listener training is an important but underinvestigated area. Basic information is not yet available in this area. For example, "what is the impact of knowledge of the results on the listener's ability to understand severely dysarthric speech?" The few studies that have been done in the area of listener performance, sought to examine the stability of intelligibility measures (Yorkston and Beukelman, 1983). Therefore, no feedback was given to the judges in terms of knowledge of results. Partners who receive their "training" in a natural setting most frequently do have information about what the speaker is intending to say. A second clinically important question would appear to be, "Is there an interaction between familiarity of the partner and the particular pattern of characteristics of dysarthric speech?" Are some particular features of the speaker's production more conductive to listener success than others? The issue of listener training is especially critical for the partners of individuals with acquired dysarthria. These partners are faced with the difficult task of accommodating to a rather sudden onset disorder.

Toward an intelligibility-based model of intervention

Clinicians face a number of tasks when managing the communication needs of dysarthric individuals. Assessment of the severity and nature of the disorder is certainly one of those tasks. Evaluation of the impact of factors that have the potential of improving speech intelligibility is another. Thus far in this chapter, a number of factors such as reduction in speaking rate, semantic context, and palatal lift fitting have been shown to impact intelligibility in some dysarthric speakers. When investigating the potential usefulness of each of these factors, an attempt must be made to keep all other variables constant. However, in natural communication situations, factors that influence speech intelligibility often occur in combination and may interact with one another in complex ways. Therefore, it is probably artificial to study any single factor in isolation. Instead, the purpose of the following case presentations will be to examine the combined impact of selected factor on the word intelligibility of severely dysarthric individuals.

The first case illustrates the combined impact of semantic context and partner familiarity on the word intelligibility of ND, a 57-year-old woman with cerebral palsy, who at the time of the examination lived at home with her mother and sister. She communicated via a Morse code-based augmentative communication device but also used natural speech extensively with her sister and mother in many situations. Results of word intelligibility judged with and without semantic context are displayed in Figure 4. A

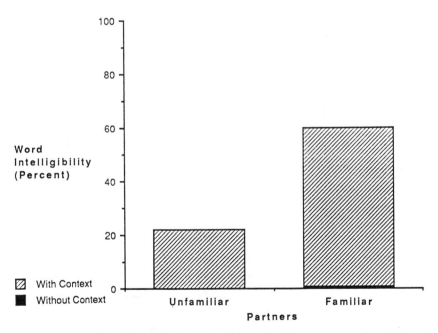

Figure 4. *Word intelligibility scores with and without context for ND, a 57-year-old woman with cerebral palsy. Judges for the task are either familiar or unfamiliar with the speaker.*

review of this figure suggests that ND's speech is severely dysarthric with unfamiliar partners understanding no words and her sister understanding one percent of words that are judged without semantic context. When context is added, scores change dramatically. Note that the unfamiliar judge's scores improved from zero to 22 percent with context. Even more dramatically, the familiar partner's scores improved from one to 60 percent correct. Thus, for this severely dysarthric speaker, adding the factor of familiarity alone resulted in only an extremely small and clinically unimportant improvement in word intelligibility scores (1 percent); adding context alone with unfamiliar judge resulted in slightly more improvement (22 percent); but combining the factors of familiarity and context resulted in a substantial and, perhaps, functionally important increase in word intelligibility. These data help to explain, at least in part, why her family members rarely utilize the augmentative communication device when communicating with ND and also why those unfamiliar with ND rely almost exclusively on the device in nearly every communicative interaction.

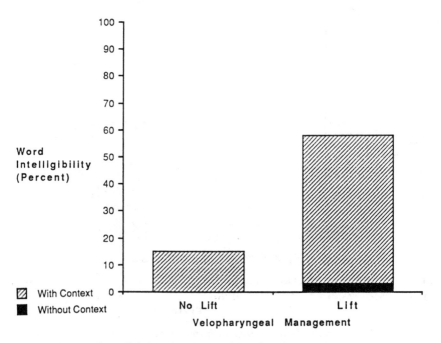

Figure 5. *Word intellibility for CM with and without semantic context. Samples were produced either with a palatal lift of without it.*

The second case illustrates the combined impact of context and palatal lift fitting on word intelligibility of CM, 22-year-old woman eight years post onset closed head injury who was described in the earlier discussion of palatal lift fitting. At the time of this evaluation, she communicated via pointing to letters on an alphabet board. Figure 5 illustrates her word intelligibility (with and without semantic context). First, the sample was recorded without a palatal lift and later with the palatal lift in place. Note that with no lift or context, judges understand none of the words. When the lift was added but judges are given no context, intelligibility improved but only very slightly (to 3 percent correct). When context is added (no palatal lift), there is an improvement to 15 percent correct; however, a much more dramatic improvement is noted when two factors are combined (60 percent correct). Each factor independently contributes in a relatively modest improvement in intelligibility which may or may not be important clinically. However, taken together the palatal lift and context result in a substantial increase in word intelligibility scores.

Information related to the factors or combination of factors that may impact intelligibility in natural communication settings is of great clinical importance. The clinical intervention process may be analogous to a scale with the heavy weight of severe motor impairment on one side tipping the scale in the direction of non-functional, unintelligible speech. The clinical intervention process involves identifying and implementing as many factors as possible that may impact intelligibility. In other words, it involves addition to the scale as many small weights as we can identify to counterbalance the heavy impairment. We have few intervention tools that are powerful enough to bring about important changes in functional performance if used in isolation. Although no single intervention is completely effective, a sufficient number of "small" interventions can accumulate to tip the balance in the favor of intelligible speech. In the case just described, the palatal lift alone was not sufficient to bring about important changes in overall performance. Only when combined with other factors did clinically important changes occur. Of course, it is important to understand what factors in isolation bring about small improvements in intelligibility. But it is also important to realize that it is the combining of factors where the true clinical benefit lies.

References

Barlow, S.M. & Abbs, J.H. 1986. "Fine force and position control of select orofacial structures in the upper motor neuron syndrome." *Experimental Neurology* 94, 699-713.

Beukelman, D.R. and Yorkston, K.M. 1980. "Influence of passage familiarity on intelligibility estimates of dysarthric speech." *Journal of Communication Disorders* 13, 33-41.

———. 1979. "The relationship between information transfer and speech intelligibility of dysarthric speakers." *Journal of Communication Disorders* 12, 189-196.

Beukelman, D.R., Yorkston, K.M. & Tice, R. 1988. *Pacer/Tally.* Tucson: Communication Skill Builders.

Darley, F.L., Aronson, A.E., & Brown, J.R. 1975. *Motor Speech Disorders.* Philadelphia: Saunders.

Dowden, P.A., Yorkston, K.M., & Stoel-Gammon, C. 1987. "Speech intelligibility of augmented system users: Effects of context." *American Speech and Hearing Association* 29:10.

Enderby, P.M. 1983. *Frenchay Dysarthria Assessment.* Boston: College-Hill Press.

Hanson, W., & Metter, E. 1983. "DAF speech rate modification in Parkinson's Disease: A report of two cases." In W. Berry (ed.), *Clinical Dysarthria*, 231-254. Boston: College-Hill Press.

———. 1980. "DAF as instrumental treatment for dysarthria in progressive supranuclear palsy: A case report." *Journal of Speech & Hearing Disorders* 45, 268-276.

Johns, D. & Darley, F. 1970. "Phoneme variability in apraxia of speech." *Journal of Speech and Hearing Disorders* 13, 556-583.

Kent, R.D., Weismer, G., Kent, J.F., & Rosenbek, J.C. 1989. "Toward phonetic intelligibility testing in dysarthria." *Journal of Speech and Hearing Disorders*, 54, 482-499.

Platt, L., Andrews, G., & Howie, P.M. 1980. "Dysarthria of adult cerebral palsy. II. Phonemic analysis of articulation errors." *Journal of Speech & Hearing Disorders* 23, 41-55.

Platt, L., Andrews, G., Young, M., & Quinn, P. 1980. "Dysarthria of adult cerebral palsy. I. Intelligibility and articulatory impairment." *Journal of Speech and Hearing Disorders* 23, 28-40.

Till, J.A., & Toye, A.R. 1988. "Acoustic phonetic effects of two types of verbal feedback in dysarthric subjects." *Journal of Speech & Hearing Disorders* 53, 449-458.

Yorkston, K.M., & Beukelman, D.R. 1983. "The influence of judge familiarization with the speaker on dysarthric speech intelligibility." In W. Berry (ed.), *Clinical dysarthria*, 154-164. Boston: College Hill Press.

———. 1981. "Communication efficiency of dysarthric speakers as measured by sentence intelligibility and speaking rate." *Journal of Speech and Hearing Disorders* 46(3), 296-301.

———. 1978. "A comparison of techniques for measuring intelligibility of dysarthric speech." *Journal of Communication Disorders* 11, 499-512.

Yorkston, K.M., Beukelman, D.R. & Bell, K. 1988. *Clinical Management of Dysarthric Speakers*. Boston: College-Hill Press.

Yorkston, K.M., Beukelman, D.R. & Traynor, C.D. 1984. *Computerized assessment of intelligibility of dysarthric speech*. Austin, TX: Pro-ed.

————. 1988. "Articulatory adequacy in dysarthric speakers: A comparison of judging formats." *Journal of Communication Disorders* 21, 351-361.

Yorkston, K.M., Beukelman, D.R., Honsinger, M.J., and Mitsuda, P.A. 1989. "Perceived articulatory adequacy and velopharyngeal function in dysarthric speakers." *Archives of Physical Medicine and Rehabilitation* 70(4), 313-317.

Yorkston, K.M., Dowden, P.A., & Honsinger, M. 1988. "Natural speech as a component of augmentative communication systems." *Augmentative and Alternative Communication* 4(3), 156.

Yorkston, K.M., Hammen, V., & Minifie, F. 1988. *Modification of Phoneme Production in Response to Listener Misunderstanding: A perceptual and acoustic analysis*. A paper presented at the Biennial Clinical Dysarthria Conference, San Diego, CA.

Yorkston, K.M., Hammen, V., Beukelman, D.R., & Iraynor, C. 1990. "The effect of rate control on the intelligibility and naturalness of dysarthric speech." *Journal of speech and Hearing Research*, 55, 225-230.

Yorkston, K.M., Honsinger, M.J., Beukelman, D.R., & Taylor, T. 1989. "The effects of palatal lift fitting on the perceived articulatory adequacy of dysarthric speakers." In K. M. Yorkston and D.R. Beukelman (eds.), *Recent Advances in Clinical Dysarthria*, 85-98. Boston: College-Hill Press.

Chapter 8

EPG-based description of apraxic speech errors

W. Hardcastle and S. Edwards
University of Reading

Introduction

The traditional taxonomy for adult acquired speech and language disorders distinguishes dysarthria from aphasia and these two disorders from apraxia (Darley, 1982; Johns and Darley, 1970). Dysarthria is usually described as a disorder occurring subsequent to motoric abnormalities of the speech musculature including increase or decrease in muscular tone, changes in control of the speed of muscular movements, impaired coordination of muscular systems or involuntary movements such as tremor (Kent, 1990). Such disturbances may produce phonetic disorders of speech. Depending on the severity of the disorder, and the particular speech variables affected, adverse effects on intelligibility may result. Aphasia, typically resulting from lesions to cortical or sub-cortical areas, unlike dysarthria, affects higher levels of language processing; primarily the phonological, semantic and/or syntactic levels. Phonological errors in aphasia have been called literal or phonemic paraphasia and are said to be characteristic of types of aphasia resulting from a posterior lesion. Commonly occurring speech errors in literal paraphasia are segmental substitutions, i.e. the substitution of one phoneme for another. These substitutions are not random, they usually differ from the target phoneme by no more than one phonetic feature (usually the place of articulation feature, see Blumstein, 1973) and are said to be due to "errors of selection from an internal phonemic and lexical store" (Mlcoch and Noll, 1980: 224).

Segmental substitutions, however, also occur in verbal apraxia or apraxia of speech, a disorder frequently associated with anterior lesions or Broca's-type aphasia and described by Rosenbek, et al. (1984) as "an impairment of the capacity to form vocal tract configurations and to move from one sequence to another for volitional speech production, in the absence of motor impairments for other responses of the same musculature". The apraxic substitutions are said to have a motoric origin rather than a phonological or linguistic origin, and will tend to be anticipatory and sequential in nature (Mlcoch and Noll, 1980: 224). The differential diagnosis of the apraxic type disorder is, however, frequently problematic. One of the difficulties lies in the nature of the traditional assessment techniques used by the clinician to diagnose apraxia of speech. Such assessment procedures require the clinician to identify speech errors as "substitutions, simplifications, distortions, omissions, additions" etc of speech sounds (see e.g. Darley, 1984) on the basis of impressionistic auditory judgements. However, as has been frequently pointed out elsewhere (e.g. Hardcastle, 1987) such analyses are not only relatively unreliable, but they give no precise indication of the nature of the error itself. Perceived substitutions or distortions may, for example, have very different origins depending on which articulatory organs are involved, how the error is manifested, the context in which it occurs, etc. Given more precise information on the articulatory activities that produce the error and the relationship between these activities and the perceived acoustic result, we would then be in a better position to assess the underlying reason for the error. Thus a /k/ heard in initial position in a word like "tick" may have a number of different interpretations. One possibility is that the /k/ phoneme has been wrongly selected from a phoneme "store" at a hypothetical higher-level linguistic encoding stage in the generation of the utterance, and has been produced correctly as far as appropriate vocal tract configurations for a velar stop are concerned. Such an explanation would presuppose an information processing model of language production which assumes that phonemic errors arise at an earlier or higher level of production than, for example, phonetic errors. Suppose, however, that both the /t/ gesture for the target initial stop and the /k/ gesture for the word final stop were both specified correctly at some stage in the generation and execution process but, because of some fault in the serial ordering of these gestures, the /k/ gesture is executed prematurely, possibly even overlapping with the /t/ gesture. A double alveolar/velar gesture may result sounding, however, more like a /k/ than a /t/. This would then be seen primarily as a problem in lower-level sequencing of articulatory gestures rather than as an incorrect selection of phonemes. It could thus be viewed as a motoric problem. Although these two speculative interpretations are quite different and may relate to quite different neural functions, the end acoustic result, the perception of a substitution error (the /k/ for the /t/) is the same. An auditory-based judgment, therefore, may not be very illuminating, because it does not reveal the intricate events that take place during speech production, the complex overlapping movements of the articulators (e.g. coarticulation) and the transitional movements between target vocal configurations. An instrumental analysis, however, may reveal these fine details of activities which, when abnormal, may be crucial diagnostically. For example, a detailed observation of a patient's tongue activity in words like "tick" may indicate a tendency towards double articulatory patterns in many similar environments which may provide additional supporting evidence for the second explanation offered above. It is difficult, therefore, on the basis of auditory identification alone to distinguish those substitutions which may have some motoric origin (e.g. be due to faulty interarticulator phasing, abnormal anticipatory coarticulation etc.) i.e. characteristic of apraxia, from those which are unrelated to any motoric impairment, and can be regarded as phonemic substitutions.

Recent instrumental investigations have contributed greatly to our knowledge of the nature of speech errors in apraxia. Physiological studies of articulatory activity such as the x-ray microbeam study of Itoh and Sasanuma (1984) found evidence of temporal discoordination among several articulators such as the velum, lip, tongue and larynx. They found, for example, that the velum was generally lowered earlier than normal for the apraxic subjects, although patterns were inconsistent. These errors were compared with those from Wernicke's- type aphasias,which were construed as being due not to inexact velar movements but rather to movements appropriate to another phoneme. Acoustic studies also have substantiated the view that apraxia is primarily a disorder of timing and the integration of movements of the articulatory system. Kent and Rosenbek (1983) identified a number of acoustic characteristics of the disorder including slowed speaking rate accompanied by lengthening of both transitional and steady states of the acoustic signal, relative flattening of prosodic contrasts, slow and inaccurate movements of articulators, initiation difficulties and discoordination of voicing with other articulators. Other acoustic studies (e.g. Ziegler and von Cramon, 1986; Tuller and Story, 1987) found evidence of abnormal anticipatory coarticulation patterns in some apraxic speakers. Duffy and Gawle (1984) measured vowel duration preceding voiced and voiceless consonants and found apraxics in general differentiated the duration in the same way as normals but with some overlap in values and considerable variability. The abnormal distribution of values was interpreted by the authors as being a consequence of generally shortened vowels in a context of poor precision of temporal control, but with accurate phonological selection of the voicing feature. Evidence for this temporal variability has been found also in studies of VOT distinctions in apraxic speakers (e.g. Itoh et al., 1982).

The general picture of verbal apraxia that emerges from these studies is of a disturbance in the high level(s) of speech organization particularly in motor programming, selection and sequencing of speech sounds (Rosenbek et al., 1984). Articulatory errors that occur have been grouped into two main types (see Mlcoch and Noll, 1980); "preprogramming" errors (such as segmental substitutions, influenced by anticipatory or carryover assimilations as well as errors due to mistimings and abnormal phasing between articulators) and errors due to impaired sensory feedback information which principally affects fricatives, affricates and other complex consonants. These two groupings are reminiscent of Luria's distinction between efferent and afferent motor aphasia — efferent characterized by transitional difficulties including the inability to move from one speech segment to the next and afferent characterized by a difficulty in discriminating and selecting the kinesthetic images of speech sounds (i.e. the distinctive features of each sound such as placement, manner, voicing). (Luria, 1973; Luria and Hutton, 1977).

An adequate model of speech production would need to take account of all these different aspects of apraxia. It is therefore clearly necessary to have more detailed descriptions of the sensori-motor abnormalities that occur in apraxia and the perceptual consequences of these abnormalities. A technique which has considerable potential for offering new insights into the nature of speech errors in apraxia is Electropalatography (see Hardcastle et al., 1989; Hardcastle, 1987; Edwards and Miller, 1989). The technique records spatial and temporal details of tongue contact with the hard palate during continuous speech, thus providing qualitative and quantitative data on a feature which has considerable phonetic relevance for studies of apraxia, namely the place of articulation.

Electropalatography

In the present EPG system, the subject wears a thin acrylic plate moulded to fit tightly against the hard palate and containing 62 silver or gold electrodes mounted on the lingual surface. When contact occurs between the tongue and any of these electrodes a signal is conducted via lead-out wires to an external processing unit that enables patterns of contact to be stored in a microprocessor and displayed on a video monitor screen. Permanent records of the contact patterns can be obtained from a computer printout (for further, more detailed analysis (see Figure 1).

The 62 electrodes are arranged according to a predetermined scheme on the surface of each plate in eight horizontal rows (for details, see Hardcastle et al., 1989). The scheme used to place the electrodes is based on readily-identifiable anatomical landmarks and enables comparisons in contact patterns to be made between subjects. Contact patterns from the control group of normal speakers were used as a baseline with which to compare the patterns produced by speech-disordered subjects. Prior to each recording session, the subjects wear a dummy plate without any electrodes but of the same thickness (i.e. approx. .8mm) as the real plate for increasing periods of time including at least one 2 hour period, so as to become accustomed to the feel of the device in the mouth.

An acrylic plate used for EPG is shown in Figure 1 together with a schematic representation of a single palatal frame and a sequence of contact patterns which occurred during a normal speaker's production of the word "kitkat". The schematic representation shows the palate divided up into three convenient reference zones based on phonetic place categories; Rows 1-3, the alveolar zone; Rows 4-5, the palatal zone; and Rows 6-8, the velar zone. In the computer printout for the word "kitkat" sampling rate is 100 Hz and the sequence of contacts is read from left to right. Various phonetic characteristics of the utterance can be noted from the pattern of contact: the full velar stop pattern for the initial /k/, (frames 119-130), the close vowel configuration with extensive contact along both sides of the palate for the /ɪ/ vowel, alveolar stop pattern for /t/ (144-147), velar stop pattern for the word medial /k/ (147), double alveolar/velar stop pattern for the medial stop (147) and word final alveolar stop pattern (180-186). From these complete printouts for all items in the corpus an analysis was made of each apraxic subject's patterns of contact for a variety of speech sounds.

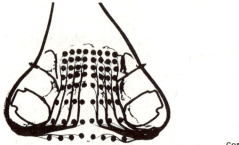

Acrylic plate for EPG

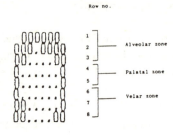

Computer display of 62 electrodes
on plate

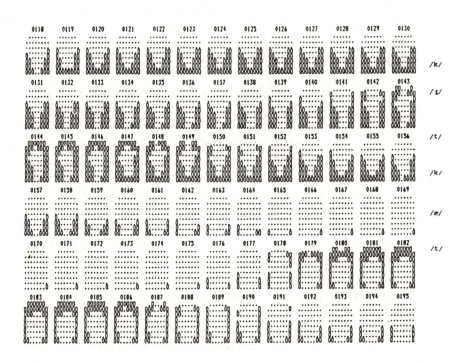

Figure 1. *An acrylic plate used for EPG with a computer display of 62 electrodes arranged into eight rows and three reference zones. The EPG printout is for the word "kitkat" and lingual contact is shown by the zeros. Sampling interval is 10 ms.*

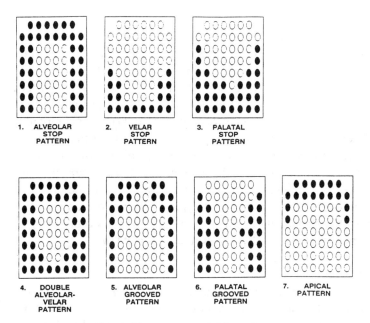

Figure 2. *Seven identifiable quasi-static EPG patterns.*

Speech production is essentially a dynamic process and this is reflected in the changing patterns of contact as illustrated in Figure 1. However, even in connected speech, it is possible to identify a limited number of quasi-static contact patterns that may be associated with a specified phase during production of a particular sound or class of sounds. This is particularly the case with lingual obstruent sounds (oral stops, fricatives and affricates) which are the main focus of interest in this paper. An extensive analysis of EPG patterns for four normal speakers has revealed a set of seven quasi-static patterns which seem to characterize the typical spatial "target" for the lingual obstruents and for the lateral approximant /l/. These quasi-static patterns constitute a useful baseline in the description of pathological speech as we shall see later.

The seven quasi-static spatial configurations are illustrated in Figure 2. The description of each, together with the lingual movements that may be inferred from them are indicated in the Figure:

Pattern 1: Alveolar stop pattern

In this configuration, lingual contact is maintained along the sides of the palate and across the alveolar ridge (usually Rows 1 and 2 but may be as far back as Row 4). The contact is usually complete in the centre part of the alveolar region. The amount of contact along the sides may vary with the vowel environment, there being a tendency towards a greater amount of lateral contact in a close front vowel environment (e.g. /i/) when compared with, say, an open vowel environment (e.g. /a/). One can infer that the tongue body is in a relatively raised, forward position (probably by the action of the posterior and central parts of the genioglossus muscle) and the tip/blade of the tongue is in a raised position (by the action of, say, the superior longitudinalis muscle). This configuration typically occurs during the closure phase of an alveolar nasal or oral stop, but it may also occur during a lateral approximant /l/ in a close front vowel environment /i/.

Pattern 2: Velar stop pattern

This configuration is characterized by complete contact across the posterior part of the palate at the juncture of the hard and soft palates (usually Row 8). Minimal lateral contact occurs, usually no more forward than Row 5. The tongue body is raised probably by action of the inferior longitudinal, bunching the central part of the body up towards the rear, and by the styloglossus and palatoglossus raising the rear sides of the tongue body. The raised body configuration typically occurs during the closure phase of velar nasal and oral stops when occurring in a relatively low and back vowel environment (e.g. in words like "core" or "car").

Pattern 3: Palatal stop pattern

This is similar to pattern 2 but the area of contact is further forward and generally more extensive. Central contact may reach as far forward as Row 5 and lateral contact as far forward as Row 3 or 4. The same muscles as in achieving pattern 2 are presumably involved but also perhaps the genioglossus posterior may bring the tongue slightly more forward. The pattern occurs during the closure phase of /k/ in close, front vowel environments (i.e. /i/, /e/ etc.)

Pattern 4: Double alveolar-velar pattern

This pattern is like a combination of 1 and 2 with complete closure at the front and rear of the palate and along both sides. The body of the tongue is raised and retracted at the same time as the tip/blade is raised. Muscle forces involved in achieving this configuration presumably include the styloglossus and inferior longitudinalis (raising the body towards the back) and the superior longitudinalis (raising the tip/blade). Some activity by the palatoglossus may keep the sides raised to ensure contact along the upper gums. The configuration may occur, typically, for short periods of time, during stop sequences such as /kt/, /tk/ in words like "cocktail", "catkin" etc.

Pattern 5: Alveolar grooved pattern
This pattern is characterized by lateral contact along the length of the palate and incomplete contact across the anterior part of the alveolar ridge (usually Rows 1 and 2). A gap occurs in the central part of the alveolar contact area with typically 1-3 electrodes remaining untouched. This configuration, occurring typically during the stricture phase of /s/, requires a complex interaction of most tongue muscles, the superior longitudinalis and anterior genioglossus to control the height of the central part of the tip/blade, the verticalis to flatten and the transversus to raise the sides slightly, while the body of the tongue is raised and positioned anteriorly. The amount of lateral contact may vary with the vowel environment as was the case with Pattern 1.

Pattern 6: Palatal grooved pattern
This pattern has lateral contact usually up to about Rows 2 or 3 and a slight narrowing in the central, post-alveolar part of the palate (Rows 4-5). The groove thus produced is wider and more retracted than in Pattern 5. The tongue tip may be down or raised slightly toward the alveolar ridge (but not touching it in the midline). Contraction of the palatoglossus and styloglossus is probably mainly responsible for this configuration, while the anterior genioglossus keeps the tip down to prevent contact with the alveolar ridge. This configuration occurs during the stricture phase of the palato alveolar fricative /ʃ/.

Pattern 7: Apical pattern
The apical pattern involves full contact across the alveolar ridge (typically rows 1-3) with little or no lateral contact. Occasionally some minimal contact may occur down one or both sides as far as Rows 4 or 5. The tongue gesture producing this configuration is probably an apical gesture with the

rest of the tongue in a concave configuration when viewed sagitally. Raising the tongue tip to make contact with the alveolar ridge is accomplished primarily by contracting the superior longitudinalis muscle. The configuration is typical of many articulations of the lateral /l/, particularly in open or back vowel environments.

It is useful to use these seven quasi-static patterns as a basis of comparison for identifying the place of articulation abnormalities in pathological speech (see e.g. Hardcastle et al, 1985; Hardcastle et al, 1989). For example, dysarthric speech is frequently characterized by target undershoot as a result of muscular weakness and may be manifested by incomplete closure in the EPG patterns. Specific examples of such abnormal spatial representations are illustrated in Figure 3 which shows incomplete closures at the alveolar and velar regions instead of the complete closures required for quasi-static Patterns 1 and 2. In both these cases the target articulation was initial /t/ and post-vocalic /k/ and the point is that the abnormal spatial patterns shown in Figure 3 do not occur in a normal speaker's production of these stops. These can be regarded as examples of *spatial distortions* of target gestures.

Other types of disorders illustrated by the EPG technique include timing problems (abnormal transitions between articulatory targets, abnormally long closure phases for stops etc.) and problems of variability either spatially or temporally.

EPG is thus a useful technique for describing spatial and temporal details of a range of sounds, particularly lingual obstruents. The present paper includes a detailed description of the patterns of lingual contact produced by four apraxic speakers. Differences from the normal patterns are described in terms of six identifiable types of errors:

1. *Misdirected articulatory gestures*
In a misdirected articulatory gesture the patterns of contact themselves for the gestures are normal, i.e. they are readily identifiable as one of the 7 quasi-static patterns (see above) but they occur in an inappropriate place in the target utterance. For example, a velar stop pattern (Pattern 2) may occur just prior to, simultaneously with, or immediately after an alveolar stop pattern (Pattern 1) in a situation where Pattern 1 only would have been normal. Such misdirected articulatory gestures are relatively common errors in our data but they are not always detected auditorily. There are numerous cases where the misdirected gesture occurs during the closure

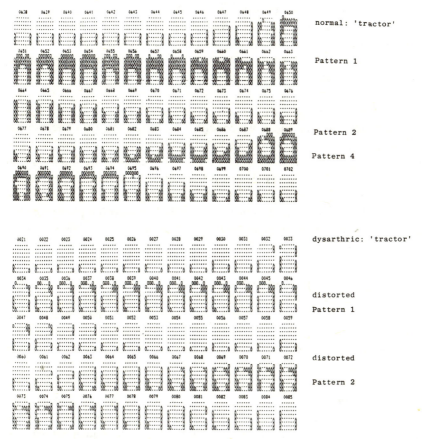

Figure 3. *EPG patterns for the word "tractor" as produced by a normal and dysarthric speaker.*

phase of a stop where no acoustic energy and thus no audible cues are present. In other cases they are heard variously as substitutions or distortions of phoneme targets. It is tempting to speculate on the possible reasons for such misdirected articulatory gestures occurring: (1) They may result from a phoneme selection problem, e.g. the velar stop instead of the alveolar stop is selected for the utterance. (2) They may be the consequence of a co-ordination/phasing problem between different articulatory organs (larynx, tongue, soft palate, lips, etc) or different parts of the same organ (tip/blade versus main body of tongue) or (3) They may result from a problem in the serial ordering of articulatory gestures for an utterance. It is suggested that some insight into which of these explanations may be the most appropriate for a given case may come from a detailed analysis of the EPG data such as that presented below.

2. *Distorted spatial patterns*

Distorted patterns are those which differ qualitatively from the normal appropriate quasi-static pattern. Such distorted patterns occur frequently in the speech of dysarthrics (see above) but some examples are found also in the apraxic data. They can be assumed to result from neuromuscular weakness, incoordination or general motoric mismanagement. Perceptually the distorted EPG patterns are frequently identified as distorted phonemes but many distorted patterns remain undetected by auditory subjective judgement.

3. *Omission of target gestures*

These are cases in which an expected quasi-static pattern appropriate for a particular target sound is missing from the record. Perceptually this phenomena is often heard as an abnormally produced target sound or as a reduction in a cluster but often subtle changes occur in the contact pattern but are not heard.

4. *Seriation problems*

These may take the form either of abnormal transitional timing between successive articulatory targets or as abnormal spatial sequencing of gestures. Abnormal timing may be manifested by longer than normal closure phases of stops or audible releases of the first element in stop-stop or stop-liquid sequences which normally involve closer coarticulation. For example the /kt/ sequence in a word such as "cocktail" may be produced with the velar stop being audibly aspirated before the alveolar stop onset. (Thus [kʰɒkʰtʰeɪl]). A normal production of this sequence would involve quasi-static Pattern 4 (double alveolar/velar configuration) and no audible aspiration of [k]. Abnormal spatial sequencing of gestures may occur in stop consonant sequences such as /tk/ or /kt/ in words like "catkin", "acting" etc where the normal alveolar-velar or velar-alveolar gesture sequence is reversed. Such cases of metathesis in the data are relatively uncommon but they do occur. They are frequently not detected auditorily.

5. *Repetitions of patterns*
Discrete patterns, (usually) normal spatially, may be repeated as in stuttering. The repeated items are usually one sound or syllable in length (as in ideopathic stuttering) but, unlike those in ideopathic stuttering they may be repeated only once. These stuttering-like repetitions as well as other disfluency features such as repetitions of elements similar to the target have frequently been noted in the literature on apraxia and are seen as part of the general tendency of articulatory "groping" or "sound searching" (Johns and Darley, 1970) in the patients. EPG analysis allows one to examine closely the various components in the non-fluent episode, to determine for example whether the reiterated items are similar to the target. Are they, for example likely to involve schwa-type vowels as claimed by Van Riper (1971) for ideopathic stuttering ?

6. *Abnormal temporal and spatial variability*
EPG analysis facilitates the quantification of variability by measuring various aspects of successive repetitions of the same target utterance, the same target sound in different environments or the same target utterance on different occasions. Excessive variability has frequently been linked with apraxia (see e.g. Ziegler, 1987) and may be seen as an indication of lack of articulatory co-ordination.

Examples of all these types of errors will be discussed in the following analysis of the data. All types of errors are to be expected in the data but they may not be evenly distributed. One patient may show a greater tendency towards misdirected articulations while another may show more repetitions. It is instructive to examine how these types of errors cluster in the four different speakers, and how they are manifested precisely in the data for each subject so as to identify which errors are common to all and which might serve as useful indices for differential diagnosis.

The experiment

Subjects

The subjects were four male patients all in their 60s who had suffered left hemisphere CVAs. According to their speech therapist all originally presented with aphasia and apraxia of speech. In each case the aphasia had largely resolved and the patient was left with some difficulty in speech production. Apraxia of speech was diagnosed in each case. Data from a control group of four normal adult speakers (see Hardcastle et al, 1985) were used as a basis for comparison with the experimental subjects and the errors are grouped according to the six types described above.

Corpus

A protocol was prepared consisting of the following main components:

A. *Single word list.* A word list was compiled containing all the lingual consonants of English in a variety of different vowel environments and occurring both syllable initially and finally. The list also included a number of complex consonant sequences such as /tk/, /kt/, /st/ both within and across morpheme boundaries (see Appendix A). Each word was produced as a single utterance and was preceded by the indefinite article (or when this was semantically inappropriate, the definite article). The reason for the article was to prevent coarticulatory effects spreading from one word to the next and to provide a consistent baseline for EPG records for the word initial consonants. The list was designed to give an overall picture of the types of errors that occurred. At least two repetitions of the list were obtained on two separate occasions.

B. *Multiple repetition task.* Four words, taken from the full word list (A) were repeated a minimum of 4 times at a slow rate and then 4 times at a fast rate. The four words were "cocktail, kitkat, clock and headlight". This task was designed to measure variability in articulation for the two different rates.

C. *Connected speech task.* Four words were selected from the word list (A) for each subject. The subject was instructed to compose and produce a sentence with each of the words in turn. The rationale behind this task was to elicit errors that could be attributed to cognitive and linguistic factors.

D. *Non-verbal tasks.* A variety of non-verbal tasks were included in the protocol including alternating movements of tongue tip and back of tongue; tongue tip to alveolar ridge; repetitions of these movements to varying rhythmic patterns. Each activity was performed with and without voice (see Appendix A). These non-verbal tasks were designed to test the motoric ability of each subject to perform relatively complex sequencing gestures in the absence of linguistic cognitive processing. Some of the results of this task have been presented elsewhere (Edwards and Miller, 1989) and will not be reported in detail here. The non-verbal tasks were not carried out on Subject T.

E.   *Voicing distinctions.* A number of minimal pairs were devised illustrating the voicing distinction in initial plosives e.g. "tier", "deer" (Appendix A). The randomized list was produced by each subject at least 5 times and VOT values measured from the acoustic signal. These VOT results will be presented in a forthcoming paper.

Procedure

All subjects were fitted with an acrylic plate for EPG and recordings were made of sections A, B, C, and D of the corpus. It was not possible to record section D (non-verbal tasks) for subject T. Auditory-based phonetic transcriptions were made of all items produced and full EPG print-outs obtained for all items. The results that follow are based on these print-outs.

Results

Subject L

The EPG analysis of subject L's errors revealed the following:

1.   *Misdirected articulatory gestures*: The misdirected articulatory gestures made by this speaker can be subdivided into 3 types. The first type of error involved the alveolar stop pattern being produced instead of a target bilabial or velar and there are frequent examples of this in the data: e.g. "dark" produced as [da:t] "shark" as [ʃa:t] and "tip" as [tʰɪt]. In all cases, the word final consonant was produced with the normal alveolar stop pattern (Pattern 1, above) which in fact occurred frequently elsewhere for this subject also in word initial position. About 75% of these misdirected alveolar patterns occurred in words already containing an alveolar stop, either preceding or following the substituted element. The occurrence of the misdirected articulatory gestures was variable; e.g. out of four attempts at the word "dark" two were produced normally with a velar stop pattern and two with a misdirected alveolar stop pattern. The misdirected pattern in all cases was identical to the alveolar stop pattern produced normally by the subject on the two other occasions.

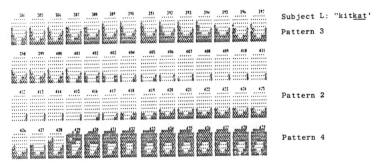

Subject L: "kit<u>kat</u>'
Pattern 3

Pattern 2

Pattern 4

Figure 4. *EPG patterns for the second syllable in the word "kitkat" as produced by subject L.*

The second type of misdirected production error occurred far less frequently than the above examples of alveolar stop pattern and involved a misdirected velar pattern. Examples were found in the production of "witchcraft" and "kitkat". In "kitkat" the misdirected velar stop pattern occurred simultaneously with the alveolar (see Figure 4). This double articulation pattern which is quite different from the errors involving one configuration was rare for this subject occurring only three times and each time in the word "kitkat".

The third subtype of misdirected patterns was similar to that of the quasi-static Pattern 7 (the apical pattern) and occurred in the subject's production of the word "mouse" heard as [naʊs]. The initial sound of the word had a similar configuration to the EPG pattern that occurred initially for this subject's normal production of "leg". It is interesting to note that one perceptual substitution made by this subject is [n] for [l] in "headlight". Whereas this subject has a general tendency for a perceptual substitution to affect place of articulation only it will be noted that this, in contrast, seems to affect manner. It may be a significant factor in explaining this substitution that both these substituted [n]s share with [l] a similar EPG contact pattern, the apical pattern 7, which, in the case of /n/ is different from a normal speaker's. This speaker's idiosyncratic pattern for /n/ is seen also in "knot" (see Figure 5 which shows this subject's EPG patterns for the three words "knot", "leg" and "mouse" as being the apical Pattern 7 and different from the target /d/ in "dart". A more normal production of /n/ would use pattern 1, as for /d/). It was also noted that, for this speaker, there was little evidence of sensory feedback monitoring taking place. In almost all cases the misdirected patterns were not corrected.

2.   *Distorted spatial patterns.* Distorted patterns occurred only on the fricative targets. The pattern for [ʃ] was more retracted than the normal palatal grooved Pattern 6 (see Figure 6 for "fish") and both [s] and [z] were abnormally asymmetric with lack of lateral contact on the left velar region and on the right alveolar (see Figure 7 for "racer"). These distorted spatial patterns were quite consistent for this speaker and were the only examples of distortions in his data. Thus for this speaker, /s/ and /ʃ/ seemed to present special production problems. This is not altogether surprising as the alveolar and palato-alveolar fircatives can be regarded as relatively complex sounds in terms of the precise co-ordination needed for their production involving the three physiological systems; the laryngeal (to control voicing), respiratory (to regulate air-flow) and articulatory (to control tongue position and configuration).

3.   *Omissions of target gestures.* Omitted target gestures frequently involved the second element in clusters or the fricative release phase of affricates. Thus "clock" was once produced as [kʰɒk] and "deckchair" as [dɛtʰdɛtʃeə]. In both cases no trace of the omitted element was present in the EPG signal. Such cases of omissions were clearly audible. They were rare in the data.

4.   *Seriation problems.* For this speaker, seriation problems were confined to abnormal transitions between elements in clusters and sequences such as, for example /tk/ produced consistently with a delay between the [t] release and the [k] closure (heard as [tʰk]). This occurred in most repetitions of words such as "kitkat", "catkin" (see Figure 8). But transitional movements in the velar, alveolar sequence [kt] or [kd] or [kl] were usually normal with a double alveolar-velar pattern present when the sequence occurred word medially (see Figure 9 for "tractor"). In initial position in sequences such as /kl/ in "clock" the delay between release of the stop and onset of the [l] alveolar contact was within normal limits. It seems then that the alveolar, velar transitional movement caused more of a problem for this subject than the reverse velar, alveolar sequence.

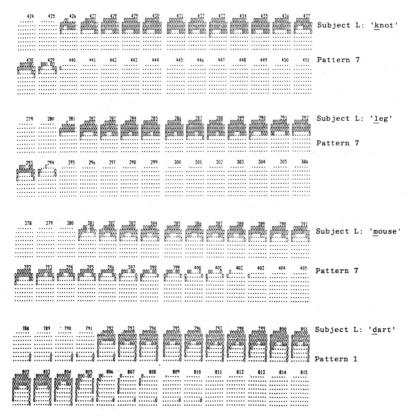

Figure 5. *EPG patterns for the subject L's attempts at the initial sounds in the words "knot", "leg", "mouse" and "dart".*

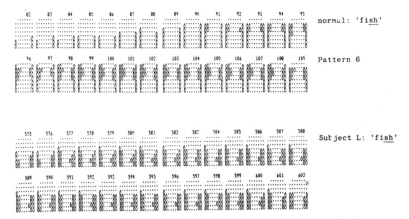

Figure 6. *EPG patterns for the palato-alveolar fricative in the word "fish" as produced by a normal speaker and subject L.*

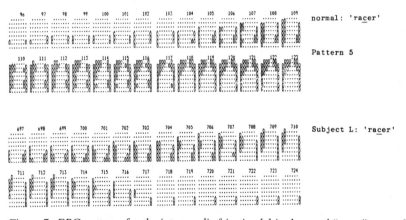

Figure 7. *EPG patterns for the intervocalic fricative [s] in the word "racer" as produced by a normal speaker and by subject L.*

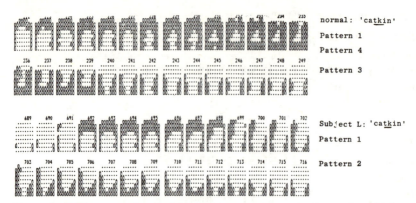

Figure 8. *EPG patterns for the intervocalic stop sequence in the word "catkin" as produced by a normal speaker and by subject L.*

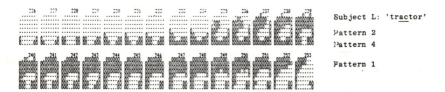

Figure 9. *EPG patterns for the /kt/ sequence in "tractor" as produced by subject L.*

5. *Repetitions.* There were a number of instances where syllables were repeated. In disyllabic words the repeated syllable could be either the first or second syllable (e.g. [dɛtʰdetʃɛə] "deckchair", [kʰɪtʰkʰætkʰæt]) "kitkat". The repeated syllable was usually identical to the subject's final version of the target, at least as far as the EPG patterns were concerned but one exception was "tractor" produced as [tʰɪtʰɛktæktə] where the EPG contact for the vowel in the repeated syllable was different from the first attempt. It could be argued in fact that the more open configuration of the repeated syllable brought the vowel closer to the target [æ]. This type of "groping" articulatory pattern where successive attempts move closer to the target articulation has frequently been noted in the literature on apraxia (see Johns and Darley, 1970; Trost and Canter, 1974), but was not frequent in the single word productions of this speaker.

6. *Variability*. Variability involving misdirected articulatory patterns was evident in the repetition task (speech task 2 in the corpus, Appendix A) particularly for item "headlight". The variations included [hɛdwɔɪlaɪt], [hɛdəlaɪt] and [lɛdəlaɪt]. Variability in transitional timing was not so evident in this subject but there was some spatial variability (see e.g. 3 repetitions of "clock" in Figure 10).

Subject M

1. *Misdirected articulations*. As with subject L there were numerous examples of misdirected articulations in M's data. However in contrast to subject L almost all M's misdirected articulations resulted in a double alveolar-velar pattern. The double articulation pattern typically occurred in words containing both a velar and an alveolar target articulation. For example the initial stops in "ticking" and "kitkat" were both produced with a double alveolar velar pattern (see Figure 11 for "kitkat"). The tendency towards a double articulation pattern was also evident in the /kt/ and /kd/ sequences in words like "tractor", "weekday" etc. The first element in the medial stop sequence in these words was usually released with audible aspiration by M and the second, syllable initial, element was frequently produced with a double articulation pattern.

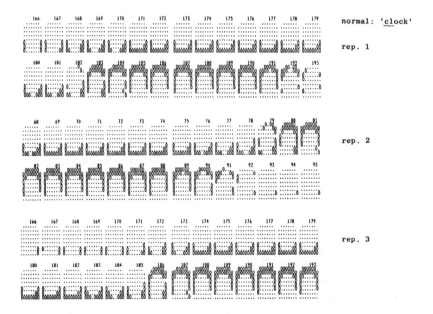

normal: 'clock'

rep. 1

rep. 2

rep. 3

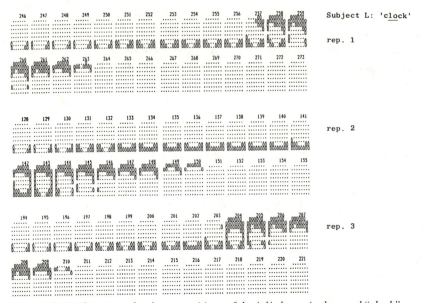

Figure 10. *EPG patterns for three repetitions of the /kl/ cluster in the word "clock" as produced by a normal speaker and by subject L.*

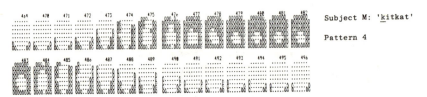

Figure 11. *EPG patterns for the initial stop in the word "kitkat" as produced by subject M.*

Figure 12 shows an example of this in the medial stop sequence of the word "weekday". The normal subject coarticulates the velar and alveolar gestures, with the alveolar gesture already completed by the time of the velar release (frame 339). Subject M abnormally releases the first, spatially normal, velar stop (at frame 484) with audible aspiration, then produces, as the initial consonant element in the second syllable, a double articulation pattern. Such a release of the /k/ with audible aspiration could occur in a normal speaker's over careful production of this word, but in such a case an alveolar stop pattern would always be used for the second element in the

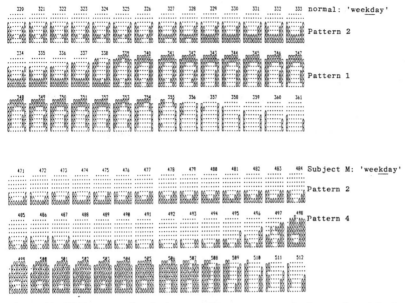

Figure 12. *EPG patterns for the intervocalic stop sequence in the word weekday" as produced by a normal speaker and by subject M.*

sequence rather than a double alveolar-velar pattern such as M's. This is therefore seen as an example of a misdirected articulatory gesture.

Sometimes these double articulation patterns were heard as /t/, other times as /k/. The initial stop in "tickling" for example was heard as /k/ although there was clearly alveolar closure in the EPG records. These perceived substitutions are therefore quite different from those noted as subtype 1 in subject L's data where no double alveolar velar pattern was evident. These also illustrate how a speaker's poor intelligibility may arise from different causes.

These misdirected articulatory patterns of M are reflected also in his non-verbal data. He had considerable difficulty with the [təkə] sequence task producing very often alveolar stop patterns instead of the velar, and frequently the alveolar-velar double articulation.

2. *Distorted spatial patterns.* As with subject L, these were confined largely to alveolar and palato-alveolar fricatives. Asymmetrical patterns were evident in M's data mainly for /ʃ/ with a skewed pattern similar to L's [s] (see Figure 13 for "bush"). These palato-alveolar fricatives were trans-

cribed as [ʃˢ] i.e. as an [ʃ] with an alveolar fricative colouring. The target alveolar fricatives also were generally produced asymmetrically and with abnormally close constriction in the palatal region i.e. Rows 4-6 (Figure 14). The auditory impression was within normal limits.

3.   *Omission of target gestures.* There are no examples of omission of target gesture in M's data. Any omitted elements noted, for example such as omission of the alveolar element in /tk/ sequences such as "kitkat", "cat-kin" etc are quite normal dialectal variants for this speaker.

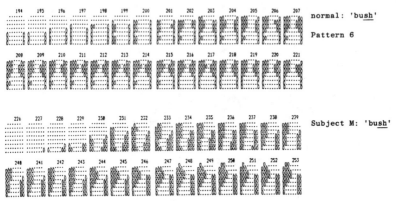

Figure 13. *EPG patterns for the palato-alveolar fricative in "bush" as produced by a normal speaker and by subject M.*

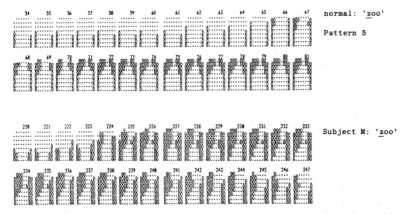

Figure 14. *EPG patterns for /z/ in "zoo" as produced by a normal speaker and by subject M.*

4. *Seriation problems*. As with subject L, most stop consonant sequences were produced by releasing the first element with audible aspiration. Thus all the repetitions of "kitkat" were produced with either the medial /t/ omitted or produced with aspirated alveolar stop or double alveolar-velar closure. In sequences such as the medial /kl/, /kd/, /kʃ/ etc. the first stop was released before onset of the gesture for the second element began, and there was a relatively long delay between the two elements. This may have been the result of a slower, more deliberate articulation rate overall. The ordering of the alveolar and velar gestures in some sequences such as the initial /kl/ sequence in "clock" caused some difficulties. Of the four repetitions of "clock" (see Figure 15) two showed no velar closure, one showed

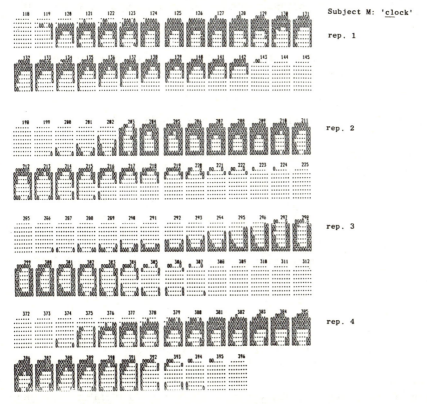

Figure 15. *EPG patterns for four repetitions of the /kl/ sequence in "clock": Subject M.*

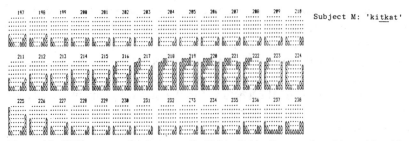

Figure 16. *EPG patterns for intervocalic /tk/ in "kitkat" as produced by subject M.*

simultaneous onset of alveolar and velar stop patterns and one showed velar onset followed by alveolar closure (for normal pattern, see Figure 10 above). One of the repetitions with no velar closure was transcribed with a lateral fricative [ɬ]. All the others were heard as /kl/. The ordering of elements seems to be a problem also in one repetition of "kitkat" (Figure 16) where a velar constriction (at frame 215) preceded the alveolar constriction in the word medial sequence rather than vice versa.

5.   *Repetitions.* There were no examples of repetitions in M's data.

6.   *Variability.* Variability was particularly noticeable in the transitions between elements in sequences such as the /tk, kt, kl/ etc. and in the occurrence of the misdirected articulatory gestures. Figure 15 above showed four repetitions of "clock" each pattern showing both temporal and spatial variability

Subject T

1.   *Misdirected articulatory gestures.* Subject T showed numerous examples of misdirected articulatory gestures particularly in word initial position. In some cases (e.g. "deer" in Figure 17) a velar stop pattern occurred followed by a brief period of double alveolar velar articulation then an alveolar stop pattern.

The whole complex stop phase thus produced was variously transcribed as [ĝd] or [d] and was very much longer than a normal initial stop. In other cases a double alveolar-velar phase persisted for a considerable time (210 ms in "tickling" see Figure 18) and appeared almost like a prolongation of the closure phase described in the stuttering literature as a block (Edwards and Hardcastle, 1987). This example is interesting also as it

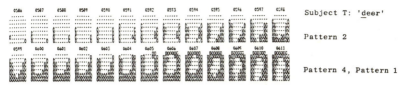

Figure 17. *EPG patterns for subject T's attempt at the initial stop in "deer".*

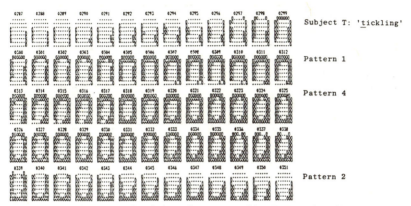

Figure 18. *EPG patterns for the initial stop in "tickling" as produced by subject T.*

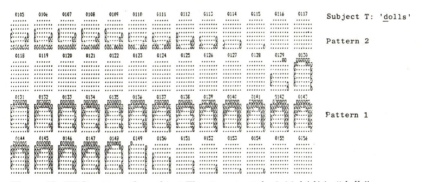

Figure 19. *EPG patterns for subject T's attempts at the initial /d/ in "dolls".*

begins with a normal alveolar stop pattern and the velar contact occurs about 190 ms after onset of the closure phase. In "dolls" a misdirected velar stop pattern occurred also, but in this case it was released with audible aspiration to be followed immediately after by a normal alveolar stop pattern (see Figure 19). Misdirected articulatory gestures occurred also for target

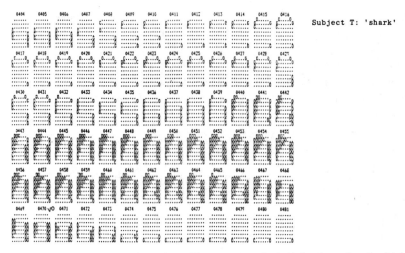

Subject T: 'shark'

Figure 20. *EPG patterns for subject T's attempt at the initial palato-alveolar fricative in* "shark".

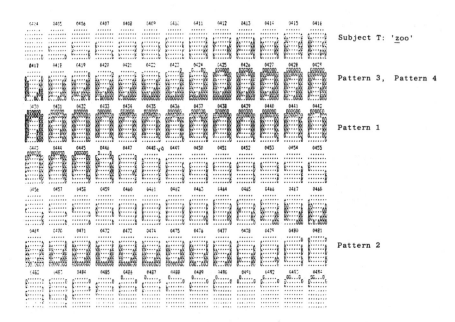

Subject T: 'zoo'

Pattern 3,   Pattern 4

Pattern 1

Pattern 2

Figure 21. *EPG patterns for subject T's /z/ in* "zoo".

fricatives. The target palato-alveolar fricative /ʃ/ in the words "sheep" or "shark" was often initiated by a misdirected alveolar grooved pattern (see Figure 20) an alveolar stop pattern or a velar stop pattern. In target "zoo", transcribed [degzu] the complex misdirected articulatory sequence began with a velar stop pattern, brief simultaneous alveolar-velar double articulation, alveolar stop pattern, then velar stop pattern (see Figure 21). Although T's data showed many examples of misdirected articulatory gestures, in all achieved cases the target articulation was finally produced successfully. Thus a target alveolar stop gesture for words like "dart, dolls" etc was eventually correctly produced by T after a variety of misdirected gestures. In cases where the double alveolar-velar pattern occurred, this was either released and a fresh attempt at the correct target made (as in "tickling") or the velar component was released leaving a normal alveolar stop pattern. In only one case (target "hats") did the incorrect target gesture remain undetected by T. In this word a velar stop pattern was produced instead of the alveolar stop. It is tempting to speculate therefore for subject T that he is using an intact sensory monitoring system to detect errors in production at least in initial position and to take the necessary steps to immediately correct them. Of course, the reasons why the errors occurred in the first place are the subject for speculation and will be discussed in the final part of this paper.

2. *Distorted spatial configurations.* As with the other subjects discussed above, T's spatial patterns were quite normal apart from the fricatives where similar abnormalities occurred. The palato alveolar fricative was produced with a skewed asymmetric pattern very similar to subject M's above (see e.g. "shark" Figure 20 above). The alveolar fricative [s] was usually produced by T with slight asymmetry and minimal lateral contact.

3. *Omission of target gestures.* No omissions were noted in T's data. Both elements in sequences such as stop-fricative, stop-stop etc were produced although usually with abnormally long transitions.

4. *Seriation problems.* Seriation problems were manifested in T's data both by abnormal temporal transitions between elements in consonant sequences and by misordering of articulatory gestures. Transitions between stop-stop sequences such as /kt, tk, kd/ etc were usually produced with the first element released, and abnormally long delays occurred in /kl/ sequences such as "clock" (see Figure 22). Abnormal sequencing of articulatory gestures was evident in some examples of stop-stop sequences

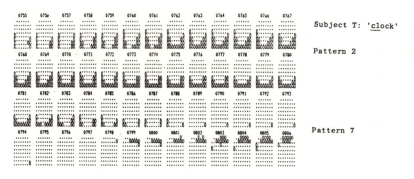

Figure 22. *EPG patterns for subject T's /kl/ in "clock".*

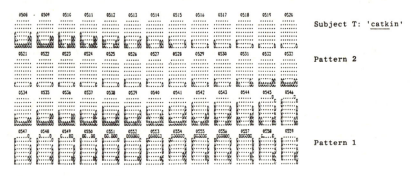

Figure 23. *EPG patterns for the first syllable in subject T's production of "catkin".*

such as the /tk/ in "catkin". In a number of cases involving velar and alveolar stop gestures, the ordering of the gestures was reversed. Thus in one repetition of "catkin" the /k/ gesture in the word medial sequence preceded the /t/ gesture (see Figure 23)

5. *Repetitions*. Stuttering like symptoms occurred frequently in T's speech as with subject L. So-called core components of stuttering — elemental repetitions and prolongations (Wingate, 1964) occurred frequently in T's speech. The prolongations involved primarily increased duration of nasals and fricatives as well as increased closure phases for stops. Repetitions involving syllables or monosyllabic words occurred frequently but usually, unlike idiopathic stuttering, only one repetition was produced and this involved either the target syllable itself or a syllable similar to it except for the final consonant segment in the syllable (e.g. [lɛg lɛg; lɛd lɛg; liːk liːf]).

In all cases where the first attempt at the target word was incorrect, a real word was in fact produced rather than a neologism. This may reflect a mild lexical selection problem in this patient. Elemental repetitions of CV sequences occurred also and here the vowel was similar both perceptually and in terms of contact patterns to the target vowel (cf: elemental repetitions in ideopathic stuttering where, according to Van Riper, 1971, a schwa type vowel usually occurs).

6.   *Variability*. As with the other subjects, T's EPG patterns showed considerable spatial and temporal variability. In successive repetitions of the same word, variability in timing, e.g. duration of stop closure phases was particularly noticeable, and on repetitions of the same word on separate occasions a variety of misdirected articulatory patterns occurred. Examples of this type of variability described in Hardcastle (1987) included the following variants at the onset of target word "shark": alveolar grooved onset followed by distorted palato-alveolar grooved pattern; velar stop pattern followed by alveolar stop pattern, alveolar grooved pattern then alveolar stop pattern for /ʃ/; essentially normal pattern except for distorted palato-alveolar grooved pattern for /ʃ/. In such cases the variability was confined to the presence and type of misdirected articulation; where a distorted pattern occurred (such as the production of target /ʃ/) it was relatively consistent in spatial configuration. There was considerable variability also in the manifestation of the same target phonemes in different environments. Thus target /s/ was sometimes produced with a relatively normal alveolar grooved pattern, but on other occasions with a misdirected, velar stop or alveolar stop pattern. No consistent pattern, for example a specific contextual effect, was noted in such cases.

Subject S

(Many of the characteristics of subject S's patterns during verbal and non-verbal tasks have been discussed at length in Edwards and Miller, 1989).

1.   *Misdirected articulatory gestures*. Misdirected articulatory gestures were relatively common in S's data. The overall auditory impression was one of frequent "groping" gestures in successive attempts at achieving the correct target articulation. Most of the misdirected gestures occurred in initial word position and most involved alternating velar and alveolar stop patterns. These patterns were frequent and rapid and often remained unde-

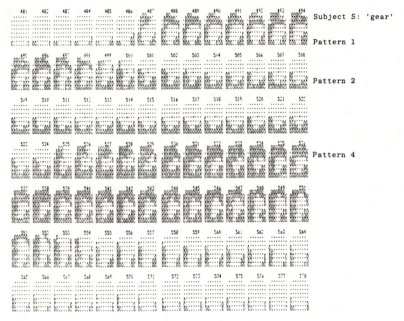

Figure 24. *EPG patterns for subject S's attempts at the initial /g/ in "gear".*

tected by the listener. There were many examples of extraneous alveolar stop gestures occurring in inappropriate places. In target "gear" he begins with a normal alveolar stop pattern (although perhaps spatially a little asymmetrical) then a velar stop pattern and another alveolar stop pattern occurring simultaneously resulting in a double alveolar velar pattern (see Figure 24). Such sequences were common in S's data, and it seemed reasonable to consider the alveolar stop patterns as fortuitous gestures rather than "phoneme substitutions".

2. *Distorted target gestures.* Most spatial configurations were normal although there was a tendency towards increased contact on the left side of the palate resulting in asymmetrical contact patterns for many of the spatial targets such as the alveolar stop pattern and the alveolar fricative pattern. As seen in Figure 24, this asymmetry led to abnormal lateral release for some stop patterns, although these were normally identified as stops rather than lateral fricatives. One example of the lateral release leading to an erroneous judgement by the listener was target "tier" heard as [kʰiə]

although there was an obvious alveolar stop pattern. However, decreased contact in the palatal region on the right hand side (with possibility of some lateral release of the airstream) was observed. This, coupled with a slight narrowing in the velar region may have led to the perceptual judgement [kʰ]. Some of the asymmetrical contact patterns such as the partial gesture on the left hand side of the alveolar ridge (see discussion in Edwards and Miller, 1989) would be regarded as abnormally distorted versions of the alveolar stop pattern. Alveolar fricatives also were produced with asymmetrical patterns.

3. *Omissions of target gestures.* Omissions of target gestures were rare for this subject.

4. *Seriation problems.* Seriation problems emerged in the non-verbal data for this subject. Whereas there was relative uniformity of timing for simple repetitive movements such as tongue tip to alveolar ridge, problems of transition emerged in the more complex [təkə] repetition task. Although the overall time frame for the different components of the sequence seemed relatively constant, the contact patterns during the non-contact periods and during the on-and off-glides to the articulatory closures showed considerable instability. The suggestion from both the verbal and non-verbal data for this subject is that he "knows" the target but has difficulty "in attaining the spatial configurations and in controlling the several movement parameters involved in effecting a smooth transition from one position to another" (Edwards and Miller, 1989: 122).

5. *Repetitions.* Numerous repetitions and similar disfluency features occurred in S's data. Typically, having made an error, subject S makes further attempts at the target word resulting in multiple syllable repetitions. Often when the word is finally produced correctly subject S continues with further attempts at the target.

6. *Variability.* Considerable spatial and temporal variability is evident in the word repetition task. Most of the spatial variability involves misdirected gestures which occurred unpredictably in successive repetitions of the same word. Temporal variability involved abnormally long durations for some repetitions of stop closures.

Table 1: *Summary of articulatory errors as revealed by EPG*

Error type	Subjects			
	L	M	T	S
Misdirected gesture	occasional: alv. stop pattern most frequent. Usually uncorrected	frequent: all patterns incl. many alv.-vel. double art.'s	frequent: all patterns incl. many alv-vel. double art.'s	frequent: mostly word initial, frequent alv. stop patterns
Spatial distortion	asymmetrical /s/, retracted /ʃ/	asymmetrical /s/ and /ʃ/ with close stricture	asymmetrical /s/ and ʃ/	asymmetrical /s/ and some alv. stops
Omission	occasional mainly second element in clusters	no examples	no examples	rare
Abnormal seriation				
a. long transitions	within alv.-vel. sequences	within alv.-vel. and vel.-alv. sequences	within alv.-vel. and vel.-alv. sequences	within alv.-vel. and vel.-alv sequences
b. metathesis	no examples	occasional	occasional	no examples
Repetition	occasional: 1st or 2nd syllable in disyllabic words	rare	occasional: syllables	frequent: multiple syllable repetitions
Variability				
a. spatial	high	low	high	high
b. temporal	low	high	high	high
c. type of misdirected gesture	high	high	high	high

Summary of results

Table 1 gives an overall view of how the six main error groups are manifested in the EPG patterns of the four test subjects.

As can be seen in the Table, all subjects show evidence of misdirected articulatory gestures, that is, gestures that are normal in their spatial configuration but are produced in inappropriate places. There is abundant evidence from these data that the tongue can be regarded as consisting of two separately controllable systems, the tip/blade system and the body system and the misdirected gestures frequently resulted in a simultaneous alveolar/velar stop pattern (i.e. Pattern 4, above), most often occurring in syllable initial position. The misdirected gesture often occurred prior to the onset of the target gesture (e.g. in Figures 17,19) but sometimes after onset of the target (e.g. Figure 18). In some cases the misdirected gesture was audibly released prior to the correct target articulation (e.g. in Figure 19) giving the impression of disfluency or "groping" for the target. In some cases a number of misdirected gestures are produced rapidly in succession (as e.g. in Figure 21). In almost all these cases of misdirected gestures, however, the spatial configurations, at least as far as tongue contact patterns are concerned, are not distorted. Unlike the case of dysarthric speech (see above) the patterns of the misdirected gestures are appropriate for particular speech sounds and usually conform to the quasi- static Patterns 1-7 described above.

For subject L, however, the misdirected gestures function differently from those for the other subjects. Firstly they are predominantly alveolar stop gestures and they are typically not corrected. Double articulation patterns are rare, only occurring in word final position in the one word "kitkat". The result of the uncorrected misdirected alveolar stop gestures is frequent perceptual substitutions (mainly /t/ for /k/). It is tempting to regard these misdirected gestures as errors of phoneme selection at a relatively high level in the speech production process. There does not seem to be any obvious motor involvement and often there are no clear contextual effects operating ("shark" [ʃaːt]). The interpretation of these errors as selection errors receives further support from the production of "mouse" as [nəʊs] with an apical pattern (Pattern 7) for /n/ rather than the more normal Pattern 1 (alveolar stop pattern). At first sight this could be regarded as a spatially abnormal production of an alveolar nasal/oral stop pattern. However, for this subject the pattern for the [n] in [nəʊs] is identical to his /n/

pattterns elsewhere (see Figure 5) and are perceived as normal /n/s. It may simply be, of course, that the difference between Subject L and the other three, at least as far as misdirected gestures is concerned, lies in the operation of sensory feedback. It could be argued for example that Subject L has impaired self-monitoring, allowing errors to proceed uncorrected whereas the more normal feedback functioning in the other subjects results in frequent corrections, retrials etc. leading to the different patterns for the misdirected gestures (simultaneous alveolar/velar patterns, for example).

The results show that, although the misdirected gestures are not in themselves spatially abnormal, all subjects have consistently distorted patterns for fricatives. These distorted patterns produced by all subjects, in addition, are remarkably similar. The /s/ target for all is produced with an asymmetric configuration skewed to the right. The asymmetrical pattern is also seen in some palato-alveolar fricatives particularly in subjects T and M. It is tempting to identify this as a slight motoric problem for these patients which is only evident during the production of relatively complex sounds such as fricatives and affricates.

Omissions of target gestures are relatively uncommon in the data with only subject L showing any clear evidence of this by omitting the second element in some complex clusters. Seriation problems, on the other hand, occurred frequently in all four subjects. Transition between stop sequences was delayed for all subjects although for subject L the transition problem was evident only for alveolar/velar sequences. Incorrect sequencing of gestures occurred in a few cases for subjects M and T with metathesis of the /t/ and /k/ gestures in words like "kitkat", "catkin".

All subjects except M showed disfluency features in their data. The disfluency features took various forms, including prolongations, repetitions and audible misdirected gestures. Many stops showed prolongation of the closure phase and sometimes a misdirected articulatory gesture occurred during the prolongation (see e.g. the initial /t/ closure phase in "tickling" for subject T, Figure 18). Repetitions included repeated sounds or CV syllables (such as subject L's production of tractor, see above) or repeated CVC syllables (e.g. subject L's [kʰɪtʰkʰætkʰæt]. In these cases, the repeated item is similar to the target element and either preceeded or followed it. There are cases, however, which could be regarded as disfluencies where an extra syllable or sound occurs which is different from the target item. Such cases are usually the result of misdirected articulatory gestures (e.g. [gədɒlz] for "dolls" in Figure 19). A succession of these misdirected gestures or the elemental repetitions mentioned probably contribute to the subjective impression of "sound searching" or "groping" said to be characteristic of some apraxic patients (see above) and may be indicative of motoric mismanagement in these subjects.

All subjects showed considerably more variability both temporally and spatially than the four normal subjects. This was particularly noticeable in the production of complex clusters and sequences such as the /tk, kt, kl/ etc in the data. Variability is seen by some authors as being characteristic of poor co-ordination (e.g. Ziegler, 1987).

Relationship between EPG patterns and speech intelligibility

The relationship between EPG patterns such as those presented in this paper and speech intelligibility has both theoretical and clinical significance. All subjects themselves claimed they had a problem with speech sound production although the EPG errors observed in the data affected the speech output in different ways. Firstly there are perceived phonemic substitutions. These were heard clearly in subject L's speech as incorrect phonemes (e.g. "tip" as [tʰɪt], "shark" as [ʃaːt] etc). When these substitutions occurred word finally, they would frequently pass unnoticed as they differed from the target in only one or two phonetic features (in the examples above the substitutions are both voiceless stops, only the place is different). In initial position, however, they were easily identifiable and may affect overall intelligibility if frequent enough (e.g. [naʊs] for "mouse", [lɛdlaɪt] for "headlight" etc.). We have attributed these substitutions to misdirected articulatory gestures which remain uncorrected. If the error is corrected rapidly as often happens with the other subjects, intelligibility is only minimally affected. If the error is not corrected rapidly there may be a long period of repetitive "sound searching" which could affect intelligibility.

A variety of abnormal EPG patterns appear to affect perception only minimally. The double articulation pattern so common with all subjects except subject L was sometimes transcribed as a double stop [ĝd] but most frequently it was identified as a normal alveolar stop. Also there were frequent cases in the data of clear misdirected target gestures which remained undetected by the listener. These undetected misdirected target gestures were usually velar stop patterns such as "catkin" produced by subject T as [kʰætʰəkʰɪn]. Figure 23 shows the first syllable of T's production with the second velar stop pattern remaining undetected (for further examples of this phenomenon see Hardcastle, 1987). This is important clinically as it shows that EPG might reveal an underlying motoric mismanagement problem which may not have been detected by an auditory analysis alone. Spatial distortions also occur in the EPG data but only for fricatives. Most of the fricatives produced by the subjects were judged perceptually to be within normal limits although their patterns of EPG contact are clearly deviant. All showed a distinctive skewed asymmetric pattern for /s/ and sometimes for /ʃ/ which has not been seen in normal subjects, although it should be emphasized that the normal data available are as yet quite limited. It seems therefore that some EPG spatial abnormality is tolerated for lingual fricative sounds. From the clinical point of view, however, once again the EPG analysis has revealed motoric abnormalities that would not have been detected from an auditory-based analysis alone.

It is arguable that the error type most likely to affect intelligibility is variability of target achievement. Where errors are consistent the listener can construct a systematic framework for interpretation but where errors involve both temporal and spatial aspects and vary from one production to another, the listener needs to constantly update his interpretation to make it plausible.

Conclusions

The data collected from these subjects demonstrate how electropalatography can reveal the complexity and variation of errors found in apraxic speakers. Of the six types of errors discussed, only four were found in all subjects. The misdirected articulatory patterns accounted for the majority of errors in all four subjects but they all had some examples of distorted configurations, especially for alveolar and for palato-alveolar fricatives. All subjects exhibited variations in both spatial and temporal aspects of production. The data also support earlier evidence (Hardcastle et al., 1985) that consonant clusters presented more problems for the speakers than singleton consonants, with some subjects increasing the delay between the two elements of the cluster, one subject reversing the order and one subject omitting the second element.

Thus although clinically, all four subjects were described as apraxic it can be seen that each had an individual profile of error types. By exposing the data to detailed examination, it has been possible to highlight both the multiplicity of error types and also tendencies for some errors to occur more frequently. The first two types of error, *misdirection* and *distortion* (both of which occurred in all speakers) can be viewed as evidence of loss or interference with the speakers' ability to achieve the correct articulatory posture for a speech sound. The underlying reason for a misdirected gesture may be a selection problem (as proposed for subject L) or a motor mismanagement problem (as proposed for the other subjects). Where the error is described as *misdirected* a clear but inaccurate position is seen whereas for errors described as *distortion* the articulatory posture fails to match either the target or to resemble any other recognizable configuration.

Only one subject (L) had examples of omission and it is therefore not seen as typical of the apraxic data. However other difficulties in the production of consonant clusters were observed in the subjects. Subject L was also the only one to repeat syllables although T's prolongations of the closure phase of stops were perceived as being similar to non-fluent features of stuttered speech. It is possible, that, given more subjects, certain typical subgroups of speakers might emerge.

These analyses have revealed a variety of errors produced by these apraxic speakers. Detailed EPG analyses give information about one aspect of intelligibility, the accuracy of tongue contact configurations which, for these speakers, was a major feature of their disordered speech but, as we have seen above, contributed in varying degrees to unintellibility. If these results can be replicated in other apraxic speakers, a profile of speech errors will emerge which will be far more detailed than previously available. Similar information has also been gained from other disordered speakers. At Reading, EPG analyses have been used with dysarthric speakers (Hardcastle et al, 1985), a child with a developmental articulatory disorder (Gibbon and Hardcastle, 1987) and children with repaired cleft palates (Hardcastle et al, 1988). In all cases, the detailed information gained from EPG has revealed features which have not been apparent when using traditional auditory analysis. Errors which are undetected by the ear, may be as theoretically important as those which are obvious to the listener and expose problems of production for the speaker with reduced intelligibility.

Acknowledgments

Special thanks are due to Nik Miller at Frenchay Hospital, Bristol for providing most of the subjects for this research and for assisting with the experiment. Thanks are due also to Rosemarie Morgan Barry for assisting with the analysis of subject T's data. Part of the work was funded by the British Medical Research Council (grant no. G8201596N).

Appendix A

Protocol used for subjects L, M, and S. (For subject T, a more extensive word list was used (see Hardcastle, 1987) and no non-verbal tasks were included.).

1. *Single word lists*

Set A (single lingual consonants)
All items were preceeded, where grammatically appropriate, by the definite or indefinite article.
"a dart, a tip, a deer, a leg, a chain, a shark, a key, the dolls, a book, a car, a beak, a knot, the dark, a tick, near, see, she, a key, a tier, a leer, a gear, a cheer, a deer, the sun, a mouse, a fish, a zoo, a sheep, a brush, a seed, a shop, a racer, a leaf."
Set B (consonant sequences both within and across morpheme boundaries)
"a cocktail, a kitkat, a clock, a headlight, a tractor, a weekday, a tickling, a deckchair, the witchcraft, a bookshop, a star, a box, the hats, a squashkit, a skirt, a catkin".

2. *Repetition task*

4 repetitions (slow rate, then fast) of
"a cocktail, a kitkat, a clock, a headlight".

3. *Compose and produce sentences with each of 4 words selected from Set A above*

4. *Non-verbal tasks*

(a)   Tongue tip to alveolar ridge. Even rhythm
(b)   Tongue tip to alveolar ridge. Short-long rhythm
(c)   Alternating alveolar-velar contact
(d)   Tongue tip to alveolar ridge + voice- tə, tə, tə etc.
(e)   Tongue tip to alveolar ridge + voice. Short-long rhythm
(f)   Velar contact + voice kə, kə, kə etc.
(g)   Alternating tə kə tə kə
(h)   Tongue movement to rhythm of "Baa baa black sheep".
(i)   t to rhythm of "Baa baa black sheep".

(j) Tongue movement to rhythm of "What shall we do with the drunken sailor".

(k) Tongue movement with voice to rhythm of "What shall we do with the drunken sailor".

Protocol for measuring voicing distinctions (VOT measurements)

5 repetitions of list: "curl, deer, girl, pin, tier, bin, chain" (= dummy item).

References

Blumstein, S. 1973. *A Phonological Investigation of Aphasic Speech*. The Hague: Mouton.

Darley, F.L. 1982. *Aphasia*. New York: Saunders.

Darley, F. 1984. "Aphasia of speech: a neurogenic articulation disorder." *Treating Articulation Disorders: For Clinicians by Clinicians*, ed. by H. Winitz. Baltimore: University Park Press.

Darley, F., Aronson, A. and Brown, J. 1975. *Motor Speech Disorders*. Philadelphia: Saunders.

Duffy, J.R. and Gawle, C.A. 1984. "Apraxic speakers' vowel duration in consonant-vowel-consonant syllables." *Apraxia of speech: Physiology, Acoustics, Linguistics, Management*, ed. by J.C. Roesnbek, M.R. McNeil and A.E. Aronson, 167-196. San Diego: College-Hill Press.

Edwards, S. and Hardcastle, W.J. 1987. "Linguistic profiling of stuttering behaviour." *Progress in the Treatment of Fluency Disorders*. ed. by L. Rustin, D. Rowley and H. Purser, 61-83. London: Taylor and Francis.

Edwards, S. and Miller, N. 1989 "Using EPG to investigate speech errors and motor agility in a dyspraxic patient". *Clinical Linguistics and Phonetics* 3, 111-126.

Gibbon, F. and Hardcastle, W. 1987. "Articulatory description and treatment of 'lateral /s/' using Electropalatography: a case study." *British Journal of Disorders of Communication* 22, 203-217.

Hardcastle, W.J. 1987. "Electropalatographic study of articulation disorders in verbal dyspraxia." *Phonetic Approaches to Speech Production in Aphasia and Related Disorders*, ed. by John H. Ryalls, 113-136. Boston: Little, Brown and Co.

Hardcastle, W., Jones, W., Knight, C, Trudgeon, A., and Calder, G. 1989. "New developments in electropalatography: a state-of-the-art report." *Clinical Linguistics and Phonetics* 3, 1-38.

Hardcastle, W.J., Morgan-Barry, R.A. and Clark, C.J. 1985. "Articulatory and voicing characteristics of adult dysarthric and verbal dyspraxic speakers: an instrumental study." *British Journal of Disorders of Communication* 20, 249-270.

Hardcastle, W.J., Morgan Barry, R.A. and Nunn, M. 1988. "Instrumental articulatory phonetics in assessment and remediation: case studies with the Electropalatograph." *Cleft Palate: Case Studies in the Treatment of Communication Disorders*, ed. by J. Stengelhofen, 136-164. Edinburgh: Churchill Livingstone.

Itoh, M. and Sasanuma, S. 1984. "Articulatory movement in apraxia of speech." *Apraxia of Speech: Physiology, Acoustics, Linguistics, Management*, ed. by J.C.

Rosenbek, M.R. McNeil and A.E. Aronson, 135-166. San Diego: College Hill Press.

Itoh, M., Sasanuma, S., Tatsumi, I., Murakami, S., Fukusako, Y. and Suzuki, T. 1982. "Voice onset times characteristics in apraxia of speech." *Brain and Language* 17, 193-210.

Johns, D.F. and Darley, F.L. 1970. "Phonemic variability in apraxia of speech." *Journal of Speech and Hearing Research* 13, 556-585.

Kent, R.D. 1990. "The acoustic and physiologic characteristics of neurologically impaired speech movements." *Speech Production and Speech Modelling*, ed. by W. Hardcastle and A. Marchal, 365-401. Dordrecht: Kluwer.

Kent, R.D. and Rosenbek, J.C. 1983. "Acoustic patterns of apraxia of speech." *Journal of Speech and Hearing Research* 13, 556-583.

Luria, A.R. 1973. *The Working Brain: An Introduction to Neuropsychology*. Baltimore: Penguin.

Luria, A.R. and Hutton, T.J. 1977. "A modern assessment of the basic forms of aphasia." *Brain and Language* 4, 129-151.

Mlcoch, A.G. and Noll, J.D. 1980. "Speech production models as related to the concept of apraxia of speech." *Speech and Language: Advances in Basic Research and Practice*, ed. by N.J. Lass, 201-238. New York: Academic Press.

Rosenbek, J.C., Kent, R.D. and LaPointe, L.L. 1984. "Apraxia of speech: an overview and some perspectives." *Apraxia of Speech: Physiology, Acoustics, Linguistics Management*, ed. by J.C. Rosenbek, M.R. McNeil and A.E. Aronson, 1-72. San Diego: College Hill Press.

Trost, J. and Canter, C. 1974. "Apraxia of speech in patients with Broca's aphasia." *Brain and Language* 1, 63-80.

Tuller, B. and Story, R.S. 1987. "Anticipatory coarticulation in aphasia." *Phonetic Approaches to Speech Production in Aphasia and Related Disorders*, ed. J.H. Ryalls, 243-256. Boston: Little, Brown and Co.

Van Riper, C. 1971. *The Nature of Stuttering*. Englewood Cliffs. N.J.: Prentice-Hall.

Wingate, M.E. 1964. "A standard definition of stuttering." *Journal of Speech and Hearing Disorders* 29, 484-489.

Ziegler, W. 1987. "Phonetic realization of phonological contrast in aphasic patients." *Phonetic Approaches to Speech Production in Aphasia and Related Disorders*, ed. by J.H. Ryalls, 163-169. San Diego: College-Hill.

Ziegler, W. and Von Cramon, D. 1986 "Disturbed coarticulation in apraxia of speech: acoustic evidence." *Brain and Language* 29, 34-474.

Chapter 9

Prospects for neurophysiological approaches to the study of speech intelligibility

S.M. Barlow
Indiana University

Introduction

Considering the prospects of applying neurophysiological techniques to the study of speech intelligibility is a radical concept that, upon initial inspection of current electrophysiological and signal processing technologies, appears totally out of the question as a feasible investigative tool. As Larson (1988) summarized in a recent review of the neural control of vocalization,

> "We know almost nothing about those aspects of vocalization related to human speech and singing. We cannot even be sure about exactly where in the brain such functions are controlled-whether it is in the neocortex, supplementary cortex, anterior cingulate gyrus, or in subcortical structures."

A growing number of neuroscientists and physiologists are entering the emerging discipline of vocal tract neurophysiology with the common objective of determining the neural mechanisms that underlie speech production in normal and disordered systems. Obviously, the nervous system, including central and peripheral mechanisms, is at the heart of the speech production process. The activity of the human brain in the programming, selection, and sequencing of vocal tract muscles for speech is considered by many to represent the pinnacle of phylogenetic elaboration. Numerous signal transformations are hypothesized to occur between neuronal firing (CNS programming structures) and intelligible speech including program selection, specification of appropriate neural networks and relays (i.e., corticomotoneurons), controlled inhibition, gating of appropriate sensory mechanisms, enabling of feedback and predictive neural mechanisms, directing outputs along final common pathways to selected effector muscle groups, and generation of active forces and subsequent movements to accurately modify the acoustic tuning properties of the vocal tract. Since there are many structures and dozens of muscle groups along the vocal tract, timing becomes an important factor to maintain coordination between structures (i.e., larynx and velopharynx). While these elements of neuromotor control are widely recognized in the neuroscience literature in the context of movement generation, it remains a conundrum as to exactly where in the brain some of these functions may occur and the relative timing of such operations for speech.

Neurophysiologic recordings from CNS in humans

It seems unlikely in the future that single unit recordings, microstimulation, and tract tracing techniques, as performed in contemporary neurophysiology laboratories, will occur in awake humans for the explicit purpose of determining the neural control of speech production. Possibilities certainly exist whereby certain neuron recording and stimulation techniques may be used in awake humans during the course of neurosurgical procedures primarily intended to remedy a medical problem. The scope of such exploratory investigations would be limited by the extent of the surgical field and restorative process.

An example of a neurophysiological recording made as part of stereotactic surgery is available from the recent work of McClean, Dostrovsky, Lee, and Tasker (1990). Multi-unit and single-unit recording of neurons located in the ventral posterior medial nucleus of the thalamus (VPM) were obtained simultaneous with the speech acoustic signal while subjects produced two or three repetitions of the syllables "apa", "ata", "aka", and isolated productions of the vowels in the words "hot", "who", and "he". McClean et al. (1990) found that somatosensory neurons in VPM with receptive fields on the lips and tongue manifested increased activity in association with a variety of orofacial speech movements. For example, gestures involving bilabial lip contact during production of the "p" sound in "apa" consistently elicited activity in VPM neurons with receptive fields on the lips.

The results of McClean et al. (1990) confirm the notion that afferent information transmitted by the trigeminal nerve during speech (Johansson, Trulsson, Olsson, and Abbs, 1988; Nordin and Thomander, 1989) is encoded by neurons in VPM.

Animal studies of central brain structures involved in vocalization

Vocalization is regarded as an integral part of human speech and many types of animal communication. Effective vocal behavior is characterized by coordinated actions of muscles located within respiratory and laryngeal systems (Larson and Kistler, 1986). For the most part, the actual neural substrate and mechanisms underlying this complex coordination process remain unknown (Larson, 1988). The complexity of the motor behavior, the elaboration of the neural substrate potentially involved in vocalization shown in Figure 1, and the lack of an animal model with comparable levels of verbal communication skills are significant factors that have impeded progress in understanding the neural control of speech and the neuromotor factors especially important in generating intelligible speech (Jurgens, 1987).

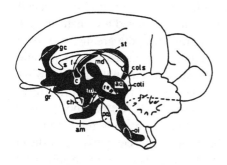

am = amygdala;
aq = periaqueductal gray;
c = anterior commissure;
ch = chiasma opticum;
coli = inferior colliculus;
cols = superior colliculus;
f = fornix;
gc = gyrus cinguli;
gr = gyrus rectus;
m = mammillary body;
md = mediodorsal thalamic nucleus;
oi = inferior olive;
po = pontine gray;
re = reticular formation of midbrain;
s = septum;
st = stria terminalis

Figure 1. *Sagittal section through squirrel monkey brain with projection of all brain structures yeilding vocalization when electrically stimulated (effective areas in full black).* (Jurgens, 1987; permission granted).

Nonetheless, scientists have begun to probe questions surrounding the loci of neural control of oral communication in a variety of species. The entry point for a number of investigators seems to involve the localization of brain structures involved in vocalization. Results from early investigations revealed that electrical stimulation of the midbrain periaqueductal gray (PAG) in anesthetized preparations produced a variety of rhythmic breathing and/or vocalization-like behaviors in the chimpanzee (Brown, 1915), monkeys and cats (Magoun, Atlas, Ingersoll, and Ranson, 1937), and other animals (see review by Larson, 1988). From a neuroanatomic standpoint, the PAG is strategically located to receive inputs from the limbic system and the diencephalon, and project outputs to the reticular formation, nucleus retroambiguus, and nucleus ambiguus (Holstege, 1987).

Neural control of vocalization in monkey

Investigations by Larson and colleagues (DeRosier, West, and Larson, 1988; Larson, 1985, 1988; Larson & Kistler, 1986) have provided important neurophysiologic information on the organization and contribution of midbrain periaqueductal gray neurons to vocalization in the behaving monkey. Electrical stimulation of the midbrain periaqueductal (PAG) elicited phonation closely resembling that naturally produced by such animals. Stimulation in the rostral periaqueductal gray elicited a greater percentage of clear calls whereas stimulation of caudal areas elicited rough sounding calls or barks (Larson, 1988). Recordings made from single neurons within the PAG in one monkey demonstrated increased firing rates prior to the onset of laryngeal electromyographic activity or vocalization (Larson, 1985). The activation patterns of some PAG neurons were related to vocal initiation, vocal intensity, and coordination of muscle subsystems during vocalization (Larson, 1988; Larson & Kistler, 1986). Some examples of excitatory and inhibitory activity patterns recorded from neurons within the dorsolateral PAG are shown in Figure 2.

    Let us digress and stretch our imagination a bit at this juncture. If one could devise a method for characterizing the intelligibility of a monkey vocalization, then it may be possible to alter activity patterns of certain PAG neurons during vocalization through the use of controlled microstimulation, thus affecting the quality of conditioned vocalizations and change the degree of intelligibility of the animal generated vocalization. This type of

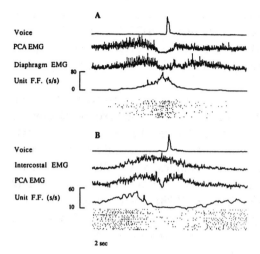

In both A and B, the top trace shows averaged rectified vocal activity. In A, the second trace is averaged, rectified EMG from the posterior cricoarytenoid (PCA) muscle and the third is from the diaphragm. The fourth trace is unit firing frequency (F.F.). Below the fourth trace is a raster display of unit activity for each of the 20 trials comprising the average of the above traces. In B, the second trace is intercostal muscle EMG, whereas the third trace is from the posterior cricoarytenoid muscle. The time sweep is 2 s for A and B. The lineup point for the averages was at the onset of vocalization. For both A and B, the averages are from 20 different vocalizations

Figure 2. *A and B: Ensemble averages of vocal, electromyographic (EMG), and unit activity for two cells recorded from the periaqueductal gray in monkey.* (Larson, 1988; permission granted).

experiment may help determine which of the many vocal parameters exert the most significant influences on call intelligibility. Obviously a bark or coo may not carry much meaning in human speech, but a considerable amount of information could be gained regarding the underlying neural control of the entire vocal tract during relatively simple call generation.

Another promising observation made by Larson (1985) is that spectrographic evidence indicated that vocalizations elicited by electrical stimulation of the PAG are acoustically similar to vocalizations produced naturally by a monkey. It is conceivable that under these recording and analysis conditions, a comparison of the spectral architecture could be made between the natural and electrically elicited vocalization as future studies progress to include other brain structures such as ACC, MI, and SMA. Larson (1985) also demonstrated that the EMG profiles of the chest, larynx, face and tongue for the electrically elicited and natural vocalization were highly similar.

In summary, the PAG can be characterized as a population of cells whose constitutent subsets differentially affect various groups of muscles and thus the *quality* of vocalization. Since the effect of a single periaqueductal gray neuron on vocalization or muscle is likely to be small, it would be desirable to study larger samples of simultaneously active periaqueductal gray cells in order to provide a more complete picture of their function during vocalization (Larson, 1988). These observations have implications for the intelligibility of call or speech production. Certain types of neurological voice disorders may result from inappropriate action of groups of periaqueductal gray neurons.

Lower motor neurons

Neurons from the neocortex project directly to the nucleus ambiguus (and other bulbar nuclei serving the vocal tract) in humans and chimpanzees, but not in monkeys or cats (Kuypers, 1958a,b,c). Zealear and Larson (1987, 1989) recorded the activity of motoneurons in the nucleus ambiguus that innervate the thyroarytenoid muscle. Several patterns of unit activity were observed including those most related to swallowing, respiration, and vocalization. It is unknown how the activity of other laryngeal motor neurons with projections to the other laryngeal muscles behave during vocalization.

Neural control of vocalization in cat

Recently, awake cats have been used to study neural mechanisms underlying conditioned vocalization (Farley, Barlow, and Netsell, 1989, 1990). Single unit recordings from the parabrachial nucleus (PBN) and simultaneous electromyographic recordings of laryngeal, respiratory, and mandibular muscle activity were made during production of instrumentally conditioned vocalizations. The parabrachial nucleus, located inferior and posterior to the inferior colliculus and proximal to the trigeminal motor nucleus, has connections with several brainstem nuclei involved in the control of respiration and vocalization in mammals. Farley et al. (1990) have noted in a preliminary report the presence of considerable PBN activity during the respiratory cycle and licking (following the food reward for vocalizing). During vocalization, some neurons within the PBN show increases in firing rate (Figure 3). This activity increase, for at least some PBN units, is modifiable by auditory feedback. Other PBN responses include strong inhibition during the vocalization phase, or activity increases preceding the onset of vocalization. These results suggest that the parabrachial region's involvement in vocal control is very complex, involving the convergence of respiratory, vocalization-related, acoustic, and possibly somatosensory influences (Farley et al., 1990).

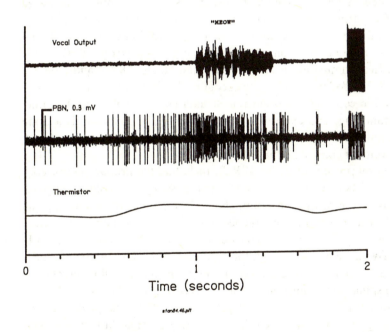

Figure 3. *Raw time domain waveforms of vocal unit activity for a cell recorded in the parabrachial nucleus, and output from an anemometer (respiratory phase) during call production in a conditioned cat. The top trace shows a "meow" production followed by a conditioning pure tone signal* (Farley, Barlow, & Netsell, 1990; reprinted with permission).

Cortical and subcortical brain structures important for speech

A brief overview is included in the following sections to identify and high-light some of the brain structures hypothesized to be of importance in the neural control of vocalization and the production of intelligible speech. A more exhaustive review can be found elsewhere (see Barlow and Farley, 1989).

Cerebral cortex

Many discussions of motor control often start with the role of the motor cortex. Like peeling the rind from an orange, the convolutions of the cerebral cortex were undoubtedly some of the first structures subject to investigation by neuroscience pioneers. Investigators sparked controversy with clinical and experimental evidence implicating that the lateral convexities of the precentral cerebral cortex were somehow involved in generating movements based upon observations in epileptic humans (Jackson, 1874), or by direct electrical stimulation in dog (Fritsch and Hitzig, 1870), and monkey (Ferrier, 1873). Today, it is widely recognized that many distributed systems located in cerebral and brainstem structures are involved in the intiation, programming, and execution of movement. The following is a brief review of some key neural structures considered essential to a model of speech movement control and intelligibility.

The lateral precentral cortex (LPC), including the primary motor cortex (MI), consists of Brodmann's area 4 and possibly the posterior strip of area 6. This region of the cerebrum, shown in Figure 4, represents a summing point or a "node" of convergence for several cortical and subcortical efferents, and, pallidal and somatosensory inputs by way of the VL thalamus. By virtue of its location, the LPC is strategically situated to operate as an "entry point" to the final common pathway, providing direct connections to spinal and brainstem motor neurons (Kuypers, 1964, 1973; Phillips and Porter, 1977). Recent investigations of corticofacial projections in monkey using electrophysiologic (Huang, Sirisko, Hiraba, Murray and Sessle, 1988; Huang, Hiraba and Sessle, 1989) and neuroanatomic tract tracing techniques (Jenny and Saper, 1987) suggest that corticofugal inputs to the facial motor nuclear region are direct and predominantly contralateral in nature. A large proportion of these corticobulbar projections are known to originate from the rostral bank of the central sulcus and the convexity of the

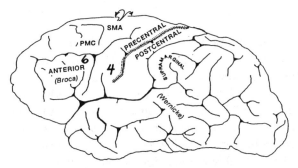

Figure 4. *Schematic subdivision of the sensory and motor cortices based upon Brodmann's areas. Primary motor and premotor regions of cerebral cortex indicated by numerals 4 and 6 respectively.*

precentral cortex (Kuypers, 1981). Electromyographic activity evoked by intracortical microstimulation (ICMS) was characterized by latency values ranging from 10 to 45 milliseconds for the face, jaw, and tongue muscles (Huang et al., 1988). The findings from ICMS studies suggest the face motor cortex is organized to coordinate the activity of numerous muscles within the face, jaw, and tongue. It is important to remember that the origins of fibers constituting the pyramidal tract are not restricted to the LPC, but rather include portions of the parietal and postcentral brain sites (Granit, 1977).

The postcentral gyrus of the cerebrum, shown in Figure 4, constitutes the primary receiving areas for somatosensory information originating from primary muscle afferents and mechanoreceptors located within skin, joints, and muscle (Mountcastle, 1957). The primary receiving areas of primate somatosensory cortex (SI) are extensively interconnected (Pandya and Kuypers, 1969; Jones and Powell, 1970) and somatotopically organized (Kaas, Nelson, Sur, Lin, and Merzenich, 1979; Merzenich, Kaas, Sur, and Lin, 1978; Paul, Merzenich, and Goodman, 1972). Tract tracing methods applied to the study of primate SI have led to the identification of subareas 3a, 3b, 1, 2, and 5 (see Evarts, 1981a; Merzenich et al., 1978). Each of these subareas receives different types of somatosensory information. Area 3a responds to stimulation of group I muscle afferents (derived from muscle spindles encoding position and velocity), area 3b is activated by slowly adapting mechanoreceptors in the skin, area 1 is activated by rapidly adapting cutaneous mechanoreceptors, and area 2 is primarily activated by joint movements.

One of the classic concepts concerning the cortical control of movement is that "premotor" areas exist in the frontal lobe that have bilateral and direct access to the primary motor cortex (Von Bonin and Bailey, 1947; Matsumura and Kubota, 1979; Muakkassa and Strick, 1979; Pandya and Vignolo, 1971). These "premotor" areas are thought to contribute to the organization of skilled movement and the programming of motor cortex output. Tract tracing techniques (horseradish peroxidase) in primates (Muakkassa and Strick, 1979) revealed the location of four spatially separate and somatotopically organized premotor areas with projections to the primary motor cortex, including (1) the inferior limb of the arcuate sulcus (caudal bank), (2) rostrally in the supplemental motor area, (3) rostrally in the ventral bank of the cingulate sulcus, and (4) the lateral bank of the inferior precentral sulcus. The densest projections originate from the premotor cortex (PMC) and the supplementary motor area (SMA). These premotor areas represent important elements in parallel pathways that influence motor cortex output and motor behavior. Of special note is the fact that the SMA contains a somatotopic representation of vocal tract structures (Brinkman and Porter, 1978; Muakkassa and Strick, 1979). This feature combined with its strategic position as one of the primary premotor inputs to MI is reason to hypothesize a special role for SMA in speech motor programming.

Subcortical-thalamo-cortical relations

An important question in movement control concerns how two of the major subcortical motor systems, the cerebellum and the basal ganglia, differentially influence premotor and motor cortex. Efferents originating from cerebellar, pallidal, and nigral nuclei are highly segregated, manifesting little overlap in their projections to the ventrolateral thalamus (Mehler, 1971; Kuo and Carpenter, 1973; Carpenter, Nakano, and Kim, 1976; Kim, Nakano, Jayarman, and Carpenter, 1976; Percheron, 1977; Stanton, 1980; Kalil, 1981; DeVito and Anderson, 1982; Asanuma, Thach, and Jones, 1983b).

There are at least two major cerebellothalamic systems that influence separate cortical areas, including APA (PMC) and MI (Schell and Strick, 1984; Sasaki, Jinnai, Gemba, Hashimoto, and Mizuno, 1979; Sasaki,

Kawaguchi, Oka, Sakai, and Mizuno, 1976). Rostral portions of the deep cerebellar nuclei project to the motor cortex via the nucleus ventralis posterior lateralis pars oralis (VPLo), and caudal portions of the deep cerebellar nuclei project to the PMC via area X of the thalamus.

Arising from the basal ganglia are two sets of efferents from the internal segment of the globus pallidus (GPi) that project to the SMA via the nucleus ventralis lateralis pars oralis (VLo) and nucleus ventralis lateralis pars medialis (VLm) (Nauta and Mehler, 1966; Kuo and Carpenter, 1973; Kim et al., 1976; DeVito and Anderson, 1982; Kusama, Mabuchi, and Sumino, 1971; Percheron, 1977; Jones, Wise, and Coulter, 1979; Kalil, 1981; Asanuma, Thach, and Jones, 1983a). Nigrothalamic projections originate from the pars reticulata segment of the substantia nigra (SNpr) and terminate in two subdivisions of the ventrolateral thalamus including the nucleus ventralis anterior magnocellularis (VAmc) and nucleus ventralis lateralis pars medialis (VLm) (Carpenter and McMasters, 1964; Carpenter and Strominger, 1967; Carpenter and Peter, 1972; Carpenter et al., 1976; Carpenter, Carleton, Keller, and Conte, 1981).

Anatomical evidence in monkey indicates that the somatotopic organization of the pallidonigral and cerebellar systems are maintained in their thalamic projections. For example, the "face" representation in SNpr projects to a "face" representation in VLm which in turn projects to the "face" representations in the SMA. In a similar fashion, "face" efferents from caudal regions of the deep cerebellar nuclei projecting to area X of the thalamus have access to neurons in the face representation of the motor cortex.

Therefore, the cerebellum, thalamus, and certain subcortical nuclei form parallel pathways to motor and premotor cortical areas that are hypothesized to contribute to the programming of skilled movement and the sequencing of motor tasks. As shown in Figure 5, outputs from the cerebellum and basal ganglia form three parallel systems of subcortical efferents to the ventrolateral thalamus that project, in a segregated fashion, to motor and premotor areas of the cerebrum (Schell and Strick, 1984). One parallel pathway originates in the caudal portions of the deep cerebellar nuclei and most directly influences the PMC. A second pathway originates in SNpr and GPi with direct access to SMA. The third pathway originates in rostral portions of the deep cerebellar nuclei and most directly influences the primary motor cortex.

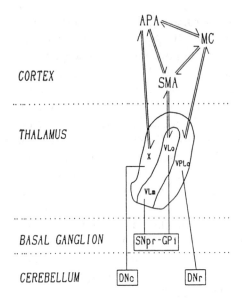

This diagram shows: (1) the pathway from caudal portions of the deep cerebellar nuclei (DNc) to area X and arcuate premotor area (APA, analogous to PMC in humans), (2) the pathways from the pars reticulata of the substantia nigra (SNpr) and the internal segment of the globus pallidus (GPi) to VLm and VLo and the supplementary motor area (SMA), (3) the pathway from rostral portions of the deep cerebellar nuclei (DNr) to VPLo and the motor cortex (MC), and (4) the reciprocal connections between the MC, APA, and SMA.

Figure 5. *Subcortico-Thalamo-Cortical Relations. Summary of anatomic relations between cerebellar and basal ganglia efferents and motor and premotor cortical areas in primates* (from Schell & Strick, 1984).

Brainstem nuclei

Speech production requires the activity of several cranial nerves (including CN V, VII, VIII, IX, X, XI, and XII) whose nuclei are located in the pontine and medullary regions of the brainstem. Speech is also dependent on spinal nerves located in the cervical and thoracic segments for control of the diaphragm and muscles of the chest wall during speech breathing. A number of these nuclei are known to receive direct inputs from sensorimotor cortex, frontal cerebral cortex, and other relay nuclei located within the brainstem. The presence of some of these relay nuclei have been confirmed using horseradish peroxidase (HRP) transport from the nucleus ambiguus and retrofacial nucleus in the cat (Yoshida, Mitsumasu, Hirano, Morimoto, and Kanaseki, 1987) and bat (Kobler, 1983). Although numerous brainstem regions were labeled in these studies, including contralateral NA cell columns, three regions had the most consistent inputs to NA and/or RFN; the nucleus tractus solitarius (NTS), which is a primary target for sensory feedback from the larynx, the parabrachial nucleus (PBN), which is involved in the central pattern generator for respiration and may perform second order sensory processing on somatosensory information from the larynx (Farley, Barlow, and Netsell, 1990), and a small area of the periaqueductal gray (PAG) near the inferior colliculus. The PAG has been implicated in the coordinated activation of vocal tract structures during call production in primates and is likely an important neural structure for human speech. Portions of the lateral pontine and medullary reticular formation project to several brainstem motor nuclei and therefore may provide a mechanism for coordinating the function of different vocal tract systems during call production (Thoms and Jurgens, 1987). Although the NTS and PBN have identified roles in metabolic respiration, it appears that both may be important in the sensorimotor control of vocalization.

Summary of brain structures important for speech

From this brief overview, it becomes readily apparent that the neuroanatomy and neurophysiology of speech bears a degree of complexity far beyond our present level of understanding. To understand speech intelligibility in neurophysiologic terms is to understand the underlying substrata that mediates selection and sequencing of hundreds of muscles along the vocal tract in delicate balance and time. A probable "road map" for a general neural control model of limb movement is shown in Figure 6 (adapted from Allen and Tsukahara, 1974; Kubota, 1984).

342   STEVEN M. BARLOW

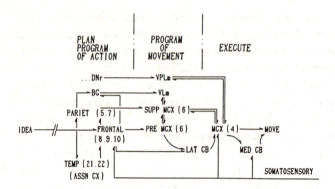

KEY: BG=basal ganglia,
DNr=dentate nucleus of cerebellum,
FRONT=frontal cortex (areas 8, 9 and 10),
LAT CB=lateral cerebellum,
MED CB=medial cerebellum,
MCX=motor cortex (area 4),
PARIET=parietal cortex (areas 5 and 7),
PRE MCX=premotor cortex (area 6),
SUPP MCX=supplementary motor cortex (area 6),
TEMP=temporal association cortex (areas 21 and 22),
VLm=medial part of the ventral lateral thalamic nucleus,
VPLm=medial part of the ventral posterior lateral thalamic nucleus

Figure 6. *Pathways for planning, control, and execution of voluntary movement* (modified from Allen & Tsukahara, 1974; Kubota, 1984).

Neurology of vocal control

Lateral precentral cortex (LPC)

The cerebral motor representation of the larynx lies in the most inferior part of the lateral precentral gyrus just above the Sylvian fissure (Jurgens, 1982). Electrical stimulation of this area in humans results in phonation (Foerster, 1936; Penfield and Bordley, 1937). Penfield and Roberts (1959) found that electrical stimulation of the precentral gyrus in either hemisphere of epileptic patients elicited vocalization. Similar studies in anthropoid apes also elicited phonation by electrical stimulation of the precentral gyrus. Mutism has been reported following damage to Broca's area (Aronson, 1980). Bilateral lesions in the primary motor cortical larynx area in humans results in an almost complete loss of voluntary phonatory control with little or no modulation of vocal fundamental frequency and intensity (Leicester, 1980). Moreover, an abnormally low vocal fundamental frequency (Kammermeier, 1969; Mysak, 1959), reduced air flow through the larynx during phonation due to overadduction (von Leden, 1968), and excessive breathiness during transitional phases between voiced segments severely limits utterance length and speech intelligibility. Reduced rates of laryngeal adduction (Darley, Aronson, and Brown, 1975) and decreases in the rate of force change and velocity of orofacial structures typifies the articulatory dynamics of individuals with the upper motor neuron syndrome (Barlow and Abbs, 1986). These observations support the hypothesis that the overlapping representation of laryngeal and supralaryngeal structures in the sensorimotor cortex probably serves to coordinate articulatory and phonatory activity in speech (Jurgens, 1982).

Supplementary motor area (SMA)

The supplementary motor area (SMA) occupies the medial portions of area 6 and is generally considered to function in programming motor sequences, including preparatory states for forthcoming movements (Wiesendanger, Hummelsheim, and Bianchetti, 1985; Kornhuber and Deecke, 1965; Roland, 1985; Roland, Larsen, Lassen, and Skinhoj, 1980; Orgogozo and Larsen, 1979; Brinkman, 1984). This region of the brain is also implicated in the control of posture, gating motor cortical reflexes, and initiating motor cortex output and movement (Brinkman and Porter, 1978; Pandya and Vignolo, 1971; Tanji, Taniguchi, and Saga, 1980; Wiesendanger, Seguin, and Kunzle, 1973).

The SMA, among other areas of the cerebral cortex, is considered an important region for speech motor control and vocalization (Penfield and Welch, 1951). Penfield and Roberts (1959) considered the SMA to be of special importance for the programming and execution of speech. The SMA, containing a somatotopic representation of vocal tract structures (Brinkman and Porter, 1978; Muakkassa and Strick, 1979), is strategically situated as one of the primary premotor inputs to MI for speech motor programming.

Recently, neuroimaging techniques have provided new and exciting data on the activity of motor areas of the brain, including the SMA, during speech motor processing in normal and neurologically impaired speakers. For example, data generated from computerized axial tomography (CAT) and regional cerebral blood flow studies (rCBF) support the hypothesis that the SMA functions as a premotor input to the MI, via Broca's area, for speech production in normal speakers (Gelmers, 1983; Jonas, 1981, 1987; Larsen, Skinhoj, Soh, Endo, and Lassen, 1977; Lassen, Ingvar, and Skinhoj, 1978; Roland, Skinhoj, Larsen, and Lassen, 1977; Roland et al., 1980). The SMA appears to be directly involved in the planning of *propositional* speech. In fact, small lesions limited to the SMA have been found to cause a pure disorder of speech initiation (Freedman, Alexander, and Naeser, 1984). The left SMA, more than the right SMA, is active during the formulation of novel speech. The output from the left SMA is processed by the ipsilateral Broca's area before being received by both the left and right MI for execution of the motor plan. Additional evidence that the SMA is involved in speech motor planning versus motor execution is realized from the observation that rCBF increases are found in the SMA while normal subjects think about counting without actually speaking (Lassen et al., 1978). Consistent with their hypothesized role as motor executors, both Broca's area and MI show no increases in rCBF during this task. These observations are somewhat at odds with an earlier notion in which the SMA, contrary to Broca's and Wernicke's areas, was hypothesized to be more involved in actual modulation of speech output than in ideational formulation (Botez and Barbeau, 1971).

If the left SMA is damaged, the normal sequences of events for propositional speech are impaired or impossible (Brown and Perecman, 1985). However, in the presence of left SMA damage, *nonpropositional* speech remains intact since the adequate stimuli have direct access to MI from subcortical centers. In fact, if the left SMA is sufficiently damaged, it may be impossible for the subject to inhibit nonpropositional speech (swearing, etc.) (Jonas, 1987). Therefore, the SMA also plays an important inhibitory role in selectively gating inputs to MI that would otherwise disrupt an ongoing speech motor program.

Cerebellum (CB)

The cerebellum, a part of the brain in all vertebrates, serves as an important brain center for postural control of the body as well as initiation, coordination, learning, and execution of voluntary movements (Botterell and Fulton, 1938; Brooks and Thach, 1981; Chambers and Sprague, 1955; Chan-Palay and Palay, 1987; Thach, 1970) and speech motor control (Holmes, 1922a, b, 1939; Kornhuber, 1977). Lesions of the cerebellum and/ or its connections via the cerebellar peduncles result in a very distinct sounding dysarthria called "ataxic dysarthria" (Brown, Darley, and Aronson, 1970; Darley, et al., 1975; Kent and Netsell, 1975; Kent, Netsell, and Abbs, 1979; Netsell, 1982). The voice of ataxic speakers is characterized by excessive variations in fundamental frequency (f_o) and intensity. This is accompanied by significant reductions in displacement velocity of the lips and jaw during speech production (Hirose, Kiritani, Ushijima, and Sawashima, 1978; Kent et al., 1975; Netsell and Kent, 1976). Although the gross features of speech coordination are preserved, significant timing errors between labial-mandibular, lingual, velopharyngeal, laryngeal, and respiratory subsystems contribute to the distorted, inebriated sound associated with ataxic dysarthria.

Cerebellar lesions in monkeys have been reported to influence several aspects of phonation including intensity, the modulation of fundamental vocal frequency, and duration (Larson, Sutton, and Lindeman, 1978). In comparing the effects between cerebellar and limbic cortex lesions on vocal performance, Larson et al. (1978) noted that the nature of the cerebellar involvement in vocal control is fundamentally different from that exerted by other neural areas based upon the characteristics of vocalization following brain lesions. For example, the anterior cingulate gyrus may be in a direct pathway for the initiation of vocalizations. Disruption of the anterior cingulate cortex is known to cause mutism and vocal initiation disorders (Sutton, Larson, and Lindeman, 1974). According to Larson et al. (1978) cerebellar lesions have a much different effect on vocalizations. They reported that that

"vocal intensity was reduced, f_o was changed, vocal duration was affected, or complex relations between intensity and f_o were altered. However, frequency of occurrence of vocalizations did not change. These data suggest that the cerebellum is to some extent involved in the modulation and control of pitch and intensity parameters of vocalization. It would not appear that the cerebellum is involved in the initiation of vocalizations as may be the case for the anterior cingulate gyrus." (p.16).

Anterior cingulate cortex (ACC)

The exact nature of the influences by the ACC on the initiation or motor control of human vocalization and speech remain unknown. Direct electrical stimulation of the anterior cingulate cortex in monkeys has been reported effective in evoking vocalization in the form of species-specific call types (Jurgens, 1987; Jurgens and Ploog, 1970; Jurgens and von Cramon, 1982; Kaada, 1951; Robinson, 1967; Smith, 1945). The responsive substrate consists of the precallosal cingulate gyrus and the supracallosal cingulate cortex at the level of the genu of the corpus callosum (Jurgens, 1983) and has been found to share reciprocal connections with the primary face motor cortex (Jurgens, 1976, 1982; Muakkassa and Strick, 1979). Fibers from the ACC also project to the homologue of Broca's area and SMA in monkeys (Muller-Preuss and Jurgens, 1976). Bilateral destruction of the anterior cingulate cortex in monkeys does not impair spontaneous "affective" calls or electrically elicited calls but severely impairs conditioned, "learned vocalizations" (Aitken, 1981; Jurgens, 1983; Kirzinger and Jurgens, 1982; Ploog, 1979, 1981; Sutton, Larson, and Lindeman, 1974; Trachy, Sutton, and Lindeman, 1981).

A comparison of the effects of cingular lesions in animals and humans reveals that in both cases, motor skills, general learning capability, and emotional reaction seem to be intact, however, the learned control of emotional reactions is severely impaired (Jurgens and Pratt, 1979). In humans, bilateral lesions in the anterior cingulate gyrus have been reported to cause akinetic mutism (Barris and Schuman, 1953; Brown, 1979; Nielsen and Jacobs, 1951).

Netsell (1984) hypothesized that damage to the limbic system, including the anterior cingulate cortex, effectively prevents the engagement of the neocortical system for purposes of ideational or propositional speech. Larson (1988) stated that cortical control of vocalization during propositional speech appears to be a relatively recent phylogenetic development compared with subcortical mechanisms present in other animals. Humans with cortically projecting ACC lesions would be unable to invoke the "analytic" power of the neocortical system and, thus, have problems in elaborating thought and translating it to articulate speech. These same individuals, with intact inferior ACC projections, might be capable of automatic speech and the affective/emotive vocalizations that characterize most of the nonhuman primate repertoires.

Basal ganglia (BG)

Lesions involving the substantia nigra in the squirrel monkey are associated with reductions in vocal fundamental frequency (Kirzinger and Jurgens, 1985). Voice characteristics of human subjects with lesions of the basal ganglia (Parkinson's disease PD) include breathiness, roughness, hoarseness, tremulousness, reduced pitch range, and inappropriate modal speaking pitch (Grewel, 1957a, 1957b; Logemann, Fisher, Boshes, and Blonsky, 1978, Darley, Aronson, and Brown, 1969), and limited vocal intensity range (Canter, 1963, 1965). See Ramig (this volume) for a more complete discussion of laryngeal dysfunction in PD individuals.

In Parkinson's disease, the rapid alternating adjustments in position of the vocal folds associated with phonatory onset and offset during connected speech is particularly impaired (Ludlow, 1976, 1981; Ludlow and Bassich, 1981). The rate of laryngeal abduction was particularly impaired in hypokinesia associated with Parkinson's disease, while the rate of adduction was not (Ludlow, 1976).

Physiologic studies of orofacial structures in PD patients generally indicate that aberrations in voluntary movement control and speech intelligibility may result from (1) involuntary tremor, (2) voluntary movement initiation delays related to the synchronizations of voluntary muscle activity with the excitatory phase of the tremor cycle (Hunker, 1984), and (3) labial hypertonus as inferred from EMG (Leanderson, Meyerson, and Persson (1971) or increased muscle stiffness (Hunker, Abbs and Barlow, 1982; Caligiuri, 1989).

The variations in symptomatology and motor impairment reported among dysarthric individuals with involvement of the basal ganglia is expected given the complex pharmacology and anatomical relations among the groups of nuclei comprising this region of the brain. The term *basal ganglia* refers to a group of anatomically and functionally related nuclei, including the striatum (caudate nucleus and the putamen), the globus pallidus, the substantia nigra, and the subthalamic nucleus (see comprehensive review by DeLong and Georgopoulos, 1981). Disease or damage to select nuclei or groups of nuclei located in the basal ganglia have been associated with some of the classic motor symptoms, including dyskinesia, tremor, and rigidity. Damage to the subthalamic nucleus and the striatum are associated with the dyskinesias. According to DeLong et al.:

"Rigidity more clearly appears to be related to striatal (putaminal) dysfunction that results in abnormal pallidal output" (1981: 1050).

For some conditions, a coexisting alteration in neural function of other
brain areas is required. For example, resting tremor appears to require
combined manipulation of basal ganglia and cerebellar connections (De-
Long and Georgopoulos, 1981).

Therefore, the basal ganglia is collection of nuclei, which for the most
part, maintain the segregation of influences from the sensorimotor and
frontal association areas. An experimental model of the effects of basal
ganglia activity on parameters of speech output, including intelligibility,
would necessarily require a consideration of the contribution of individual
nuclei and combinations of coexisting alterations in other brain relays given
the variety of motor symptoms observed in patients and experimental animal models with lesions of the basal ganglia.

Periaqueductal gray (PAG)

Both specialized calls and spontaneous vocalizations are abolished following lesions to the PAG and lateral tegmentum (Adametz and O'Leary,
1959, in cats; Jurgens and Pratt, 1979, in squirrel monkey; Larson and Kistler, 1984, in maccaque monkey). Interposed between the cingular cortex
and nucleus ambiguus, the PAG has been hypothesized to serve integrative
functions in the coordination of several muscle systems in the monkey
including, respiratory, laryngeal, velopharyngeal, and orofacial (Jurgens
and Pratt, 1979; Larson and Kistler, 1984). Because of this complex
neuroanatomic relation, lesions of the dorsolateral PAG would be expected
to have devastating effects on interstructure coordination (turning muscles
on and off at correct times) along the vocal tract (Larson, 1988).

Relations between motor output and speech intelligibility

To the author's knowledge, there are only two published studies that have
specifically examined the relation between subsystem motor physiology and
a standardized measure of *overall* speech intelligibility. The first such investigation involved the parameterization of force and movement control in a
group of five patients with a congenital form of the upper motor neuron
syndrome — UMN-S (Barlow and Abbs, 1986). These patients exhibited

significant reductions in the rate of force change during the production of a *"ramp-and-hold"* compression force control task using the upper lip, lower lip, tongue tip, and jaw. The inability of these UMN-S patients to "turn-on" select orofacial muscles was paralleled by commensurate reductions in displacement velocity for nonspeech tasks requiring precise adjustments in articulatory position. Pearson product linear correlation coefficients, derived from a comparison between the average rate of force change and the average displacement velocity, ranged from 0.640 to 0.987 among the four orofacial structures studied. Therefore deficits in generating the dynamic phase of a "ramp-and-hold" forcing function are predictive of the degree of impairment in driving an affected articulatory structure through an appropriate velocity operating range. The dynamic parameters derived from the force and displacement waveforms sampled from the four orofacial structures were related to a quantitative measure of overall speech intelligibility. As shown in Figure 7, patients with severe neuromotor con-

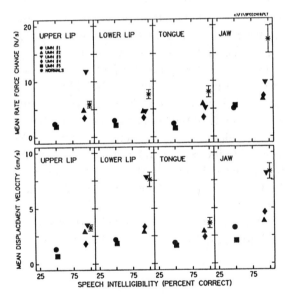

Figure 7. *The relations between the average rate of force change (upper panels) and speech intelligibility, and mean displacement velocity (lower panels) and speech intelligibility by orofacial structure for each UMN-S patient is shown. Control group means and 99% confidence intervals are indicated by asterisks and vertical bars* (Barlow & Abbs, 1986; permission granted).

trol impairments had substantially lower intelligibility scores than those with milder force and velocity control deficits. The UMN-S patients with good intelligibility scores (approximately 91 to 95 percent correct), performed rather poorly on the ramp-and-hold force and position control tasks using orofacial structures, often times only capable of 50 percent of the expected value. This observation provides evidence in support for neural reorganization to achieve compensatory action among structures of the vocal tract to maintain a high level of speech intelligibility.

The second investigation involved more detailed analyses of "ramp-and-hold" force dynamics in the upper and lower lip of normal and traumatically brain injured (TBI) adults (Barlow and Burton, 1988; 1990). The parameters of force control analysis included the peak of the first derivative of force (dF/dt^{max}), peak force during the ramp phase, mean force during hold phase, and measures of variability during incremental periods of the hold phase. Although the nature of force control impairments among the TBI subjects was different from those manifested by the congenital UMNS patients described above, the relation between the degree of impairment on force control parameters associated with the "ramp-and-hold" task and *overall* speech intelligibility was maintained.

These studies have been useful in mapping the distribution and nature of motor impairments among orofacial systems in individuals with neurological involvement. Experience gained from these experiments and others have advanced our understanding of the biomechanical properties of the orofacial mechanism (Muller, Milenkovic, and MacLeod, 1985; Barlow and Muller, 1990) and contributed to the development of specialized transduction and digital signal processing algorithms (Barlow, Suing, Grossman, Bodmer, and Colbert, 1989). Our studies have fallen short of establishing cause-effect relations between fine motor control impairments of a single structure (i.e., anterior tongue) and degradation of individual items in the phonetic inventory (i.e., articulatory gestures involving /t/, /d/, /s/, and /z/).

Future directions

Intelligibility measures are needed that extend auditory-perceptual assessment tools of *overall* communicative effectiveness to emphasize the *efficiency and relative communicative power associated with the activity of indi-*

vidual vocal tract structures. Fractionation of the intelligibility code according to the place of articulation along the vocal tract would be a useful first step in quantifying the relations between subsystem pathophysiology and speech performance. This would mean the development of intelligibility protocols comprised of syllables or words targeted to reflect the action of a primary articulator or structure. A number of interesting hypotheses could then be subjected to formal tests relating individual parameters of force and movement control among individual articulatory structures to these hybrid measures of speech intelligibility. The prospects to undertake such a set of experiments is more exciting than ever due, in part, to the vastly improved methods of neuroimaging available to the speech physiologist.

Obviously, our understanding of brain mechanisms involved in the control of speech is almost nonexistent, and at best, extremely limited when considering call production in animal models. Animal vocalization studies need continued support to firmly establish the neural substrate required for propositional and nonpropositional vocal/verbal behavior. It seems within the realm of these experiments to develop a measure of vocalization quality or "*intelligibility*". More use of the well developed science of acoustics could be used to augment perceptual measures of animal call quality or "*intelligibility*". This inclusion into the experimental design would help identify the salient parameters of vocalization and the underlying controlling neural substrate. The use of microstimulation, macrostimulation, spike triggered averaging (STA), evoked potentials, brain imaging of metabolic activities, tract tracing, and monitoring physiologic outputs (EMG, force, movement, voice, etc) will continue to be important tools for the neuroscientist.

Mathematical modeling efforts are needed to merge the neurophysiologic, kinematic, and intelligibility data to begin simulating the properties of neural networks, muscle systems, synthesized resultant speech acoustics, and machine speech recognition (intelligibility). Given the lack of an animal model with speech (as defined in human terms), the application of computer science to incorporate empirical data collected from neurophysiological studies of vocalization in cat and monkey, subsystem motor physiology in humans, acoustics, and perception, may represent the only common ground available to bridge the gap between the neuron, speech motor control, and intelligibility. Development of a such a computer model may be extremely useful in determining how speech intelligibility may be preserved by compensatory neural actions.

Acknowledgements

This work was supported in part by a grant from the the Moody Foundation of Galveston, Texas (88-46). Reprint requests should be sent to Dr. Steven M. Barlow, Department of Speech and Hearing Sciences, Indiana University, Bloomington, Indiana 47405.

Abbreviations

ACC	anterior cingulate cortex
APA	anterior premotor area
CNS	central nervous system
CAT	computerized axial tomography
EMG	electromyography
GP_i	globus pallidus internal division
HRP	horseradish peroxidase
ICMS	intracortical microstimulation
LPC	lateral precentral cortex
MI	primary motor cortex
NA	nucleus ambiguus
NTS	nucleus tractus solitarius
PAG	periaqueductal gray
PBN	parabrachial nucleus
PD	Parkinson's disease
PMC	premotor cortex
rCBF	regional cerebral blood flow
SI	primary somatosensory cortex
SMA	supplementary motor area
SN_{pr}	substantia nigra pars reticulata
STA	spike triggered averaging
UMN-S	upper motor neuron syndrome
VA_{mc}	ventralis anterior magnocellularis nucleus of thalamus
VL	ventralis lateralis nucleus of thalamus
VL_m	ventralis lateralis pars medialis nucleus of thalamus
VL_o	ventralis lateralis pars oralis nucleus of thalamus
VPL_o	ventralis posterior lateralis pars oralis nucleus of thalamus
VPM	ventral posteromedial division of ventral posterior nucleus of thalamus

References

Adametz, J., & O'Leary, J.L. 1959. "Experimental mutism resulting from periaqueductal lesions in cats." *Neurology* 9, 636-642.

Aitken, P.G. 1981. "Cortical control of conditioned and spontaneous vocal behavior in rhesus monkeys." *Brain and Language* 13, 171-184.

Allen, G.I., and Tsukahara, N. 1974. "Cerebrocerebellar communication systems." *Physiology Review* 54, 957-1006.

Aronson, A. 1980. *Clinical Voice Disorders*. New York: Thieme-Stratton, 77-126.

Asanuma, C., Thach, W.T., & Jones, E.G. 1983a. "Distribution of cerebellar terminations in the ventral lateral thalamic region of the monkey." *Brain Research Reviews* 5, 237-265.

————. 1983b. "Anatomical evidence for segregated focal groupings of efferent cells and their terminal ramifications in the cerebellothalamic pathway of the monkey." *Brain Research Reviews* 5, 267-297.

Barlow, S.M., & Abbs, J.H. 1986. "Fine force and position control of select orofacial structures in the upper motor neuron syndrome." *Experimental Neurology* 94, 699-713.

Barlow, S.M., & Burton, M. 1988. "Orofacial force control impairments in brain injured adults." *Abstracts Association for Research in Otolaryngology* 11, 218.

————. 1990. "Ramp-and-hold force control in the upper and lower lips: Developing new neuromotor assessment applications in traumatically brain injured adults." *Journal of Speech and Hearing Research* 33, 660-675.

Barlow, S.M. and Farley, G. 1989. "Neurophysiology of speech." In D. Kuehn, M. and J. Baumgartner (Eds.), *Neurobiology of Speech, Language and Hearing*. Boston: Little, Brown and Company, 146-200.

Barlow, S.M., & Muller, E.M. 1991. "The relation between interangle span and in vivo resultant force in the perioral musculature." *Journal of Speech and Hearing Research* 34, 252-259.

Barlow, S.M., Suing, G., Grossman, A., Bodmer, P., & Colbert, R. 1989. "A high-speed data acquisition and protocol control system for vocal tract physiology." *Journal of Voice* 3, 283-293.

Barris, R.W., & Schuman, H.R. 1953. "Bilateral anterior cingulate gyrus lesions." *Neurology* 3, 44-52.

Botez, M. I., & Barbeau, A. 1971. "Role of subcortical structures and particularly of the thalamus, in the mechanisms of speech and language." *International Journal of Neurology* 8, 300-320.

Botterell, E.H., & Fulton, J.F. 1938. "Functional localization in the cerebellum of primates. I. Unilateral section of the peduncles." *Journal of Comparative Neurology* 69, 31.

Brinkman, C. 1984. "Supplementary motor area of the monkey's cerebral cortex: short- and long-term deficits after unilateral ablation and the effects of subsequent callosal section." *The Journal of Neuroscience* 4, 918-929.

Brinkman, C., & Porter, R. 1978. "Supplementary motor area in the monkey: activity of neurons during performance of a learned motor task." *Journal of Neurophysiology* 42, 681-709.

Brooks, V.B., & Thach, W.T. 1981. "Cerebellar Control of Posture and Movement." In V.B. Brooks (Ed.), *Handbook of Physiology. Section I: The Nervous System. Vol. II: Motor Control.* Bethesda, MD: American Physiological Society.

Brown, J. 1979. *Neurobiology of Social Communication in Primates: An evolutionary perspective: Language representation in the brain,* ed. 1, New York, Academic Press.

Brown, J., Darley, F., & Aronson, A. 1970. "Ataxic dysarthria." *International Journal of Neurology* 7, 302-318.

Brown, J.W., & Perecman, E. 1985. "Neurological basis of language processing." In: Darby J.K. (ed.), *Speech and Language Evaluation in Neurology: Adult Disorders.* New York: Grune & Stratton, 45-81.

Brown, T.G. 1915. "Note on the physiology of the basal ganglia and midbrain of the anthropoid ape, expecially in reference to the act of laughter." *Journal of Physiology* 49, 195-207.

Caligiuri, M.P. 1989. "Short-term fluctuations in orofacial motor control in Parkinson's disease." In K. Yorkston and D. Beukelman, eds. *Recent Advances in Clinical Dysarthria.* College Hill Press, Boston, 199-212.

Canter, C.J. 1963. "Speech characteristics of patients with Parkinson's disease: I. Intensity, pitch, and duration." *Journal of Speech Hearing Disorders* 28, 221-229.

———. 1965. "Speech characteristics of patients with Parkinson's disease: II. Physiological support for speech." *Journal of Speech Hearing Disorders* 30, 44-49.

Carpenter, M. B., Carleton, S. C., Keller, J. T., & Conte, P. 1981. "Connections of the subthalamic nucleus in the monkey." *Brain Research* 224, 1-29.

Carpenter, M. B., & McMasters, R. E. 1964. "Lesions of the substantia nigral in the rhesus monkey. Efferent fiber degeneration and behavioral observations." *American Journal of Anatomy* 114, 293-320.

Carpenter, M.B., Nakano, K., & Kim, R. 1976. "Nigrothalamic projections in the monkey demonstrated by autoradiographic techniques." *Journal of Comparative Neurology* 165, 401-416.

Carpenter, M.B., & Peter, P. 1972. "Nigrostriatal and nigrothalamic fibers in the rhesus monkey." *Journal of Comparative Neurology* 144, 93-116.

Carpenter, M.B., & Strominger, N.L. 1967. "Efferent fiber projections of the subthalamic nucleus in the rhesus monkey. A comparison of the efferent projections of the subthalamic nucleus, substantia nigra, and globus pallidus." *American Journal of Anatomy* 121, 41-72.

Chambers, W.W., & Sprague, J.M. 1955. "Functional localization in the cerebellum. II. Somatotopic organization in cortex and nuclei." *Arch. Neurol. Psychiatry* 74, 653-680.

Chan-Palay, V., & Palay, S.L. 1987. "Cerebellum." In G. Adelman (ed.), *Encyclopedia of Neuroscience.* Birkhauser Boston, 194-198.

Darley, F.L., Aronson, A.E., & Brown, J.R. 1969. "Differential diagnostic patterns of dysarthria." *Journal of Speech and Hearing Research* 12, 246-269.

———. 1975. *Motor Speech Disorders.* Philadelphia: W. B. Saunders Company.

DeLong, M.R., & Georgopoulos, A.P. 1981. "Motor functions of the basal ganglia." In V.B. Brooks (ed.), *Handbook of Physiology: The Nervous System II: Motor Control.* Bethesda: American Physiological Society, 1017-1061.

DeRosier, E.A., West, R.A., & Larson, C.R. 1988. "Comparison of single unit discharge properties in the periaqueductal gray and nucleus retroambiguus during vocalization in monkeys." *Abstracts Society for Neuroscience* 14, 1237.

DeVito, J.L., & Anderson, M.E. 1982. "An autoradiographic study of efferent connections of the globus pallidus in Macaca mulatta." *Experimental Brain Research* 46, 107-117.

Evarts, E.V. 1981a. "Role of motor cortex in voluntary movements in primates." In V. B. Brooks (ed.), *Handbook of Physiology. Section I: The Nervous System. Vol II: Motor Control.* Bethesda, MD: American Physiological Society.

Farley, G.R., Barlow, S.M., & Netsell, R. 1989. "Conditioned cats as models for studying neural mechanisms of vocalization." *Abstract for American Speech, Hearing and Language Association (ASHA)* 31, 153.

———. 1990. "Unit activity in parabrachial regions during cat vocalizations." Invited paper presented to the UCLA Conference on Neurological Disorders of Laryngeal Function.

Ferrier, D. 1873. "Experimental researches in cerebral physiology and pathology." *Western Riding Lunatics Asylum Medical Report* 3, 30-96.

Foerster, O. 1936. "Motorische Felder und Bahnen." *Handbuch der Neurologie* VI: 1.

Freedman, M., Alexander, M.P., & Naeser, M. A. 1984. "Anatomic basis of transcortical motor aphasia." *Neurology* 34, 409-417.

Fritsch, G., & Hitzig, E. 1870. "Über die elektrische Erregbarkeit des Grosshirns." *Archives of the Anatomy and Physiology Wiss. Medicine* 37: 300-332. (Translated by G. von Bonin. In W. W. Nowinski (ed.), *The Cerebral Cortex*, Springfield, IL: Charles C. Thomas, 1960, 73-96.)

Gelmers, H.J. 1983. "Non-paralytic motor disturbances and speech disorders: the role of the supplementary motor area." *Journal of Neurology, Neurosurgery, and Psychiatry* 46, 1052-1054.

Granit, R. 1977. *The Purposive Brain.* Cambridge, MA Press.

Grewel, F. 1957a. "Classification of dysarthrias." *Acta Psychiatr. Neurol. Scand.* 32, 325-337.

———. 1957b. "Dysarthria in post-encephalitic parkinsonism." *Acta Psychiatr. Neurol. Scand.* 32, 440-449.

Holstege, G. 1987. "The final common pathway in vocalization in cat." *Abstracts Society for Neuroscience* 13, 855.

Hirose, H., Kiritani, S., Ushijima, T., & Sawashima, M. 1978. "Analysis of abnormal articulatory dynamics in two dysarthric patients." *Journal of Speech and Hearing Disorders* 43, 96-105.

Holmes, G. 1922a. "Clinical symptoms of cerebellar disease and their interpretation: The Croonian Lectures. III." *Lancet* 2, 59-65.

———. 1922b. "Clinical symptoms of cerebellar disease and their interpretation: The Croonian Lectures. IV." *Lancet* 2, 111-115.

———. 1939. "The cerebellum of man." *Brain* 62, 1-30.

Huang, C.-S., Hiraba, H., & Sessle, B.J. 1989. "Input-output relationships of the primary face motor cortex in the monkey." *Journal of Neurophysiology* 61, 350-362.

Huang, C.-S., Sirisko, M.A., Hiraba, H., Murray, G.M., & Sessle, B. J. 1988. "Organization of the primate face motor cortex as revealed by intracortical microstimulation and electrophysiological identification of afferent inputs and corticobulbar projections." *Journal of Neurophysiology* 59, 796-818.

Hunker, C.J. 1984. "Parkinsonian resting tremor and its relationship to movement initiation." Doctoral dissertation, Univ. of Wisconsin, Madison. (University Microfilms No. 84-10772).

Hunker, C.J., Abbs, J.H., & Barlow, S.M. 1982. "The relationship between parkinsonian rigidity and hypokinesia in the orofacial system: a quantitative analysis." *Neurology* 32, 755-761.

Jackson, J.H. 1874. "On the anatomical and physiological locaization of movements in the brain." *British Medical Journal*, September 26, 1874. [In *Selected Writings of John Hughlings Jackson*. New YHork: Basic Books, 1958, 37-76.]

Jenny, A. B., & Saper, C. B. 1987. "Organization of the facial nucleus and corticofacial projection in the monkey: a reconsideration of the upper motor neuron facial palsy." *Neurology* 37, 930-939.

Johansson, R.S., Trulsson, M., Olsson, K.A., & Abbs, J.H. 1988. "Mechanoreceptive afferent activity in the infraorbital nerve in man during speech and chewing movements." *Experimental Brain Research* 72, 209-214.

Jonas, S. 1981. "The supplementary motor region and speech emission." *Journal of Communication Disorders* 14, 349-373.

———. 1987. "The supplementary motor region and speech." In E. Perecman (ed.), *The Frontal Lobes Revisited*, 241-250. New York: The Institute for Research in Behavioral Neuroscience Press.

Jones, E.G., & Powell, T.P.S. 1970. "An anatomical study of converging sensory pathways within the cerebral cortex of the monkey." *Brain* 93, 793-820.

Jones, E.G., Wise, S.P., & Coulter, J.D. 1979. "Differential thalamic relationships of sensory-motor and parietal cortical fields in monkeys." *Journal of Comparative Neurology* 183, 833-882.

Jurgens, U. 1976. "Projections from the Cortical Larynx Area in the Squirrel Monkey." *Experimental Brain Research* 25, 401-411.

———. 1982. "Afferents to the cortical larynx area in the monkey." *Brain Research* 239, 377-389.

———. 1983. "Afferent fibers to the cingular vocalization region in the squirrel monkey." *Experimental Neurology* 80, 395-409.

———. 1987. "Primate communication: Signaling, vocalization." In G. Adelman (ed.), *Encyclopedia of Neuroscience*. Birkhauser Boston, 976-979.

Jurgens, U., & Ploog, D. 1970. "Cerebral representation of vocalization in the squirrel monkey." *Experimental Brain Research* 10, 532-544.

Jurgens, U., & Pratt, R. 1979. "Role of Periaqueductal Grey in vocal expression of emotion." *Brain Research* 167, 367-378.

Jurgens, U., & von Cramon, D. 1982. "On the role of the anterior cingulate cortex in phonation: a case report." *Brain and Language* 15, 234-248.

Kaada, B.R. 1951. "Somato-motor, autonomic and electrocorticographic responses to electrical stimulation of 'rhinencephalic' and other structures in primates, cat and dog." *Acta Physiol. Scand. Suppl.* 83, 1.

Kaas, J.H., Nelson, R.J., Sur, M., Lin, C., & Merzenich, M.M. 1979. "Multiple representations of the body within the primary somatosensory cortex of primates." *Science* 204, 521-523.

Kalil, K. 1981. "Projections of the cerebellar and dorsal column nuclei upon the thalamus of the rhesus monkey." *Journal of Comparative Neurology* 195, 25-50.

Kammermeier, M.A. 1969. "A comparison of phonatory phenomena among groups of neurologically impaired speakers." Ph.D. dissertation, University of Minnesota.

Kent, R., & Netsell, R. 1975. "A case study of an ataxic dysarthric: cinefluorographic and spectrographic observations." *Journal of Speech and Hearing Disorders* 40, 115-134.

Kent, R., Netsell, R., & Abbs, J. 1979. "Acoustic characteristics of dysarthria associated with cerebellar disease." *Journal of Speech and Hearing Reserch* 22, 627-648.

Kim, R., Nakano, K., Jayarman, A., & Carpenter, M.B. 1976. "Projections of the globus pallidus and adjacent structures: an autoradiographic study in the monkey." *Journal of Comparative Neurology* 169, 263-289.

Kirzinger, A., & Jurgens, U. 1982. "Cortical lesion effects and vocalization in the squirrel monkey." *Brain Research* 233, 299-315.

———. 1985. "The effects of brainstem lesions on vocalization in the squirrel monkey." *Brain Research* 358, 150-162.

Kobler, J.B. 1983. "The nucleus ambiguus of the bat, Pteronotus Parnelli: peripheral targets and central inputs." Ph.D. thesis, Department of Neurobiology, University of North Carolina.

Kornhuber, H.H. 1977. "A reconsideration of the cortical and subcortical mechanisms involved in speech and aphasia." *Progress in Clinical Neurophysiology* 3, 28.

Kornhuber, H.H., & Deecke, L. 1965. "Hirnpotentialanderungen bei Wilkurbewegungen und passiven Bewegungen des Menschen: Bereitschaftspotential und reafferente Potentiale." *Pflugers Archiv. fur die Gesamte Physiologie* 284, 1-17.

Kubota, K. 1984. "An introduction to 'voluntary movement and the brain'." *Advances in Neurological Science* 28, 3-6.

Kuo, J.S., & Carpenter, M.B. 1973. "Organization of pallidothalamic projections in rhesus monkey." *Journal of Comparative Neurology* 151, 201-236.

Kusama, T., Mabuchi, M., & Sumino, T. 1971. "Cerebellar projections to the thalamic nuclei in monkeys." *Proceedings of the Japanese Academy* 47, 505-510.

Kuypers, H.G.H.M. 1958a. "Corticobulbar connexions to the pons and lower brain stem in man." *Brain* 81, 364-388.

———. 1958b. "Some projections from the peri-central cortex to the pons and lower brain stem in monkey and chimpanzee." *Journal of Comparative Neurology* 110, 221-255.

——— 1958c. "An anatomical analysis of cortico-bulbar connexions to the pons and lower brain stem in the cat." *Journal of Anatomy* 92, 198-218.

———. 1964. "The descending pathways to the spinal cord, their anatomy and function." In J. C. Eccles and J. P. Schade (ed.), *Progress in Brain Research, Organization of the Spinal Cord*, Vol. II. Amsterdam: Elsevier.

———. 1973. "The Anatomical Organization of the Descending Pathways and Their Contributions to Motor Control Especially in Primates." In J. E. Desmedt (ed.),

New Developments in Electromyography and Clinical Neurophysiology, Vol. 3. Basel: Karger.

————. 1981. "Anatomy of the descending pathways." In *Handbook of Physiology, The Nervous System. Motor Control.* Volume II, p. 597-666. Bethesda, MD: American Physiological Society.

Larsen, B., Skinhoj, E., Soh, K., Endo, H., & Lassen, N.A. 1977. "The pattern of cortical activity provoked by listening and speech revealed by rCBF measurements." *Acta Neurologica Scandinavica Supplement* 64, 268-269.

Larson, C.R. 1985. "The midbrain periaqueductal gray: a brainstem structure involved in vocalization." *Journal of Speech and Hearing Research* 28, 241-249.

————. 1988. "Brain mechanisms involved in the control of vocalization." *Journal of Voice* 2, 301-311.

Larson, C.R., & Kistler, M.K. 1984. "Periaqueductal gray neuronal activity associated with laryngeal EMG and vocalization in the awake monkey." *Neuroscience Letters* 46, 261-266.

————. 1986. "The relationship of periaqueductal gray neurons to vocalization and laryngeal EMG in the behaving monkey." *Experimental Brain Research* 63, 596-606.

Larson, C.R., Sutton, D., & Lindeman, R.C. 1978. "Cerebellar regulation of phonation in rhesus monkey (Macaca mulatta)." *Experimental Brain Research* 33, 1-18.

Lassen, N.A., Ingvar, D.H., & Skinhoj, E. 1978. "Brain function and blood flow." *Scientific American* 239, 62-71.

Leanderson, R., Meyerson, B.A., & Persson, A. 1971. "Effect of L-dopa on speech in parkinsonism." *Journal of Neurology, Neurosurgery and Psychiatry* 34, 679-681.

Leicester, J. 1980. "Central deafness and subcortical motor aphasia." *Brain and Language* 10, 224-242.

Logemann, J., Fisher, H.B., Boshes, B., & Blonsky, E.R. 1978. "Frequency and occurrence of vocal tract dysfunctions in the speech of a large number of Parkinson patients." *Journal of Speech and Hearing Disorders* 43, 47-57.

Ludlow, C.L. 1976. "Acoustic study of speech in Parkinson's disease." Paper presented at the Fall meeting of the Acoustical Society of America, San Diego.

————. 1981. "Research Needs for the Assessment of Phonatory Functions." *Proceedings of the Conference on the Assessment of Vocal Pathology* 11, 3.

Ludlow, C.L., & Bassich, C.B. 1981. *Speech and Language: Advances in Basic Research and Practice: The differential diagnosis of syndromes of dysarthria using measures of speech production*, ed. 1. New York, Academic Press.

Magoun, H.W., Atlas, D., Ingersoll, E.H., & Ranson, S.W. 1937. "Associated facial, vocal and respiratory components of emotional expression: An experimental study." *Journal of Neurology and Psychopathology* 17, 241-255.

Matsumura, M., & Kubota, K. 1979. "Cortical projection to hand-arm motor area from post-arcuate in macaque monkeys: a histological study of retrograde transport of horseradish peroxidase." *Neuroscience Letters* 11, 241-246.

McClean, M., Dostrovsky, J.O., Lee, L., & Tasker, R.R. 1990. "Somatosensory neurons in human thalamus respond to speech-induced orofacial movements." *Brain Research*.

Mehler, W.R. 1971. "Idea of a new anatomy of the thalamus." *Journal of Psychiatric Research* 8, 203-217.

Merzenich, M.M., Kaas, J.H., Sur, M., & Lin, C.S. 1978. "Double representation of the body surface within cytoarchitectonic Areas 3b and 1 in "SI" in the owl monkey (*Aotus trivirgatus*)." *Journal of Comparative Neurology* 181, 41-74.

Mountcastle, V. 1957. "Modality and topographic properties of single neurons of cat's somatic sensory cortex." *Journal of Neurophysiology* 20. 408-434.

Muakkassa, K.F., & Strick, P.L. 1979. Frontal lobe inputs to primate motor cortex: evidence for four somatotopically organized "premotor" areas. *Brain Research* 177, 176-182.

Muller, E.M., Milenkovic, P.H., & MacLeod, G.E. 1985. "Perioral tissue mechanics during speech production." In J. Eisenfeld and C. DeLisi (eds.), *Mathematics and Computers in Biomedical Application*. Amsterdam: Elsevier.

Muller-Preuss, P., & Jurgens, U. 1976. "Projections from the cingular vocalization area in the squirrel monkey." *Brain Research* 103, 29-34.

Mysak, E.D. 1959. "Pitch and duration characteristics of older males." *Journal of Speech Hearing Research* 2, 46-54.

Nauta, W.J.H., & Mehler, W.R. 1966. "Projections of the lentiform nucleus in the monkey." *Brain Research* 1, 3-42.

Netsell, R. 1982. "Speech motor control and selected neurologic disorders." In S. Grillner, B. Lindblom, J. Lubker, and A. Persson (eds), *Speech Motor Control*. New York: Pergamon Press.

———. 1984. "A neurobiologic view of the dysarthrias." In M. McNeil, J. Rosenbek, and A. Aronson (eds), *The Dysarthrias: Physiology-Acoustics-Perception-Management*. San Diego: College-Hill Press.

Netsell, R., & Kent, R. 1976. "Paroxysmal ataxic dysarthria." *Journal of Speech and Hearing Disorders* 41, 93-109.

Nielsen, J.M., & Jacobs, L.L. 1951. "Bilateral lesions of the anterior cingulate gyri." *Bull. Los Angeles Neurol. Soc.* 16, 231-234.

Nordin, M., & Thomander, L. 1989. "Infrafascicular multi-unit recordings from the human infra-orbital nerve." *Acta Physiologica Scandanavia* 135, 139-148.

Orgogozo, J.M., & Larsen, B. 1979. "Activation of the supplementary motor area during voluntary movement in man suggests it works as a supra-motor area." *Science* 206, 847-850.

Pandya, D.N., & Kuypers, H.G.J.M. 1969. "Cortico-cortical connections in the rhesus monkey." *Brain Research* 13, 13-36.

Pandya, D.N., & Vignolo, L.A. 1971. "Intra- and inter- hemispheric projections of the precentral, premotor, and arcuate areas in the rhesus monkey." *Brain Research* 26, 217-233.

Paul, R.L., Merzenich, M., & Goodman, H. 1972. "Representation of slowly and rapidly adapting cutaneous mechanoreceptors of the hand in Brodmann's Areas 3 and 1 of Macaca mulatta." *Brain Research* 36, 229-249.

Penfield, W., & Bordley, E. 1937. "Somatic motor and sensory representation in the cortex as studied by electrical stimulation." *Brain* 60, 389-443.

Penfield, W., & Roberts, L. 1959. "Speech and brain mechanisms." Princeton, NJ: Princeton University Press, 3-137.

Penfield, W., & Welch, K. 1951. "The supplementary motor area of the cerebral cortex." *Archives of Neurology and Psychiatry* 66, 289-317.

Percheron, G. 1977. "The thalamic territory of cerebellar afferents and the lateral region of the thalamus of the macaque in stereotaxic ventricular coordinates." *Journal
fur Hirnforschung* 18, 375-400.

Phillips, C.G., & Porter, R. 1977. *Corticospinal Neurons: Their Role in Movements*.
London: Academic Press.

Ploog, D. 1979. "Phonation, emotion, cognition, with reference to the brain
mechanisms involved." *Ciba Foundation Symposium* 69, 78-98.

――――. 1981. "On the neural control of mammalian vocalization." *Trends in Neuroscience* 4, 135.

Robinson, B.W. 1967. "Vocalization evoked from forebrain in Macaca mulatta."
Physiology and Behavior 2, 345-354.

Roland, P.E. 1985. "Cortical organization of voluntary behavior in man." *Human
Neurobiology* 4, 155-167.

Roland, P.E., Larsen, B., Lassen, N.A., & Skinhoj, E. 1980. "Supplementary motor
area and other cortical areas in organization of voluntary movements in man." *Journal of Neurophysiology* 43, 118-136.

Roland, P.E., Skinhoj, E., Larsen, B., & Lassen, N.A. 1977. "The role of different cortical areas in the organization of voluntary movements in man." *Acta Neurologica
Scandinavica Supplement* 64, 542-543.

Sasaki, K., Jinnai, K., Gemba, H., Hashimoto, S., & Mizuno, N. 1979. "Projection of
the cerebellar dentate nucleus onto the frontal association cortex in monkeys."
Experimental Brain Research 37, 193-198.

Sasaki, K., Kawaguchi, S., Oka, H., Sakai, M., & Mizuno, N. 1976. "Electrophysiological studies on the cerebellocerebral projections in monkeys." *Experimental Brain
Research* 24, 495-507.

Schell, G.R., & Strick, P.L. 1984. "The origin of thalamic inputs to the arcuate premotor and supplementary motor areas." *Journal of Neuroscience* 4, 539-560.

Smith, W.K. 1945. "The functional significance of the rostral cingular cortex as revealed
by its responses to electrical excitation." *Journal of Neurophysiology* 8, 241-255.

Stanton, G.B. 1980. "Topographical organization of ascending cerebellar projections
from the dentate and interposed nuclei in Macaca mulatta: an anterograde degeneration study." *Journal of Comparative Neurology* 19, 699-731.

Sutton, D., Larson, C.R., & Lindeman, R.C. 1974. "Neocortical and limbic lesion
effects on primate phonation." *Brain Research* 71, 61-75.

Tanji, J., Taniguchi, K., & Saga, T. 1980. "Supplementary motor area: neuronal
response to motor instructions." *Journal of Neurophysiology* 43, 60-68.

Thach, W.T. 1970. "Discharge of cerebellar neurons related to two maintained postures
and two prompt movements, I. Nuclear Cell Output." *Journal of Neurophysiology*
33, 527.

Thoms, G., & Jurgens, U. 1987. "Common input of the cranial motor nuclei involved in
phonation in squirrel monkey." *Experimental Neurology* 95, 85-99.

Trachy, R.E., Sutton, D., & Lindeman, R.C. 1981. "Primate phonation: anterior cingulate lesion effects on response rate and acoustical structure." *Americal Journal of
Primatology* 1, 43-55.

von Bonin, G., & Bailey, P. 1947. *The Neocortex of Macaca mullata*. Urbana: University of Illinois Press (Illinois Monograph Medical Science, Vol. 5, No. XII).

von Leden, H. 1968. "Objective measures of laryngeal function and phonation." *Ann. N.Y. Acad. Sci.* 155, 56-66.

Wiesendanger, M., Hummelsheim, H., & Bianchetti, M. 1985. "Sensory input to the motor fields of the agranular frontal cortex: a comparison of the precentral, supplementary motor and premotor cortex." *Behavioral Brain Research* 18, 89-94.

Wiesendanger, M., Seguin, J.J., & Kunzle, H. 1973. "The supplementary motor area. A control system for posture?" *Advances in Behavioral Biology* 7, 331-346.

Yoshida, Y., Mitsumasu, T., Hirano, M., Morimoto, M., & Kanaseki, T. 1987. "Afferent connections to the nucleus ambiguus in the brainstem of the cat — an HRP study." In T. Baer, C. Sasaki, and K. Harris (eds), *Laryngeal Function in Phonation and Respiration*. Boston: College-Hill Press.

Zealear, D.L., & Larson, C.R. 1987. "Microelectrode studies of laryngeal motoneurons in the nucleus ambiguus of the awake vocalizing monkey." *Abstracts Society for Neuroscience* 13, 1696.

———. 1989. "A microelectrode study of laryngeal motoneurons in the nucleus ambiguus of the awake vocalizing monkey." In Fujimura O, Saito S, (eds) *Vocal Physiology: Voice Production, Mechanisms and Functions*. New York: Raven Press.

Index